T0262040

Handbook of Regenerative Medicine and Tissue Engineering

Volume I

Handbook of Regenerative Medicine and Tissue Engineering
Volume I

Edited by **Shay Fisher**

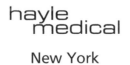

New York

Published by Hayle Medical,
30 West, 37th Street, Suite 612,
New York, NY 10018, USA
www.haylemedical.com

Handbook of Regenerative Medicine and Tissue Engineering
Volume I
Edited by Shay Fisher

© 2015 Hayle Medical

International Standard Book Number: 978-1-63241-243-0 (Hardback)

This book contains information obtained from authentic and highly regarded sources. Copyright for all individual chapters remain with the respective authors as indicated. A wide variety of references are listed. Permission and sources are indicated; for detailed attributions, please refer to the permissions page. Reasonable efforts have been made to publish reliable data and information, but the authors, editors and publisher cannot assume any responsibility for the validity of all materials or the consequences of their use.

The publisher's policy is to use permanent paper from mills that operate a sustainable forestry policy. Furthermore, the publisher ensures that the text paper and cover boards used have met acceptable environmental accreditation standards.

Trademark Notice: Registered trademark of products or corporate names are used only for explanation and identification without intent to infringe.

Printed in the United States of America.

Contents

Preface

This book has been an outcome of determined endeavour from a group of educationists in the field. The primary objective was to involve a broad spectrum of professionals from diverse cultural background involved in the field for developing new researches. The book not only targets students but also scholars pursuing higher research for further enhancement of the theoretical and practical applications of the subject.

The basic concept of regenerative medicine and tissue engineering is intriguing for physicians and scientists as it involves healing tissues or organ defects that the present medical practice finds difficult or impossible to cure. Tissue engineering involves cells, materials methods and engineering supported by appropriate physiochemical and biological factors to enhance or replace biologic functions. Regenerative medicine is a new division of medicine which aims to change the course of chronic disease and regenerate failing organ systems lost due to damage, age, disease and congenital defects. This book reflects state-of-the-art of these two disciplines at this time, as well as their therapeutic application. It discusses various topics related to stem cells in regenerative medicines. This book will prove to be a reference for physicians, scientists and students and an explanatory analysis for individuals in pharmaceuticals and biotech companies.

It was an honour to edit such a profound book and also a challenging task to compile and examine all the relevant data for accuracy and originality. I wish to acknowledge the efforts of the contributors for submitting such brilliant and diverse chapters in the field and for endlessly working for the completion of the book. Last, but not the least; I thank my family for being a constant source of support in all my research endeavours.

Editor

Stem Cells in Regenerative Medicine

The ASC: Critical Participants in Paracrine-Mediated Tissue Health and Function

Patricia Zuk

Additional information is available at the end of the chapter

1. Introduction

1.1. The adipose-derived stem cell — A pluripotent adult stem cell?

In 2001, the journal Tissue Engineering published an article describing the isolation of a population of putative multipotent stem cells from adipose tissue termed Processed Lipoaspirate Cells or PLA cells [1]. Based on isolation methods designed for the harvest of adherent, fibroblastic cells from the adipose stroma capable of adipogenic differentiation in vitro [2], this work by Zuk et al. described the differentiation of their PLA cells toward multiple mesodermal lineages, including fat, bone and cartilage. This ground-breaking article has since been followed by over 3500 studies published and available through PubMed, describing the differentiation capacity of ASCs in a variety of in vitro and in vivo model systems. Early works continued the characterization of PLA cells – now termed ASCs for Adipose-derived Stem Cells - identifying a unique CD "signature" for these cells [3]-[8] and studying their mesodermal differentiation capacity at a molecular and biochemical level [8]. Subsequent studies have since confirmed the ASC's mesodermal differentiation capacity in vitro reporting osteogenic, adipogenic, chondrogenic and skeletal myogenic capacities [9]-[20]. These works have since been expanded into in vivo translational models using a variety of animal systems for bone formation [21]-[25], cartilage [26]-[28], fat [29]-[32] and skeletal muscle [33]-[35]. In addition, recent years have presented some exciting results, expanding ASC potential to add smooth muscle [36], [37] and cardiac myogenesis [38], [39] to the growing list of ASC capacities.

With these increased capacities, it became natural to ask if the ASC possessed pluripotent potential and initial in vitro studies appeared to answer this question, reporting ectodermal [8], and endodermal differentiation [40], [41]. However, the true test of these germ line potentials still lies in the in vivo model. Consistent with the in vitro studies, numerous in vivo model systems have reported possible ectodermal and endodermal potentials, describing the repair of nervous and epithelial tissues [42], [43], together with hepatic and pancreatic regeneration [44]-[46]. With these in vivo results, combined with earlier in vitro analysis, it becomes easier to conclude that the ASC is an adult pluripotent stem cell population.

1.2. ASC-mediated tissue regeneration: Secretion of soluble factors

Despite the in vivo translational studies above suggesting that ASCs are capable of enhancing tissue healing and regeneration, many of these studies cannot confirm the direct differentiation of the ASC into a specific cell type. For example, while bone regeneration is observed upon implantation of ASCs, very few studies report the presence of the ASC within the newly formed bone. Whether this is an oversight by the research team or an indication that the ASC does not directly form part of the new tissue is unclear. It is entirely possible that the ASC does not directly differentiate into the desired regenerating tissue, but simply directs tissue formation "from the sidelines". Tissue development and healing is incredibly complex and the role of paracrine signaling is still not entirely understood. Therefore, it is possible that ASCs may be intimately involved in tissue regeneration and health through their ability to mediate the host's regenerative capacity using paracrine signaling.

Two arguments can be made in support of this theory. First, in many translational models, it does not appear that the ASC has any difficulty in surviving within the transplantation region for extended periods of time. In addition, the range of tissues capable of engrafting ASCs appears to be quite broad. Initial studies by Nolta and researchers show that systemic administration of human ASCs is followed by multi-organ engraftment in nude mice [47]. In support of this, human ASCs administered via tail vein migrate and home efficiently to multiple tissues (epithelial and endothelial) in irradiated mice [48], [49]. The specific migration of ASCs to injured tissues has also been shown by the Longaker group, who confirm the presence of ASCs specifically in parietal bone defects and their persistence as the defect heals [50]. Second, stem cells like bone marrow MSCs and ASCs are known to secrete numerous factors and cytokines, including VEGF, HGF, NGF, BDNF and multiple interleukins [49], [51]. In fact, Salgado's article calls these factors the "secretome" of ASCs. This secretome may have powerful paracrine effects on the health, repair and function of a tissue and has resulted in an exciting, new theory that proposes the ASC as a mediator of tissue regeneration through the secretion of specific soluble factors. In this regard, the ASC could be used in an incredibly broad range of applications. However, the most popular are reviewed below.

2. The use of ASCs in transplantation — Immunomodulatory and anti-inflammatory actions

Successful transplantation is reliant upon tolerance by the host's immune system. In 2000, human MSCs were transplanted into immunocompetent sheep without significant rejection [52], suggesting that adult stem cells might survive in a xenogeneic environment. Subsequent work with MSCs has described their ability to immunosuppress mixed lymphocyte reactions and to suppress stimulated T cell proliferation [53]-[55]. MSCs are also known to inhibit cytotoxic T lymphocyte toxicity [56], [57] and inhibit B cell proliferation by altering the G0/G1 transition [58]. Likewise ASC-mediated immunosuppression has been confirmed through a series of elegant in vitro experiments that describe the suppression of mixed lymphocyte reactions and/or proliferation of key immune cells like the T cell [59]-[63]. Immunosuppression has also been observed in a variety of in vivo model systems (Table 1). For example, reduced inflammatory infiltration and airspace enlargement results from the systemic administration of human ASCs to murine models of emphysema [64]. Moreover, the ASCs are capable of rescuing the suppressive effects of cigarette smoke on bone marrow hematopoietic progenitor function [64]. Experimental autoimmune hearing loss can be treated in mice through the systemic infusion of human ASCs, resulting in protection of hair cells possibly through the production of the anti-inflammatory cytokine IL10 by splenocytes [65] and decreasing the proliferation of antigen-specific Th1 and Th17 cells. Similar immunosuppression and amelioration of disease is reported upon injection of ASCs in models of rheumatoid arthritis [66] and IgA nephropathy [67], resulting in decreased inflammatory markers and Th1 cytokine activity, together with the generation of regulatory T cells capable of suppressing T cell responses. Finally significant anti-inflammatory responses are observed upon the transplantation of allogeneic murine ASCs into dystrophin-deficient mice, decreasing markers of oxidative stress and inflammation, including TNFα and IL6, decreasing production of CD3+ T cells, and enhancing the synthesis of anti-inflammatory IL4 and IL10 [68]. While these studies are supportive of the role for ASCs in modulating immune responses, what remains unknown is the mechanism. One theory proposes that cell-cell contact is required [61]. However, others dispute this finding, suggesting that it is the secretion of soluble factors by the ASC that mediates the eventual reaction by the host's immune system [69]. In support of this, inhibition of prostaglandin E2 production in ASCs by indomethacin can abolish the immunosuppressive properties of ASCs. Alternatively, neutralizing leukemia inhibitory factor has had similar effects [70]. Finally, there are those that suggest a role for IL-6 [55].

The immunosuppressive properties of ASCs may make it possible to use more xenogeneic transplantation model systems without the fear of significant immune reactions in animal hosts. Such models would allow for a more direct study of human ASCs in vivo, thus allowing researchers to more accurately predict what these cells could do clinically. An excellent review of these models can be found in a recent article by Lin et al. [81]. In this article, they present a detailed table outlining many of the recent xenogeneic model systems, such as one by Paul and colleagues [82], who perform a xenogeneic transplantation of human ASCs into myocardial infarcts produced in immunocompetent rats. Histology confirms human ASCs in the infarct region after 6 weeks, with no detectable inflammatory reaction even in the absence of immunosuppressive action. Furthermore, these animals show improvement of cardiac function and reduced infarct size, together with significant improvement in myocardial anti-inflammatory cytokine levels. The success of such xenogeneic transplantation models may be explained, in part, by the immunogenic profile of the ASC. Immunophenotyping of ASCs has not only provided researchers with a CD antigen profile but has confirmed the absence of the HLA-DR antigen on the ASC surface. Divided into classes such as HLA-A, B and C (or MHC

Author and Year (Reference)	ASC type	Disease Model	Inflammatory/Immunosuppressive action
Pinheiro et al. 2012 [68]	human	murine dystrophy	decreased CD3+ve T cells, increased IL-4, IL-10 synthesis
Payne et al. 2012 [71]	human	autoimmune demyelination – IL-4 overexpressing ASCs	increased T cell responses
Zhou et al. 2011 [65]	human	autoimmune hearing loss	secretion of IL-10, decreased proliferation of Th1, Th17 cells
Hyun et al. 2011[67],	mouse	IgA-induced nephropathy	decreased inflammatory markers, decreased Th1 activity
Schweitzer et al. 2011 [64]	human, mouse	emphysema	decreased inflammatory infiltration
Lai 2011 et al. [72]	human	systemic lupus erythamatosis	decreased Th17 production, decrease IL-17 synthesis
Zhou 2011 et al. [66]	human	rheumatoid arthritis	decreased Th1, Th17 proliferation/expansion, increased IL10 synthesis
Kuo 2011 et al. [73]	rat	hind limb allotransplantion	increased Treg proliferation
Gonzalez-Rey et al. 2010 [74], Gonzalez et al. 2009 [75]	human	rheumatoid arthritis	inhibition of CD4+ T cell proliferation, increase in IL-10 producing T cells and monocytes, stimulation of Treg cell development
Cho et al. 2010 [76]	mouse	airway allergic disease	decreased airway inflammation, shift from a Th2 to a Th1-biased immune reponse
Gonzalez-Rey et al. 2009 [77], Gonzalez et al. 2009 [78]	human	experimental colitis	decrease in Th1-driven inflammation, decrease inflammatory cytokines, increased IL-10 activity
Kim et al. 2007 [79]	human	hemorrhagic stroke	decreased brain inflammation markers
Wan et al. 2008 [59]	rat	orthotopic liver transplant	increased IL-2 and IL-10 synthesis
Constatin et al. 2009 [80]	mouse	autoimmune encephalolyelitis (multiple sclerosis)	increased Th2-type shift in cytokine production[80]

Table 1. Immunosuppressive action of ASCs

class I) and HLA-DP, DM and DR (or MHC class II), HLA receptors display proteins on the cell surface for immune surveillance. Of particular interest is the HLA/MHC class II protein, which is found on the surface of antigen-presenting cells and plays critical roles in immuno-tolerance and transplantation (for reviews see [83], [84]). The absence of this class of HLA protein may allow the ASC to evade the host's immune surveillance machinery. Of additional interest is a recent study by DelaRosa et al. [85], who note that human ASCs have lower susceptibility to natural killer (NK) cell-mediated lysis in comparison to bone marrow MSCs.

This finding may be part of the reason for xenogeneic tolerance of ASCs in that NK-ASC crosstalk does not result in immediate recognition. Continued research in this area is sure to expand the possible uses of ASCs in translational model systems.

3. Vascularization by ASCs in tissue repair

Tissue repair and regeneration is reliant upon vascularization. Newly formed tissues must have sufficient blood flow to maintain their health and support their growth. Early in vitro studies with ASCs suggest the capacity to differentiate into endothelial cells and to form vessel-like structures. For example, using simple in vitro induction conditions, ASCs express typical markers of endothelial cells, such as von Willebrand Factor (vWF) and function as endothelial cells, taking up acetylated LDL and forming tubular structures on Matrigel substrates [40], [41], [86]. Tubule formation, LDL uptake and CD31 expression by ASCs are also found upon in vitro exposure to shear stress [87], [88]. Such evidence provides strong support for the use of ASCs in the induction of vessel formation and some have attempted to isolate the specific ASC subpopulation that might be responsible for endothelial differentiation. For example, Wosnitza et al. postulate that a population of CD31-ve, S100+ve ASCs are capable of endothelial differentiation [89], while CD34-ve ASCs have been observed to undergo differentiation by others [90].

Author and Year (Reference)	ASC type	Secreted Factor
Ribeiro et al. 2012 [91]	human	VEGF, HGF, bFGF, NGF, SCF
Ii et al. 2012 [92]	human	VEGF, bFGF, SDF1α
Kim et al. 2011 [93]	human	VEGF
Lu et al. 2011 [94]	human	VEGF, HGF, BDNF, NGF
Liu et al. 2011 [95]	rat	HGF
Nie et al. 2011 [96]	rat	VEGF, HGF, bFGF
Salgado et al. 2010 [49]	human	VEGF, HGF, BDNF
Zhu et al. 2010 [97]	human	VEGF
Grewal et al. 2009 [98]	human	VEGF
Rubina et al. 2009 [99]	mouse	VEGF, HGF, bFGF, PDGFB, TGFb
Park et al. 2008 [100]	human	VEGF, HGF, PDGF
Prichard et al. 2008 [101]	rat	VEGF
Kilroy et al. 2007 [102]	human	HGF
Wang et al. 2006 [103]	human	VEGF, HGF, IGF-1
Cao et al. 2005 [41]	human	VEGF, HGF, bFGF, KGF, TGFβ
Rehman et al. 2004 [104]	human	VEGF

Table 2. Growth factor secretion by ASCs

However, the efficacy of ASCs in tissue repair may not be entirely due to their direct differentiation into endothelial lineages, but also to their secretion of paracrine factors capable of

increasing vascularization. In support of this, co-culture of ASCs with postnatal cardiomyocytes results in the formation of stable, branching CD31+ve vessel-like structures that disas-
semble in the absence of ASCs [99]. Similarly, ASC-conditioned media can induce the
formation of vessel-like tubules within Matrigel [105]. More recently, while rat ASCs express
Flt-1, CD31 and vascular endothelial cadherin, when injected into a wire injury model in the
rat femoral artery, induction of endothelial repair occurs without any observable differentiation of these ASCs into endothelial cells [106]– a finding that can be explained if repair is driven
through the production of soluble factors. In the hopes of identifying what angiogenic factors
improve a tissue's vasculature, numerous studies have characterized the secretion of growth
factors by ASCs (Table 2). Of all of these factors, perhaps the most commonly reported is VEGF,
with secretion of this factor being reported under normal culture conditions [98], hypoxic
conditions [104] in models of wound healing [96], [107] and cell-assisted lipotransfer [97]. The
ability of VEGF to stimulate neoangiogenesis is well known [108]-[110]. Consistent with this,
conditioned medium from ASCs, maintained under hypoxic culture conditions in order to
increase production of HGF, VEGF and TGFβ, has been found to increase endothelial cell (EC)
growth and reduce their apoptosis [104]. In addition, VEGF secretion by ASCs is significantly
upregulated in vitro upon metabolic induction of ischemia [111]. However, the role of other
secreted factors cannot be ruled out as suppression of HGF production by ASCs through RNA
interference significantly impairs ischemic tissue revascularization [112] and SDF-1α from
ASCs has been identified as being involved in myocardial vascularization [92]

3.1. Ischemia/ischemia-reperfusion injury

Today, there are several model systems that study the paracrine-mediated vascularization
potential of ASCs but some of the most common are: ischemia and ischemia-reperfusion (IR)
injuries, wound healing and cardiac infarct treatment. Enhanced angiogenesis within ischemic
limbs has been reported following treatment with freshly isolated ASCs (i.e. the stromal
vascular fraction) and vessels derived from these cells confirmed [113]. However, the use of
such a heterogenous population makes it difficult to confirm direct ASC involvement.
Fortunately, there have been numerous studies describing the beneficial use of cultured/
purified ASCs in the treatment of ischemia [86], [90], [93], [114]-[117]. Consistent with paracrine
action, improved vascularization within ischemic limbs has been associated with increased
levels of plasma VEGF [93]. In addition, human ASCs cultured in vitro as spheroids improve
neovascularization and limb survival when compared to the implantation of dissociated ASCs
– a finding thought to be due to the induction of vascular factors, like HGF, VEGF and bFGF,
by the hypoxic conditions of the spheroid [118]. In support of this, decreases in the ability of
ASCs to induce reperfusion in ischemic hindlimbs are observed if secretion of HGF by the ASC
is inhibited [112]. However, the role of the ASC in angiogenesis may not be restricted to their
secretion of established angiogenic factors. Transplantation of ASCs transfected with siRNA
to either MMP3 or MMP9 to ischemic hind-limbs results in lower blood flow recovery and
higher tissue injury [119], suggesting that ASCs may also promote angiogenesis through their
secretion of matrix-remodelling enzymes.

Whereas prolonged ischemia can cause significant tissue damage, there is evidence now that the reperfusion period is also associated with injury, amplified by the production of reactive oxygen species and inflammatory cascades [120]. Events such as these are a major obstacle to successful tissue transplantation. However, the ASC may ameliorate IR injury through its secretion of pro-angiogenic factors, thus increasing the density of developing capillaries within the reperfused tissue. Consistent with this, a significant increase in pro-angiogenic factors can be confirmed in IR skin flap models treated with ASCs [121]. Long-lasting improvement in cardiac function with increased angiogenesis and vasculogenesis can also be observed in IR in minipigs treated with a trans-endocardial injection of ASCs [122] and a higher number of CD31+ve and vWF+ve cells have been found in models of lung IR followed by ASC injection [123]. While the finding that ASCs can form vessel-like structures in Matrigel in vitro and re-endothelialize carotid injuries in vivo [87], [124] may suggest that the observed angiogenesis is due to differentiation by ASCs, the failure to observe significant ASC engraftment in IR models [122] again suggests that the role of ASCs may be paracrine in nature.

In addition to stimulating angiogenesis, the ASC may also lessen the damaging effects of IR through paracrine secretion of a combination of anti-inflammatory and anti-oxidant factors. The production of oxidative toxins such as free radicals and reactive oxygen species in ischemia and IR is well-established [125]-[128]. The synthesis of enzymatic anti-oxidants, such as superoxide dismutase and glutathione peroxidase, not only can be detected by proteomic analysis in ASC-conditioned media, but this media is able to protect dermal fibroblasts from oxidative damage [129]. Therefore, the ASC may be an excellent candidate for protection against oxidative damage. In support of this, Chen and co-workers, using a model of kidney IR treated with either conditioned medium from ASCs or direct injection of ASCs during reperfusion, find increased clearance of creatinine and urea from blood plasma in ASC/IR groups together with higher levels of the anti-oxidant markers NAD(P)H quinine oxidore-ductase, heme-oxygenase 1/HO-1, glutathione peroxidase and glutathione reductase [130]. Increased anti-oxidant marker levels (i.e. NAD(P)H quinine oxidoreductase and HO-1) have also been reported, together with increased eNOS expression and decreased hepatic oxidative stress versus controls upon multiple injections of ASCs in hepatic IR models [131]. These anti-oxidant actions by ASCs are not only likely to protect the reperfused tissue from oxidative damage but may also protect the ASC itself. A recent study by Suga and colleagues suggests that resident ASCs are resistant to ischemia-mediated damage, surviving within ischemic adipose grafts [132]. Moreover, this work specifically postulates that the actions of these resident ASCs may be responsible for the observed increases in vascular density and the number of new adipocytes over time. Therefore, ASCs may be resistant to the toxic environment of ischemic tissues and may retain their functional capacities, thus being able to either differentiate or secrete paracrine factors for critical for angiogenesis.

3.2. Wound healing

Paracrine action is also likely to play a significant role in the beneficial effects of ASCs in wound healing models. ASCs isolated from debrided skin are capable of producing an epithelial layer when seeded into collagen gels, together with a dermis when seeded fibrin gels are co-cultured with ASC/collagen/epithelial constructs, suggesting that the ASC would be an excellent cell source for healing skin wounds [133]. In support of this, increased collagen density has been reported in full-thickness rat skin grafts injected with ASCs [134] and Lim et al. [135] note improved wound healing rates upon implantation of ASCs. These wound healing rates are significantly higher than in controls treated with ASC extracts, suggesting that production of paracrine factors by viable ASCs are necessary in order to direct the formation of new tissue within the wound. In vitro culture of immortalized keratinocytes or dermal fibroblasts with ASC-conditioned medium results in increased proliferation of these cells, in addition to increased transcription and production of collagen type I, suggesting that secreted ASC-derived factors may ultimately influence keratinocyte-mediated healing in skin grafts [136], [137]. Finally, Jung and colleagues have reported that conditioned medium from ASCs can increase CNI, CNIII and hyaluronic acid synthesis by human dermal fibroblasts and that neutralizing antibodies to TGFβ1 can abolish this effect [138]. However, it is equally likely that improved wound-healing using ASCs is due to their secretion of angiogenic factors, thus improving healing through augmentation of vascularization. As proponents of this theory, Reichenberger et al. [139] and Gao et al. [107] report higher blood flow and skin flap survival, respectively when the flaps are combined with ASCs. In addition, Gao and colleagues report increased capillary density, together with increased expression of VEGF within the dermis in the ASC-treated groups. In support of this, increased VEGF expression and microvascular density is also measured in ASC-treated rat skin grafts [134]. Interestingly, recent studies suggest that AKT/c-myc signaling pathways may mediate increased VEGF secretion in ASCs as injection of constitutively active AKT/v-myc-expressing ASCs promote better wound healing compared to normal controls [140]. How exactly the ASC promotes wound healing is likely to be a combination of increased tissue healing and vascularization as directed by their secretion of specific paracrine factors. In support of this, GFP-labelled ASCs not only secrete the angiogenic factors VEGF, HGF and bFGF in vivo, but co-stain with keratin and CD31 in excisional wound healing models in normal and diabetic rats, possibly undergoing both epithelial and endothelial differentiation [96]. Similar differentiation by human ASCs, implanted into skin wounds via silk/chitosan scaffolds, has also been reported by Altman and colleagues [141]. Therefore, the successful use of ASCs in wound healing models may be due to their paracrine action in promoting angiogenesis by the host and their autocrine action in promoting differentiation in themselves.

3.3. Infarct treatment

In a 2007 study by Fotuhi, freshly isolated ASCs injected into porcine transmural infarcts were shown not to cause arrhythmia, bradycardia or conduction block. Moreover, these ASC-treated hearts required extra-stimuli to induce an arrhythmia, suggesting that ASCs could be used in the treatment of cardiac infarcts [142]. With in vitro studies confirming the cardiomyogenic potential of these stem cells, infarct treatment could be mediated through the differentiation of ASCs into cardiomyocytes. However, there is a debate on whether the ASC contributes directly to cardiac muscle regeneration or supports this event through the production of angiogenic growth factors and cytokines. An example of this debate can be seen in the 2007 article by Zhang et al. [143]. Rabbit ASCs injected into transmural infarcts in hearts three wks after occlusion decrease transmural scar and improve left ventricle ejection fraction (LVEF), end-diastolic pressure and myocardial performance relative to saline controls, with ASCs pre-induced with 5-azacytidine for 24 hours giving slightly better results versus untreated controls. When the infarct region is examined histologically, the ASCs form islands of cardiac tissue in and around the scar. However, all infarcts treated with ASCs also show greater capillary density, with the ASCs also differentiating into endothelial cells. Increased capillary densities/ angiogenesis have previously been reported using bone marrow mononuclear cells and endothelial progenitors and MSCs are known to cause improvement in cardiac function by incorporating into newly formed capillaries and releasing angiogenic factors [144]. Similar events may also be induced by ASCs. In support of this, mouse ASCs injected into murine infarcts take up residence in the infarct area, with EKGs showing stability of LVEF [145]. Murine ASCs [146] or rat ASCs [147] transplanted into rat infarcts result in significant improvement in heart function and tissue viability. Human ASCs not only increase peri-infarct capillary density in rat infarcts but increase numbers of nerve sprouts [148]. Finally, while Beitnes and co-workers show significant improvement in LVEF, smaller infarct sizes and increased vascularization when human ASCs are injected into infarcts in nude rats, they specifically observe an absence of ASC engraftment [149]. However, it is important to note that ASC engraftment was examined in this study 4 weeks post-transplant. It is possible that the long-term beneficial effects of ASCs on infarct treatment can result from short-term engraft-ment. In support of this, while transdifferentiation of human ASCs into cardiomyocytes or endothelial cells is also not observed in rat cardiac infarcts, the expression of VEGF, bFGF and SDF-1α can be confirmed in these hearts within the first few days of transplant and improved heart function and vascular density is ultimately observed [92]. Therefore, long-term survival of ASCs within the myocardium may not be necessary for their beneficial effects on cardiac function to be realized. Such a possibility would be extremely exciting if this treatment modality is translated into the clinic.

3.4. Other vascularization systems

In addition to wound healing, infarct treatment and ischemia-reperfusion, there are numerous other vascularization systems that might benefit from the putative angiogenic action of ASCs. Hemodynamic abnormalities may be reversed with the treatment of pulmonary arterial hypertension with ASCs through their augmented expression of HGF for angiogenesis and increased number of small pulmonary arteries [95]. Small-for-size liver injury may be treated through their secretion of VEGF. Inhibition of VEGF secretion by ASCs through RNA interference (RNAi) does not prevent apoptosis of liver sinusoidal endothe-lial cells in vitro and when cells are transplanted syngeneically results in significant disturbances to graft microcirculation, serum liver functional parameters and graft surviv-al [150]. Finally, at the cosmetic level, cell-assisted lipotransfer fat grafts survive at higher levels, are 35% larger and show increased neoangigogenesis when compared to grafts transplanted without isolated ASCs [151].

4. Neuroprotection by ASCs — Demyelination, stroke, spinal cord injury

Early translational studies do suggest that ASCs can be safely administered to nervous tissue injuries and that functional improvement is noted. Transplanted ASCs have been reported to improve functional deficits following middle cerebral occlusion or ischemic stroke [152]-[154], spinal cord contusion injury [155] and peripheral nerve gaps [156], [157]. Histologic analysis of these injury sites has suggested that ASC differentiation into neurons and/or glial cells may play a role in the functional recovery, with transplanted cells staining positively for MAP2 [153], GFAP, Tuj-1 and an oligodendrocyte marker [155]. However, this functional improvement may be due to paracrine actions on the host more than ASC differentiation, as less then 1% of transplanted ASCs can be found within a spinal contusive injury model, with those remaining appearing to be oligodendrocytes [158]. In addition, extremely low levels ASC differentiation into mature neurons is noted in a model of cerebral cortex injury [159]. However, both of these studies note significant changes in the host tissue with Nakada et al. observing improvements in microvasculature and Zhang et al. measuring increases in host oligodendrocyte formation. Therefore, like wound healing and IR models, ASCs are likely to exert paracrine actions within nervous tissue.

In 2002, Zhao et al. suggested that functional recovery in ischemic brain injury was not due to MSC differentiation but to secreted paracrine factors that act on the host [160]. A similar hypothesis has been put forth by bone marrow MSC groups who have noted increased survival and differentiation of Tuj1+ve neurons and neuroblastoma cells in co-cultures [161] and increased neuronal viability and glial cell differentiation using MSC conditioned media [162]. Consistent with this, ASC/Matrigel constructs implanted into models of mice limb re-inner-vation stimulate the regeneration of nerves and induce axon growth, likely through the expression numerous neurotrophins [163]. Moreover, enhanced nerve fiber growth is observed if the ASCs are pre-induced toward the neural lineage thus enhancing their production of brain-derived neurotrophic factor (BNDF). BDNF secretion (together with nerve growth factor/NGF and glial cell-derived neurotrophic factor/GDNF) by ASCs pre-differentiated toward a Schwann Cell (SC) phenotype is thought to be the basis for axonal regeneration in sciatic nerve gap models - although these authors speculate that this regeneration is likely due to the neuroprotective function of these three neurotrophins [164]. In support of this, studies using ASC-conditioned media appeared to further strengthen this theory. Protection against cortical and hippocampal volume loss in rats can be achieved through the infusion of ASC-conditioned medium [165]. ASC-conditioned medium containing VEGF, BDNF and NGF is shown to have a protective effect against glutamate excitotoxicity on PC12 cells (a key factor implicated in stroke and neurodegenerative diseases) and increase PC12 viability [94]. Conditioned media from pre-differentiated ASCs infused over one week into a rat model of ischemic stroke 8 days after stroke induction increases the number of CD31+ve cells [166]. Finally, functional deficits in a model of middle cerebral artery occlusion can be dramatically improved using ASC transduced to overexpress BDNF [153].

While these neurotrophic factors may act to protect neurons, ASCs may also play roles in decreasing inflammation and gliosis (i.e. glial cell-mediated scar formation) – two critical events that specifically affect healing in the both the central and peripheral nervous system. Systemic transplantation of human ASCs can attenuate cerebral degeneration in rats, reducing both brain atrophy and glial proliferation [79]. Rats implanted with ASC-derived SCs show significant locomotor function recovery compared with untreated ASCs and also reduction in gliosis [152]. Pre-differentiated canine ASCs in Matrigel scaffolds show better functional recovery and reduced fibrosis and inflammation when implanted into spinal cord injuries [167]. Decreased gliosis is also noted upon intrathecal administration of ASCs in a model of IR neuronal damage in rabbits – an event accompanied by increased expression of BDNF within the first 72 hours following ASCs administration [168]. Finally, a possible anti-inflammatory role for ASCs in sciatic nerve repair might be seen in a recent model describing possible immunosuppression of xenogeneic acellular nerve matrices combined with autologous ASCs [169]. Implantation of this construct does not result in host rejection, making it possible that peripheral nerves repair can be accomplished using commercial nerve matrices combined with the patient's own ASCs.

4.1. Controlled release from ASCs — ASCs as a cellular biopump

It is possible that the paracrine action of ASCs may be "fine-tuned" so that the ASC secretes a desired factor, hence turning the ASC into a "cellular biopump". This is not a recent concept as the engineering of numerous cell types to secrete a variety of factors has been reported in the literature for over a decade. In the field of stem cell research, bone marrow MSCs have been modified to secrete various factors, including BMP2 [170], [171], bFGF [172], IFN-β [173] and IL12 [174]. Similar to these studies, ASCs have been engineered for the delivery of BMP4 [175], BMP2 [176], [177], and BMP6 [178] in several bone regeneration models. Delivery of TGFβ2 by ASCs for the induction of chondrogenesis has been reported [179]. Adenovirally-mediated VEGF secretion by ASCs has been used to induce vascular growth in a bone defect model [180] and adipose tissue grafts [181]. Finally, as described above, BDNF delivery by transduced ASCs into a model of middle cerebral artery occlusion improves functional deficits when compared to control ASCs [153].

However, a more exciting idea might be in the engineering of ASCs in the treatment of disease. In 2007, ASCs engineered to express cytosine deaminase were found to decrease the growth of colon carcinoma cells [182]. ASCs have recently been described in the delivery of an oncolytic myxoma virus that will specifically target gliomas [183]. ASC viability is not impacted with transduction and successful cross-infection of gliomablastoma cells is observed upon 3D co-culture with glioblastoma cells, leading to their cell death. More importantly, rat survival is increased with this myxoma virus delivery, with the size of the gliomas significantly decreasing upon injection of transduced ASCs in comparison to non-transduced ASCs controls. Localization of ASCs and increased apoptosis within tumors has also been reported following intravenous or subcutaneous injection of ASCs engineered to express TRAIL, having no effect on the surrounding healthy tissue [184]. Finally, this approach may have far-reaching effects on autoimmune diseases through the delivery of interleukins and interferons. ASCs engineered to overexpress IL4 and administered at the time of T cell priming attenuate autoimmune encephalomyelitis and reduce peripheral T cell responses shifting the host pro-inflammatory response to an anti-inflammatory one [71]. With the development of inducible viral systems, there is the possibility that the ASC cellular biopump could be controlled not only at the dose level through the number of cells delivered but at the temporal level, giving clinicians more precise control over their therapeutic regimen.

4.2. ASC uses in the clinic

In light of their differentiative capacity and paracrine actions, there is great interest in the use of ASCs within the clinic. As source of regenerative stem cells, the ASC may have no equal. Bone marrow aspirates yield on average 6×10^6 nucleated cells per ml, of which, only 0.001 to 0.01% are thought to be stem cells [185], [186]. In comparison, approximately three-fold more cells can be obtained per gram adipose tissue [187] [188] with 10% of these cells thought to be stem cells [188], [189]. The abundance of ASCs within adipose tissue, combined with the relative ease of its harvest and isolation also makes the ASC a good choice for clinical work. Patient's could conceivably have their adipose tissue harvested relatively painlessly a few weeks prior to their procedure in a simple outpatient procedure, the ASCs isolated and expanded under good manufacturing protocols and then used for regenerative purposes. With the confirmed absence of HLA/MHC class II proteins and continuing xenogeneic animal models, the patient may not even need to use their own stem cells. Donated allogeneic ASC lines could be used in lieu of autologous cells without the fear of immunorejection or inflammatory complications. Such a situation might be perfect in the case of myocardial infarct treatment where a delay in treatment could have serious consequences.

The first published article using ASCs in a clinical setting was in 2004, in which freshly harvested SVF cells were combined with fibrin glue and used in the repair of a traumatic calvarial injury [190]. Three months after reconstruction, CT scans showed new bone formation within the injury. However, it is important to point out that the cells used in this study were not ASCs, purified through plastic adherence and culture time, but the SVF - a heterogenous mixture of ASCs, endothelial cells, pre-adipocytes, pericytes, fibroblasts and red blood cells. Therefore, it is difficult to attribute the observed healing to the action of the ASC itself. Since that time, other clinical studies using the SVF have been attempted [191] and a review by Casteilla et al. does an excellent job of summarizing these works [192]. It is worth noting that with the exception of some cysts and microcalcifications being observed upon breast reconstruction [193], the use of SVFs clinically has not resulted in any serious complications.

Because of its heterogeneity, clinical studies using purified ASCs have also been performed for the treatment of such disorders as critical limb ischemia and radiation therapy ([194], [195] – for a more comprehensive review, see [192]). Bone regeneration using ASCs has recently been reported in 2009 with the reconstruction of the maxilla being induced using ASC in combination with BMP2 [196]. Bony healing using BMPs has been documented in numerous translational animal models [197]-[201], making this clinical study an exciting addition to the ways bone regeneration and healing can be brought about in the clinic. However, many of these translational models fail to report the appropriate control – the amount of bone being formed just by the BMP itself. The first translational study to combine ASCs and a BMP (i.e. BMP2) failed to measure any significant improvement in bone formation when BMP2 and ASC+BMP2 groups were compared [197]. Since this study, others have appeared to suggest that BMP2 may not pro-mote the in vivo osteogneic capacity of the ASC [202] but may, in fact, may have a deleterious effect on bone regeneration [203]. Since it is not possible to perform similarly controlled studies clinically, it remains unknown if the addition of ASCs to BMP-treated scaffolds provides any more advantage. However, It is worth noting that, as with the use of SVFs, administration of ASCs into human patients has not been associated with any adverse effects [204].

The first phase I clinical trials using ASCs were not conducted on bone formation or even fat grafting but in the healing of chronic fistulae in Crohn's disease [205]-[210]. In 2005, nine rectovaginal fistulae in four patients were treated with ASCs, purified and cultured for up to one month. Of the eight fistulae examined, six showed complete healing in 8 weeks [206]. These fistulae had previously failed to heal using conventional surgical treatments, thus justifying progression to more comprehensive phase II trials. In 2009, a larger phase II trial using patients with and without Crohn's fistulae were treated with ASCs [211]. As seen with their earlier clinical trial, the majority of Crohn's and non-Crohn's fistulae were healed completely using ASCs in comparison to controls. Currently, there are three phase II clinical trials recruiting for the use of ASCs in Crohn's disease fistulae (Clinicaltrials identifiers: NCT01011244, NCT01157650, NCT00999115, http://clinicaltrials.gov/ct2/results?term=adipose+derived+cells), in addition to one phase III trial (NCT00475410) recently completed [212].

One of the reasons ASCs are considered in the treatment of Crohn's disease is their ability to suppress inflammation. This review includes numerous examples of how the ASC may be capable of suppressing the immune system and recent clinical trials have attempted to take direct advantage of this quality. The treatment of multiple sclerosis (MS) with SVFs, containing ASCs, has been described by Riordan and colleagues in 2009, with the 3 enrolled patients showing improvement in numerous functional categories including balance and coordination [213]. The use of culture expanded ASCs in autoimmune diseases like hearing loss, MS and rheumatoid arthritis was recently discussed in 2011 [214]. Prior to this, ASCs have been proposed as a viable therapy for suppression of graft vs. host disease (GVHD) [215]-[218]. Each of these studies report favorable functional outcomes and propose ASCs, or their SVF counterpart, for the treatment of immune system disorders.

The most obvious application of the ASC clinically should be in breast reconstruction. In the lab, the combination of ASC-containing SVFs with fat grafts through a protocol called cell-assisted lipotransfer has enjoyed success [151]. Clinically, treatment of facial lipoatrophy has been reported [219] and two recent trials overseas has suggested that the ASCs within the SVF are capable of increasing breast volume and improving contour 6 months post-surgery [193], [220]. However, the use of ASCs in breast reconstruction is being pursued carefully in light of recent findings that link stem cells to cancer. Bone marrow MSCs have been found to increase proliferation of breast cancer cell lines [221] and subcutaneous injection of MSCs with tumor cells can favor their growth [222]. Similar to this, ASCs can increase tumorigenesis of estab-lished breast cancer lines [223]. In this study, ASCs not only promote the growth of metastatic pleural effusion cells both in vitro and in vivo but the ASC also secretes adipsin and leptin – both of which are known to promote breast cancer growth [224]. Additional work in MSCs has documented their ability to secrete large amounts of IL-6 and the corresponding increase in the growth of estrogen receptor alpha-positive cell lines [225]. Increased expression of IL4 and IL10 have also been reported by ASCs isolated from breast cancer tissue [226], leading many to speculate that the ASC may be capable of altering the immune environment within the breast, resulting in the "protection" of the cancerous cells. Such a possibility could have far-reaching effects in the development of breast cancer and in its possible reoccurrence if ASCs are used in reconstruction. However, it is encouraging to find that cultured ASCs are resistant to the chemotherapies cisplatin, vincristine or comptothecin and that they still retain their stem cell characteristics [227]. Such findings could make it possible for a more natural reconstruction of the breast if ASCs are found not to contribute to the cancer itself.

4.3. "Paracrines gone wild" — ASCs and adipose disorders

With the proposed paracrine function of ASCs now well accepted, a re-examination of certain disorders and how the ASC might play a role might now be in order. The most obvious of these disorders would be obesity. However, studying the ASC might allow more information into lesser known dysfunctions such as lipedema and rare adipose disorders (RADs) like Dercum's and Madelung's disease. Normal fat has been described as having an anti-inflammatory milieu with adipocytes storing lipid, regulating energy metabolism, and, together with resident macrophages, secreting anti-inflammatory mediators such as IL-10 and adiponectin to protect against the possible development of inflammation-driven obesity [228]-[230]. However, with chronic nutrient overload, existing adipocytes increase their fat storage to become hypertrophic and resident pre-adipocytes (or ASCs) are thought to undergo increased differentiation to increase adipocyte number (i.e. hyperplasia). The hypertrophic adipocytes increase their secretion of "adipokines" - soluble factors known to affect angiogenesis and inflammation [231], [232]. Specifically, these adipocytes shift their adipokine production from anti-inflammatory to inflammatory, producing a series of feedback cascades that ultimately manifests in obesity [232].

Obesity has been recognized since the 1950s as a chronic state of low-level inflammation associated with excess accumulation of adipose tissue [233]. This inflammation is now thought to be a complex response to cellular events, such as hypoxia and oxidative stresses within the adipocyte. Figure 1 outlines the possible interacting events underlying obesity starting with the creation of hypertrophic adipocytes. These adipocytes become too large to be adequately supplied by the existing vasculature in the adipose depot, resulting in localized areas of hypoxia. This hypoxic state induces the production of numerous pro-inflammatory adipokines (e.g. IL1Rα, IL6, IL8, TNFα, MCP-1, leptin) and decreases the secretion of several key anti-inflammatory factors (e.g. IL10, adiponectin). Excellent reviews on these adipokines in obesity can be found in Fain et al. 2010 and Balistreri 2010. In these hypertrophic adipocytes, hypoxia is thought to induce oxidative stress [234], [235]. Oxidative stress is defined as an imbalance in the levels of reaction oxygen species (ROS) relative to the tissue's antioxidant capacity, resulting in the accumulation of oxidative products such as superoxide and hydroxyl radicals, reactive nitrogen species (RNS) and hydrogen peroxide [236]. Excess nutrients and hypertrophic adipocytes can produce ROS through: the nicotinamide dinucleotide phosphate oxidase (NOX) system [237], incomplete mitochondrial respiration due to excess free fatty acids [238] and endoplasmic reticulum (ER) stress due to excess lipid storage [239]. Both mitochondrial and ER dysfunction have been demonstrated to increase the secretion of inflammatory adipokines [239], [240] and numerous studies in obesity models and obese subjects now exist linking hypoxia, oxidative stress and inflammation (reviewed in [236]). Concomitant with the development of hypertrophic adipocytes, there is a shift within the adipose tissue from M2 macrophages, found in normal adipose tissue, to a more pro-inflammatory M1 macrophage subset [241]-[243]. This shift is likely, in part, a consequence of the production of pro-inflammatory adipokines by adipocytes – such as MCP-1, but this infiltration is also likely to be due to the death of these adipocytes [244]. Consistent with this, "crown-like" structures of macrophages are known to be associated with necrotic adipocytes in obese murine adipose tissue [242]. These macrophages may directly contribute to the production of inflammatory agents within obese adipose tissue [245]. However, they may also augment adipokine production by the adipocyte through possible cross-talk mechanisms. While these mechanisms are unclear at this point, there are many who postulate that adipocyte-macrophage interaction is the key factor in inflammation and resulting obesity [230], [246], [247].

Author & Year (Reference)	Secreted factor
Blaber et al. 2012 [267]	IFNγ, IL8, IL9, IL12, IL17, TNFα
Hsiao et al. 2012 [268]	IL6, IL8, MCP-1, MCSF, RANTES
Bhang et al. 2011 [118]	HIF1α
Salgado et al. 2010 49	TNFα, IL6, IL8
Banas et al. 2008 [269]	IL6, IL8, IL1Rα, MCP-1, GMCSF
Kilroy et al. 2007 [102]	IL6, IL8, TNFα, MCSF, GMSCF

MCSF – macrophage colony stimulating factor

GMCSF – granulocyte-macrophage colony stimulating factor

MCP-1 – monocyte chemoattractant protein 1

IFNγ – interferon gamma

TNFα – tumor necrosis factor alpha

IL - interleukin

Table 3. Secretion of Pro-inflammatory Cytokines by ASCs

So obesity results from a complex series of cellular events that ultimately increases the production of inflammatory adipokines within the tissue. These adipokines are known to further increase adipocyte hypertrophy producing a positive feedback system. This feedback system could be augmented further by the secretory activity of non-fat cells – i.e. the pre-adipocyte and even the ASC. Pre-adipocytes and adipocytes secrete many of the same pro-inflammatory factors listed above - with the exception of leptin and adiponectin, factors secreted by the adipocyte (reviewed in [235]). Furthermore, a review of the current literature

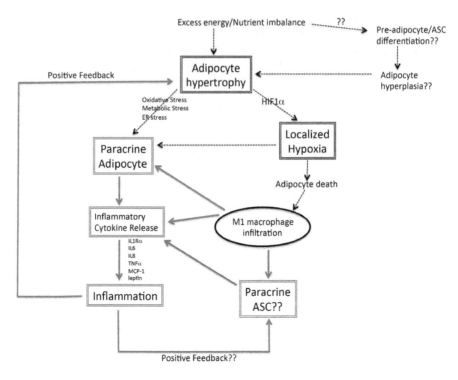

Figure 1. Possible interactions in obesity. Excess energy leads to development of hypertophic adipocytes. Hypertrophic adipocytes lead to the development of cellular stresses and hypoxia, via HIFl1α signaling, which can induce the adipocyte to release numerous pro-inflammatory cytokines. Hypoxia can also result in the death of adipocytes, inducing infiltration by pro-inflamatory/M1 macrophages into the adipose tissue. Paracrine activity by macrophages could affect the release of inflammatory cytokines from the adipocytes. In addition the macrophage may also release these cytokines directly. The resulting inflammation is likely to set up a feedback loop to enhance hypertrophic adipocyte development. The role of the ASC remains unknown in obesity but possible points of interaction could be the differentiation of ASCs, leading to adipocyte hyperplasia and the release of similar pro-inflammatory cytokines. Paracrine activity is shown as solid arrows.

turns up many studies that document the secretion of similar pro-inflammatory factors by ASCs (Table 3). It is possible that the secretion of inflammatory factors, like IL6 or TNFα, by ASCs may play a crucial role in inflammation and the development of obesity. Alternatively, it is possible that inflammation and obesity may result from "defective" ASCs that fail to secrete key anti-inflammatory factors such as IL-10 or have lost their ability to ameliorate oxidative stresses, thus allowing inflammation to go on unchecked. Unfortunately, the effect of inflammation and the ASC is under-represented in today's literature. Those studies that do exist document the inhibition of ASC adipogenesis under inflammatory conditions [248]. This is an interesting finding, as the ASC might be thought of as the logical source for adipocyte hyperplasia observed in obesity. However, if it is the paracrine activity of the ASC that plays a crucial role in the development or maintenance of obesity, then ASC differentiation capacity might be sacrificed in the name of maintaining this function. In light of what we know about adipocytes and pre-adipocytes in obesity, more in-depth studies on the ASC are certainly warranted.

A similar argument for ASCs could be made for other adipose disorders such lipedema and rare adipose disorders (RADs) such as Dercum's (aka Adiposa Dolorosa) [249] and Madelung's disease or Multiple Symmetric Lipomatosis (MSL) [250]. Lipedema (LD), or edema of the fat, is defined as the symmetrical accumulation of adipose tissue in the lower extremities [251]. Because the fat may also be painful as the disorder progresses, LD is often described in the same spectrum as Dercum's [252]. While lipedema and obesity share many similarities – leading to the misdiagnosis of lipedema in up to 15% of the population as obesity, there are some significant differences between LD and obesity. Specifically, excess fat accumulates almost exclusively in the lower limbs in LD and this adipose tissue is stubbornly resistant to loss through dieting [253]. LD is almost exclusively seen in women in their 30s or older, suggesting a hormonal component [251]. Despite these differences, the etiology of obesity and LD may share some commonalities, in that LD is thought to be mediated, in part, through hypoxia and the production of inflammatory cytokines (Figure 2). Like obesity, LD is initially characterized by adipocyte hypertrophy and hyperplasia [254], although the reason for this hypertrophy cannot be attributed to nutrient overload and currently remains unknown. This hypertrophy results in hypoxia, which is thought to result in inflammatory adipokine secretion and a putative positive feedback cascade as seen in obesity. Like obesity, LD fat is characterized by macrophage "crowns" in close association with hypertrophic and/or necrotic adipocytes [132]. These macrophages will almost certainly contribute to the inflammatory reactions occurring in LD fat. Furthermore, when examining adipose tissues isolated from Dercum's, similar immune infiltrations in association with perivascular cells and hypertrophic adipocytes are also seen, again, suggesting that LD and Dercum's may be points along the same spectrum [252]. In light of these commonalities with obesity, it would be logical to assume that the ASC would also play some critical role in mediating inflammation in LD or RADs through its production of paracrine factors. Unfortunately, these studies do not exist at this point.

Despite sharing many of the same characteristics, there are some important distinctions between obesity and LD that may also be at work. These distinctions are also likely to be found in RADs like Dercum's and Madelung's disease. Specifically, LD (and possibly Dercum's and Madelung's) is associated with defects in the microvasculature, together with lymphatic dysfunction [252]. Current theories propose that adipocyte hypertrophy leads to hypoxia, which results in increased angiogenesis. However, this angiogenesis is pathologic and the resulting capillaries are said to be "fragile" or "leaky" [255]. In support of this, perivascular cells, indicative of vascular damage, can be found in LD adipose tissue [254] and pathologic angiogenesis producing fragile capillaries have been found in many eye diseases [256], [257]. What produces this pathology is unknown but studies have shown that leptin can increase the number of fenestrations in capillaries [258] and increased plasma VEGF levels can be found in LD patients [259]. Increased plasma VEGF levels can also be found in LD patients [259], so it is possible that paracrine secretion from hypertrophic and hypoxic adipocytes could disrupt angiogenesis within LD adipose tissue. With studies showing ASCs capable of secreting

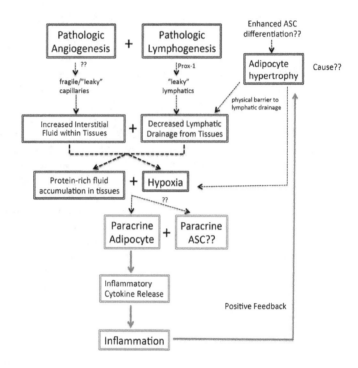

Figure 2. Lipedema. Development of lipedema may have numerous commonalities with obesity starting with the development of hypertrophic adipocytes. Howerver, causation for this is unknown at this time may involve the ASC. As with obesity, adipocyte hypertrophy can lead to the development of hypoxia and the release of inflammatory cytokines from the adipocyte. Possible release of these factors from the ASC due to hypoxia is also shown. In addition, adipocyte hypertrophy is also accompanied by the development of "leaky" capillaries and lymphatics. While the cause of pathologic angiogenesis remains unclear, a role for the gene Prox-1 is though to be involved in lymphatic pathology. Increased filtration from capillaries, combined with poor lympmhatic drainage (due to hypertrophic adipocytes and the the leaking of lymph back from the lymphatic vessel) leads to an accumulation of protein rich fluids within the tissue. Fluid accumulation and hypoxia may induce pro-inflammatory cytokine release. Other mechanisms of obesity (e.g. macrophage infiltration) are also likely to be involved. Paracrine activity is shown as solid arrows.

numerous paracrine factors, including VEGF, and inducing endothelial differentiation and vessel formation, the question of whether the ASC plays a role in this vascular pathology should be asked. The fragile capillaries allow the filtration of protein-rich plasma into the interstitial space, driving the formation of edema [255]. In the early stages of LD, lymphatic drainage can keep up [260]. However with progression of the disorder, lymphatic drainage does decrease as the patient ages [253]. Added to this, the hypertrophic adipocytes are thought to physically restrict fluid drainage and the smaller lymphatic vessels themselves are thought to become "leaky", possibly through the appearance of microaneurysms in these vessels [253]. All of this results in the accumulation of lymph within the adipose tissue. Recent studies now suggest that "lymph can make you fat" [261]. In support of this, adipogenesis in vitro increases when cells are cultured in the presence of lymph [262], [263]. Furthermore, the removal of axillary lymphs nodes in individuals with breast cancer is frequently associated with increased fat deposition within the arm [263]. More recently, mice heterozygous for a mutation in the Prox1 gene not only exhibit leaky lymphatics, but develop obesity as they age [264]-[266]. What it is in the lymph that enhances adipogenesis is unclear. It simply could be the result of edema causing hypoxia, inflammation and adipocyte hypertrophy – not unlike obesity. Alternatively, factors in the lymph could directly induce the ASC to differentiate or the mature adipocyte to store more fat. Since lymph is interstitial fluid combined with emulsified fats, non-reabsorbed proteins and immunocompetent leukocytes, any of these factors could conceivably alter the behavior of the ASC. As it stands, more studies investigating the exact consequences of lymph accumulation on ASC and adipocyte behavior are needed.

So while the mechanisms may differ at points, at the basis of obesity, LD and RADs is inflammation. How the ASC participates in this inflammation remains to be seen, but the ASC could be used in the treatment of these disorders. If inflammation results in adipocyte hypertrophy, then ameliorating this process could decrease the size and number of these cells. In this regard, the anti-inflammatory, anti-oxidant properties of ASCs could be taken advantage of and enhanced in the hopes of mitigating the damaging effects of inflammation in these adipose disorders. However, before this could be attempted, more information is definitely required on the exact roles the ASC plays in adipose tissue formation and how these roles can go wrong when adipose disorders develop.

5. Conclusion

Since 2001, the number of studies characterizing and utilizing the ASC is truly staggering. It appears that the ASC is even passing the bone marrow MSC as the preferred adult stem cell for regenerative medicine. With its ease of isolation from adipose tissue, its availability within the tissue, its long term viability in culture and its persistence when implanted in vivo, the ASC is not only a great stem cell choice for studying mechanisms in vitro but for how it can regenerate tissues in vivo. In response, the studies using ASCs are incredibly diverse and range from their direct differentiation in regenerating tissues such as bone, muscle, nerve and liver to their indirect use in mediating inflammation, protecting nervous tissue and directing vascularization and wound healing through their production of paracrine factors. Finally, a truly exciting use for the ASC may be based on this paracrine activity, in that ASC appears to be easily engineered for the delivery of key factors capable of regenerating many tissue types and maintaining their health. Only time will tell how far the ASC will go.

Abbreviations

ASC = adipose-derived stem cell; EC = endothelial cell; LD = lipedema; MSC = mesenchymal stem cell; GFAP = glial fibrillary acidic protein; HLA = human leukocyte antigen; IR = ischemia reperfusion; LVEF = left ventricular ejection fraction; MAP2 = microtubule associated protein-2; MLR = mixed lymphocyte reaction; PLA = processed lipoaspirate; RAD = rare adipose disorder; SVF = stromal vascular fraction; SC = Schwann cell; Tuj-1 = class III beta-tubulin; vWF = von Willebrand factor

Author details

Patricia Zuk*

Regenerative Bioengineering and Repair Lab, Division of Plastic Surgery, Department of Surgery, David Geffen School of Medicine at UCLA, Los Angeles, USA

References

[1] Zuk PA, Zhu, M., Mizuno, H., Huang, J.I., Futrell, W.J, Katz, A.J., Benhaim, P., Lorenz, H. P., and Hedrick, M. H. Multi-lineage cells from human adipose tissue: implications for cell-based therapies. Tissue Engineering. 2001;7:211-226.

[2] Pozanski WJ, Waheed, I., and Van, R. Human fat cell precursors: morphologic and metabolic differentiation in culture. Lab Invest. 1973;29(5):570-576.

[3] Gronthos S, Franklin DM, Leddy HA, Robey PG, Storms RW, Gimble JM. Surface protein characterization of human adipose tissue-derived stromal cells. J Cell Physiol. 2001;189(1):54-63.

[4] Mitchell JB, McIntosh K, Zvonic S, Garrett S, Floyd ZE, Kloster A, Di Halvorsen Y, Storms RW, Goh B, Kilroy G, Wu X, Gimble JM. Immunophenotype of human adipose-derived cells: temporal changes in stromal-associated and stem cell-associated markers. Stem Cells. 2006;24(2):376-385.

[5] Varma MJ, Breuls RG, Schouten TE, Jurgens WJ, Bontkes HJ, Schuurhuis GJ, van Ham SM, van Milligen FJ. Phenotypical and functional characterization of freshly isolated adipose tissue-derived stem cells. Stem Cells Dev. 2007;16(1):91-104.

[6] Zannettino AC, Paton S, Arthur A, Khor F, Itescu S, Gimble JM, Gronthos S. Multipotential human adipose-derived stromal stem cells exhibit a perivascular phenotype in vitro and in vivo. J Cell Physiol. 2008;214(2):413-421.

[7] Katz AJ, Tholpady A, Tholpady SS, Shang H, Ogle RC. Cell surface and transcriptional characterization of human adipose-derived adherent stromal (hADAS) cells. Stem Cells. 2005;23(3):412-423.

[8] Zuk PA, Zhu M., Ashjian, P., De Ugarte, D.A., Huang, J.I., Mizuno, H., Alfonso, Z.C., Fraser, J.K., Benhaim, P., Hedrick, M.H. Human adipose tissue is a source of multipotent stem cells. Mol. Biol. Cell. 2002;13:4279-4295.

[9] Hattori H, Sato M, Masuoka K, Ishihara M, Kikuchi T, Matsui T, Takase B, Ishizuka T, Kikuchi M, Fujikawa K, Ishihara M. Osteogenic potential of human adipose tissue-derived stromal cells as an alternative stem cell source. Cells Tissues Organs. 2004;178(1):2-12.

[10] Leong DT, Khor WM, Chew FT, Lim TC, Hutmacher DW. Characterization of osteogenically induced adipose tissue-derived precursor cells in 2-dimensional and 3-dimensional environments. Cells Tissues Organs. 2006;182(1):1-11.

[11] Hao W, Hu YY, Wei YY, Pang L, Lv R, Bai JP, Xiong Z, Jiang M. Collagen I gel can facilitate homogenous bone formation of adipose-derived stem cells in PLGA-beta-TCP scaffold. Cells Tissues Organs. 2008;187(2):89-102.

[12] Lee JH, Rhie JW, Oh DY, Ahn ST. Osteogenic differentiation of human adipose tissue-derived stromal cells (hASCs) in a porous three-dimensional scaffold. Biochem Biophys Res Commun. 2008;370(3):456-460.

[13] Huang JI, Beanes SR, Zhu M, Lorenz HP, Hedrick MH, Benhaim P. Rat extramedullary adipose tissue as a source of osteochondrogenic progenitor cells. Plast Reconstr Surg. 2002;109(3):1033-1041; discussion 1042-1033.

[14] Huang JI, Zuk, P.A., Jones, N.F., Zhu, M., Lorenz, H.P., Hedrick, M.H., Benhaim, P. Chondrogenic potential of multipotential cells from human adipose tissue. Plast. Reconstr. Surg. 2003; 2004; 113(2):585-594

[15] Tholpady SS, Katz AJ, Ogle RC. Mesenchymal stem cells from rat visceral fat exhibit multipotential differentiation in vitro. Anat Rec A Discov Mol Cell Evol Biol. 2003;272(1):398-402.

[16] Ogawa R, Mizuno H, Hyakusoku H, Watanabe A, Migita M, Shimada T. Chondrogenic and osteogenic differentiation of adipose-derived stem cells isolated from GFP transgenic mice. J Nippon Med Sch. 2004;71(4):240-241.

[17] Ogawa R, Mizuno H, Watanabe A, Migita M, Hyakusoku H, Shimada T. Adipogenic differentiation by adipose-derived stem cells harvested from GFP transgenic mice-including relationship of sex differences. Biochem Biophys Res Commun. 2004;319(2): 511-517.

[18] Awad HA, Wickham MQ, Leddy HA, Gimble JM, Guilak F. Chondrogenic differentiation of adipose-derived adult stem cells in agarose, alginate, and gelatin scaffolds. Biomaterials. 2004;25(16):3211-3222.

[19] Rodriguez AM, Elabd C, Delteil F, Astier J, Vernochet C, Saint-Marc P, Guesnet J, Guezennec A, Amri EZ, Dani C, Ailhaud G. Adipocyte differentiation of multipotent

cells established from human adipose tissue. Biochem Biophys Res Commun. 2004;315(2):255-263.

[20] Mizuno H, Zuk, P.A., Zhu, M., Lorenz, H.P., Benhaim, P., and Hedrick, M.H. Myogenic differentiation of human processed lipoaspirate cells. Plastic and Reconstr. Surg. 2001;109(1):199-209.

[21] Hicok KC, Du Laney TV, Zhou YS, Halvorsen YD, Hitt DC, Cooper LF, Gimble JM. Human adipose-derived adult stem cells produce osteoid in vivo. Tissue Eng. 2004;10(3-4):371-380.

[22] Yoon E, Dhar S, Chun DE, Gharibjanian NA, Evans GR. In Vivo Osteogenic Potential of Human Adipose-Derived Stem Cells/Poly Lactide-Co-Glycolic Acid Constructs for Bone Regeneration in a Rat Critical-Sized Calvarial Defect Model. Tissue Eng. 2007;13(3):619-627.

[23] Conejero JA, Lee JA, Parrett BM, Terry M, Wear-Maggitti K, Grant RT, Breitbart AS. Repair of palatal bone defects using osteogenically differentiated fat-derived stem cells. Plast Reconstr Surg. 2006;117(3):857-863.

[24] Lee JA, Parrett, B.M., Conejero, J.A., Laser, J., Chen, J., Kogon, A.J., Nanda, D., Grant, R.T., Breitbart, A.S. Biological alchemy: engineering bone and fat from fat-derived stem cells. Ann. Plast. Surg. 2003;50(610-617.

[25] Cowan CM, Shi YY, Aalami OO, Chou YF, Mari C, Thomas R, Quarto N, Contag CH, Wu B, Longaker MT. Adipose-derived adult stromal cells heal critical-size mouse calvarial defects. Nat Biotechnol. 2004;22(5):560-567.

[26] Jin XB, Sun YS, Zhang K, Wang J, Ju XD, Lou SQ. Neocartilage formation from predifferentiated human adipose derived stem cells in vivo. Acta Pharmacol Sin. 2007;28(5):663-671.

[27] Mehlhorn AT, Zwingmann J, Finkenzeller G, Niemeyer P, Dauner M, Stark B, Sudkamp NP, Schmal H. Chondrogenesis of adipose-derived adult stem cells in a polylactide-co-glycolide scaffold. Tissue Eng Part A. 2009;15(5):1159-1167.

[28] Lin Y, Luo E, Chen X, Liu L, Qiao J, Yan Z, Li Z, Tang W, Zheng X, Tian W. Molecular and cellular characterization during chondrogenic differentiation of adipose tissue-derived stromal cells in vitro and cartilage formation in vivo. J Cell Mol Med. 2005;9(4):929-939.

[29] Lu F, Gao JH, Ogawa R, Mizuro H, Hykusoku H. Adipose tissues differentiated by adipose-derived stem cells harvested from transgenic mice. Chin J Traumatol. 2006;9(6):359-364.

[30] Mizuno H, Itoi Y, Kawahara S, Ogawa R, Akaishi S, Hyakusoku H. In vivo adipose tissue regeneration by adipose-derived stromal cells isolated from GFP transgenic mice. Cells Tissues Organs. 2008;187(3):177-185.

[31] Hong L, Peptan IA, Colpan A, Daw JL. Adipose tissue engineering by human adipose-derived stromal cells. Cells Tissues Organs. 2006;183(3):133-140.

[32] Mauney JR, Nguyen T, Gillen K, Kirker-Head C, Gimble JM, Kaplan DL. Engineering adipose-like tissue in vitro and in vivo utilizing human bone marrow and adipose-derived mesenchymal stem cells with silk fibroin 3D scaffolds. Biomaterials. 2007;28(35):5280-5290.

[33] Rodriguez AM, Pisani D, Dechesne CA, Turc-Carel C, Kurzenne JY, Wdziekonski B, Villageois A, Bagnis C, Breittmayer JP, Groux H, Ailhaud G, Dani C. Transplantation of a multipotent cell population from human adipose tissue induces dystrophin expression in the immunocompetent mdx mouse. J Exp Med. 2005;201(9):1397-1405.

[34] Goudenege S, Pisani DF, Wdziekonski B, Di Santo JP, Bagnis C, Dani C, Dechesne CA. Enhancement of myogenic and muscle repair capacities of human adipose-derived stem cells with forced expression of MyoD. Mol Ther. 2009;17(6):1064-1072.

[35] Liu Y, Yan X, Sun Z, Chen B, Han Q, Li J, Zhao RC. Flk-1+ adipose-derived mesenchymal stem cells differentiate into skeletal muscle satellite cells and ameliorate muscular dystrophy in mdx mice. Stem Cells Dev. 2007;16(5):695-706.

[36] Jack GS, Almeida FG, Zhang R, Alfonso ZC, Zuk PA, Rodriguez LV. Processed lipoaspirate cells for tissue engineering of the lower urinary tract: implications for the treatment of stress urinary incontinence and bladder reconstruction. J Urol. 2005;174(5):2041-2045.

[37] Harris LJ, Abdollahi H, Zhang P, McIlhenny S, Tulenko TN, DiMuzio PJ. Differentiation of adult stem cells into smooth muscle for vascular tissue engineering. J Surg Res. 2011;168(2):306-314.

[38] Choi YS, Dusting GJ, Stubbs S, Arunothayaraj S, Han XL, Collas P, Morrison WA, Dilley RJ. Differentiation of human adipose-derived stem cells into beating cardiomyocytes. J Cell Mol Med. 2010;14(4):878-889.

[39] Planat-Benard V, Menard C, Andre M, Puceat M, Perez A, Garcia-Verdugo JM, Penicaud L, Casteilla L. Spontaneous cardiomyocyte differentiation from adipose tissue stroma cells. Circ Res. 2004;94(2):223-229.

[40] Colazzo F, Chester AH, Taylor PM, Yacoub MH. Induction of mesenchymal to endothelial transformation of adipose-derived stem cells. J Heart Valve Dis. 2010;19(6):736-744.

[41] Cao Y, Sun Z, Liao L, Meng Y, Han Q, Zhao RC. Human adipose tissue-derived stem cells differentiate into endothelial cells in vitro and improve postnatal neovascularization in vivo. Biochem Biophys Res Commun. 2005;332(2):370-379.

[42] Long JL, Zuk P, Berke GS, Chhetri DK. Epithelial differentiation of adipose-derived stem cells for laryngeal tissue engineering. Laryngoscope. 2010;120(1):125-131.

[43] Kumai Y, Kobler JB, Park H, Lopez-Guerra G, Karajanagi S, Herrera VL, Zeitels SM. Crosstalk between adipose-derived stem/stromal cells and vocal fold fibroblasts in vitro. Laryngoscope. 2009;119(4):799-805.

[44] Chandra V, Swetha G, Muthyala S, Jaiswal AK, Bellare JR, Nair PD, Bhonde RR. Islet-like cell aggregates generated from human adipose tissue derived stem cells ameliorate experimental diabetes in mice. PLoS One. 2011;6(6):e20615.

[45] Bassi EJ, Moraes-Vieira PM, Moreira Sa CS, Almeida DC, Vieira LM, Cunha CS, Hiyane MI, Basso AS, Pacheco-Silva A, Camara NO. Immune Regulatory Properties of Allogeneic Adipose-Derived Mesenchymal Stem Cells in the Treatment of Experimental Autoimmune Diabetes. Diabetes. 2012; 61(10):2534-2545.

[46] Li YY, Liu HH, Chen HL, Li YP. Adipose-derived mesenchymal stem cells ameliorate STZ-induced pancreas damage in type 1 diabetes. Biomed Mater Eng. 2012;22(1): 97-103.

[47] Meyerrose TE, De Ugarte DA, Hofling AA, Herrbrich PE, Cordonnier TD, Shultz LD, Eagon JC, Wirthlin L, Sands MS, Hedrick MA, Nolta JA. In vivo distribution of human adipose-derived mesenchymal stem cells in novel xenotransplantation models. Stem Cells. 2007;25(1):220-227.

[48] Fang B, Li Y, Song Y, Li N, Cao Y, Wei X, Lin Q, Zhao RC. Human adipose tissue-derived adult stem cells can lead to multiorgan engraftment. Transplant Proc. 2010;42(5):1849-1856.

[49] Salgado AJ, Reis RL, Sousa NJ, Gimble JM. Adipose tissue derived stem cells secretome: soluble factors and their roles in regenerative medicine. Curr Stem Cell Res Ther. 2010;5(2):103-110.

[50] Levi B, James AW, Nelson ER, Hu S, Sun N, Peng M, Wu J, Longaker MT. Studies in adipose-derived stromal cells: migration and participation in repair of cranial injury after systemic injection. Plast Reconstr Surg. 2011;127(3):1130-1140.

[51] Caplan AI, Dennis JE. Mesenchymal stem cells as trophic mediators. J Cell Biochem. 2006;98(5):1076-1084.

[52] Liechty KW, MacKenzie, T.C., Shaaban, A.F., Radu, A., Moseley, A.M., Deans, R., Marshak,D.R., Flake, A.W. Human mesenchymal stem cells engraft and demonstrate site-specific differentiation after in utero transplantation in sheep. Nat. Med. 2000;6:1282-1286.

[53] Di Nicola M, Carlo-Stella C, Magni M, Milanesi M, Longoni PD, Matteucci P, Grisanti S, Gianni AM. Human bone marrow stromal cells suppress T-lymphocyte proliferation induced by cellular or nonspecific mitogenic stimuli. Blood. 2002;99(10): 3838-3843.

[54] Krampera M, Glennie S, Dyson J, Scott D, Laylor R, Simpson E, Dazzi F. Bone marrow mesenchymal stem cells inhibit the response of naive and memory antigen-specific T cells to their cognate peptide. Blood. 2003;101(9):3722-3729.

[55] Djouad F, Plence P, Bony C, Tropel P, Apparailly F, Sany J, Noel D, Jorgensen C. Immunosuppressive effect of mesenchymal stem cells favors tumor growth in allogeneic animals. Blood. 2003;102(10):3837-3844.

[56] Angoulvant D, Clerc A, Benchalal S, Galambrun C, Farre A, Bertrand Y, Eljaafari A. Human mesenchymal stem cells suppress induction of cytotoxic response to alloantigens. Biorheology. 2004;41(3-4):469-476.

[57] Rasmusson I, Ringden O, Sundberg B, Le Blanc K. Mesenchymal stem cells inhibit the formation of cytotoxic T lymphocytes, but not activated cytotoxic T lymphocytes or natural killer cells. Transplantation. 2003;76(8):1208-1213.

[58] Corcione A, Benvenuto F, Ferretti E, Giunti D, Cappiello V, Cazzanti F, Risso M, Gualandi F, Mancardi GL, Pistoia V, Uccelli A. Human mesenchymal stem cells modulate B-cell functions. Blood. 2006;107(1):367-372.

[59] Wan CD, Cheng R, Wang HB, Liu T. Immunomodulatory effects of mesenchymal stem cells derived from adipose tissues in a rat orthotopic liver transplantation model. Hepatobiliary Pancreat Dis Int. 2008;7(1):29-33.

[60] Cui L, Yin S, Liu W, Li N, Zhang W, Cao Y. Expanded adipose-derived stem cells suppress mixed lymphocyte reaction by secretion of prostaglandin E2. Tissue Eng. 2007;13(6):1185-1195.

[61] Puissant B, Barreau C, Bourin P, Clavel C, Corre J, Bousquet C, Taureau C, Cousin B, Abbal M, Laharrague P, Penicaud L, Casteilla L, Blancher A. Immunomodulatory effect of human adipose tissue-derived adult stem cells: comparison with bone marrow mesenchymal stem cells. Br J Haematol. 2005;129(1):118-129.

[62] Wolbank S, Peterbauer A, Fahrner M, Hennerbichler S, van Griensven M, Stadler G, Redl H, Gabriel C. Dose-dependent immunomodulatory effect of human stem cells from amniotic membrane: a comparison with human mesenchymal stem cells from adipose tissue. Tissue Eng. 2007;13(6):1173-1183.

[63] Yoo KH, Jang IK, Lee MW, Kim HE, Yang MS, Eom Y, Lee JE, Kim YJ, Yang SK, Jung HL, Sung KW, Kim CW, Koo HH. Comparison of immunomodulatory properties of mesenchymal stem cells derived from adult human tissues. Cell Immunol. 2009;259(2):150-156.

[64] Schweitzer KS, Johnstone BH, Garrison J, Rush NI, Cooper S, Traktuev DO, Feng D, Adamowicz JJ, Van Demark M, Fisher AJ, Kamocki K, Brown MB, Presson RG, Jr., Broxmeyer HE, March KL, Petrache I. Adipose stem cell treatment in mice attenuates lung and systemic injury induced by cigarette smoking. Am J Respir Crit Care Med. 2011;183(2):215-225.

[65] Zhou Y, Yuan J, Zhou B, Lee AJ, Ghawji M, Jr., Yoo TJ. The therapeutic efficacy of human adipose tissue-derived mesenchymal stem cells on experimental autoimmune hearing loss in mice. Immunology. 2011;133(1):133-140.

[66] Zhou B, Yuan J, Zhou Y, Ghawji M, Jr., Deng YP, Lee AJ, Nair U, Kang AH, Brand DD, Yoo TJ. Administering human adipose-derived mesenchymal stem cells to prevent and treat experimental arthritis. Clin Immunol. 2011;141(3):328-337.

[67] Hyun YY, Kim IO, Kim MH, Nam DH, Lee MH, Kim JE, Song HK, Cha JJ, Kang YS, Lee JE, Kim HW, Han JY, Cha DR. Adipose-Derived Stem Cells Improve Renal Function in a Mouse Model of IgA Nephropathy. Cell Transplant. 2012 in press.

[68] Pinheiro CH, de Queiroz JC, Guimaraes-Ferreira L, Vitzel KF, Nachbar RT, de Sousa LG, de Souza-Jr AL, Nunes MT, Curi R. Local injections of adipose-derived mesenchymal stem cells modulate inflammation and increase angiogenesis ameliorating the dystrophic phenotype in dystrophin-deficient skeletal muscle. Stem Cell Rev. 2012;8(2):363-374.

[69] Cui L, Yin S, Yang P, Liu B, Zhang Y, Liu W, Cao YL. [Human adipose derived stem cells suppress lymphocyte proliferation induced by cellular or nonspecific mitogenic stimuli]. Zhonghua Yi Xue Za Zhi. 2005;85(27):1890-1894.

[70] Najar M, Raicevic G, Boufker HI, Fayyad-Kazan H, De Bruyn C, Meuleman N, Bron D, Toungouz M, Lagneaux L. Adipose-tissue-derived and Wharton's jelly-derived mesenchymal stromal cells suppress lymphocyte responses by secreting leukemia inhibitory factor. Tissue Eng Part A. 2010;16(11):3537-3546.

[71] Payne NL, Dantanarayana A, Sun G, Moussa L, Caine S, McDonald C, Herszfeld D, Bernard CC, Siatskas C. Early intervention with gene-modified mesenchymal stem cells overexpressing interleukin-4 enhances anti-inflammatory responses and functional recovery in experimental autoimmune demyelination. Cell Adh Migr. 2012;6(3):179-189.

[72] Lai K, Zeng K, Zeng F, Wei J, Tan G. Allogeneic adipose-derived stem cells suppress Th17 lymphocytes in patients with active lupus in vitro. Acta Biochim Biophys Sin (Shanghai). 2011;43(10):805-812.

[73] Kuo YR, Chen CC, Goto S, Lee IT, Huang CW, Tsai CC, Wang CT, Chen CL. Modulation of immune response and T-cell regulation by donor adipose-derived stem cells in a rodent hind-limb allotransplant model. Plast Reconstr Surg. 2011;128(6): 661e-672e.

[74] Gonzalez-Rey E, Gonzalez MA, Varela N, O'Valle F, Hernandez-Cortes P, Rico L, Buscher D, Delgado M. Human adipose-derived mesenchymal stem cells reduce inflammatory and T cell responses and induce regulatory T cells in vitro in rheumatoid arthritis. Ann Rheum Dis. 2010;69(1):241-248.

[75] Gonzalez MA, Gonzalez-Rey E, Rico L, Buscher D, Delgado M. Treatment of experimental arthritis by inducing immune tolerance with human adipose-derived mesenchymal stem cells. Arthritis Rheum. 2009;60(4):1006-1019.

[76] Cho KS, Roh HJ. Immunomodulatory effects of adipose-derived stem cells in airway allergic diseases. Curr Stem Cell Res Ther. 2010;5(2):111-115.

[77] Gonzalez-Rey E, Anderson P, Gonzalez MA, Rico L, Buscher D, Delgado M. Human adult stem cells derived from adipose tissue protect against experimental colitis and sepsis. Gut. 2009;58(7):929-939.

[78] Gonzalez MA, Gonzalez-Rey E, Rico L, Buscher D, Delgado M. Adipose-derived mesenchymal stem cells alleviate experimental colitis by inhibiting inflammatory and autoimmune responses. Gastroenterology. 2009;136(3):978-989.

[79] Kim JM, Lee ST, Chu K, Jung KH, Song EC, Kim SJ, Sinn DI, Kim JH, Park DK, Kang KM, Hyung Hong N, Park HK, Won CH, Kim KH, Kim M, Kun Lee S, Roh JK. Systemic transplantation of human adipose stem cells attenuated cerebral inflammation and degeneration in a hemorrhagic stroke model. Brain Res. 2007;1183:43-50.

[80] Constantin G, Marconi S, Rossi B, Angiari S, Calderan L, Anghileri E, Gini B, Bach SD, Martinello M, Bifari F, Galie M, Turano E, Budui S, Sbarbati A, Krampera M, Bonetti B. Adipose-derived mesenchymal stem cells ameliorate chronic experimental autoimmune encephalomyelitis. Stem Cells. 2009;27(10):2624-2635.

[81] Lin CS, Lin G, Lue TF. Allogeneic and Xenogeneic Transplantation of Adipose-Derived Stem Cells in Immunocompetent Recipients Without Immunosuppressants. Stem Cells Dev. 2012; 21(15):2770-2778.

[82] Paul A, Srivastava S, Chen G, Shum-Tim D, Prakash S. Functional Assessment of Adipose Stem Cells for Xenotransplantation Using Myocardial Infarction Immunocompetent Models: Comparison with Bone Marrow Stem Cells. Cell Biochem Biophys. 2011; in press.

[83] Bradley BA. The role of HLA matching in transplantation. Immunol Lett. 1991;29(1-2):55-59.

[84] Lombardi G, Lechler R. The molecular basis of allorecognition of major histocompatibility complex molecules by T lymphocytes. Ann Ist Super Sanita. 1991;27(1):7-14.

[85] DelaRosa O, Sanchez-Correa B, Morgado S, Ramirez C, del Rio B, Menta R, Lombardo E, Tarazona R, Casado JG. Human adipose-derived stem cells impair natural killer cell function and exhibit low susceptibility to natural killer-mediated lysis. Stem Cells Dev. 2012;21(8):1333-1343.

[86] Moon MH, Kim SY, Kim YJ, Kim SJ, Lee JB, Bae YC, Sung SM, Jung JS. Human adipose tissue-derived mesenchymal stem cells improve postnatal neovascularization in a mouse model of hindlimb ischemia. Cell Physiol Biochem. 2006;17(5-6):279-290.

[87] Fischer LJ, McIlhenny S, Tulenko T, Golesorkhi N, Zhang P, Larson R, Lombardi J, Shapiro I, DiMuzio PJ. Endothelial differentiation of adipose-derived stem cells: effects of endothelial cell growth supplement and shear force. J Surg Res. 2009;152(1): 157-166.

[88] DiMuzio P, Tulenko T. Tissue engineering applications to vascular bypass graft development: the use of adipose-derived stem cells. J Vasc Surg. 2012; in press.

[89] Wosnitza M, Hemmrich K, Groger A, Graber S, Pallua N. Plasticity of human adipose stem cells to perform adipogenic and endothelial differentiation. Differentiation. 2007;75(1):12-23.

[90] Planat-Benard V, Silvestre JS, Cousin B, Andre M, Nibbelink M, Tamarat R, Clergue M, Manneville C, Saillan-Barreau C, Duriez M, Tedgui A, Levy B, Penicaud L, Casteilla L. Plasticity of human adipose lineage cells toward endothelial cells: physiological and therapeutic perspectives. Circulation. 2004;109(5):656-663.

[91] Ribeiro CA, Fraga JS, Graos M, Neves NM, Reis RL, Gimble JM, Sousa N, Salgado AJ. The secretome of stem cells isolated from the adipose tissue and Wharton jelly acts differently on central nervous system derived cell populations. Stem Cell Res Ther. 2012;3(3):18.

[92] Ii M, Horii M, Yokoyama A, Shoji T, Mifune Y, Kawamoto A, Asahi M, Asahara T. Synergistic effect of adipose-derived stem cell therapy and bone marrow progenitor recruitment in ischemic heart. Lab Invest. 2011;91(4):539-552.

[93] Kim EK, Li G, Lee TJ, Hong JP. The effect of human adipose-derived stem cells on healing of ischemic wounds in a diabetic nude mouse model. Plast Reconstr Surg. 2011;128(2):387-394.

[94] Lu S, Lu C, Han Q, Li J, Du Z, Liao L, Zhao RC. Adipose-derived mesenchymal stem cells protect PC12 cells from glutamate excitotoxicity-induced apoptosis by upregulation of XIAP through PI3-K/Akt activation. Toxicology. 2011;279(1-3):189-195.

[95] Liu K, Liu R, Cao G, Sun H, Wang X, Wu S. Adipose-derived stromal cell autologous transplantation ameliorates pulmonary arterial hypertension induced by shunt flow in rat models. Stem Cells Dev. 2011;20(6):1001-1010.

[96] Nie C, Yang D, Xu J, Si Z, Jin X, Zhang J. Locally administered adipose-derived stem cells accelerate wound healing through differentiation and vasculogenesis. Cell Transplant. 2011;20(2):205-216.

[97] Zhu M, Zhou Z, Chen Y, Schreiber R, Ransom JT, Fraser JK, Hedrick MH, Pinkernell K, Kuo HC. Supplementation of fat grafts with adipose-derived regenerative cells improves long-term graft retention. Ann Plast Surg. 2010;64(2):222-228.

[98] Grewal N, Yacomotti L, Melkonyan V, Massey M, Bradley JP, Zuk PA. Freezing adipose tissue grafts may damage their ability to integrate into the host. Connect Tissue Res. 2009;50(1):14-28.

[99] Rubina K, Kalinina N, Efimenko A, Lopatina T, Melikhova V, Tsokolaeva Z, Sysoeva V, Tkachuk V, Parfyonova Y. Adipose stromal cells stimulate angiogenesis via promoting progenitor cell differentiation, secretion of angiogenic factors, and enhancing vessel maturation. Tissue Eng Part A. 2009;15(8):2039-2050.

[100] Park BS, Jang KA, Sung JH, Park JS, Kwon YH, Kim KJ, Kim WS. Adipose-derived stem cells and their secretory factors as a promising therapy for skin aging. Dermatol Surg. 2008;34(10):1323-1326.

[101] Prichard HL, Reichert W, Klitzman B. IFATS collection: Adipose-derived stromal cells improve the foreign body response. Stem Cells. 2008;26(10):2691-2695.

[102] Kilroy GE, Foster SJ, Wu X, Ruiz J, Sherwood S, Heifetz A, Ludlow JW, Stricker DM, Potiny S, Green P, Halvorsen YD, Cheatham B, Storms RW, Gimble JM. Cytokine profile of human adipose-derived stem cells: expression of angiogenic, hematopoietic, and pro-inflammatory factors. J Cell Physiol. 2007;212(3):702-709.

[103] Wang M, Crisostomo PR, Herring C, Meldrum KK, Meldrum DR. Human progenitor cells from bone marrow or adipose tissue produce VEGF, HGF, and IGF-I in response to TNF by a p38 MAPK-dependent mechanism. Am J Physiol Regul Integr Comp Physiol. 2006;291(4):R880-884.

[104] Rehman J, Traktuev D, Li J, Merfeld-Clauss S, Temm-Grove CJ, Bovenkerk JE, Pell CL, Johnstone BH, Considine RV, March KL. Secretion of angiogenic and antiapoptotic factors by human adipose stromal cells. Circulation. 2004;109(10):1292-1298.

[105] Kim Y, Kim H, Cho H, Bae Y, Suh K, Jung J. Direct comparison of human mesenchymal stem cells derived from adipose tissues and bone marrow in mediating neovascularization in response to vascular ischemia. Cell Physiol Biochem. 2007;20(6): 867-876.

[106] Takahashi M, Suzuki E, Oba S, Nishimatsu H, Kimura K, Nagano T, Nagai R, Hirata Y. Adipose tissue-derived stem cells inhibit neointimal formation in a paracrine fashion in rat femoral artery. Am J Physiol Heart Circ Physiol. 2010;298(2):H415-423.

[107] Gao W, Qiao X, Ma S, Cui L. Adipose-derived stem cells accelerate neovascularization in ischaemic diabetic skin flap via expression of hypoxia-inducible factor-1alpha. J Cell Mol Med. 2010;15(12):2575-2585.

[108] Dumont DJ, Fong GH, Puri MC, Gradwohl G, Alitalo K, Breitman ML. Vascularization of the mouse embryo: a study of flk-1, tek, tie, and vascular endothelial growth factor expression during development. Dev Dyn. 1995;203(1):80-92.

[109] Jakeman LB, Armanini M, Phillips HS, Ferrara N. Developmental expression of binding sites and messenger ribonucleic acid for vascular endothelial growth factor suggests a role for this protein in vasculogenesis and angiogenesis. Endocrinology. 1993;133(2):848-859.

[110] Tufro A, Norwood VF, Carey RM, Gomez RA. Vascular endothelial growth factor induces nephrogenesis and vasculogenesis. J Am Soc Nephrol. 1999;10(10):2125-2134.

[111] Tse KH, Kingham PJ, Novikov LN, Wiberg M. Adipose tissue and bone marrow-derived stem cells react similarly in an ischaemia-like microenvironment. J Tissue Eng Regen Med. 2012;6(6):473-485.

[112] Cai L, Johnstone BH, Cook TG, Liang Z, Traktuev D, Cornetta K, Ingram DA, Rosen ED, March KL. Suppression of hepatocyte growth factor production impairs the ability of adipose-derived stem cells to promote ischemic tissue revascularization. Stem Cells. 2007;25(12):3234-3243.

[113] Sumi M, Sata M, Toya N, Yanaga K, Ohki T, Nagai R. Transplantation of adipose stromal cells, but not mature adipocytes, augments ischemia-induced angiogenesis. Life Sci. 2007;80(6):559-565.

[114] Kondo K, Shintani S, Shibata R, Murakami H, Murakami R, Imaizumi M, Kitagawa Y, Murohara T. Implantation of adipose-derived regenerative cells enhances ischemia-induced angiogenesis. Arterioscler Thromb Vasc Biol. 2009;29(1):61-66.

[115] Miranville A, Heeschen C, Sengenes C, Curat CA, Busse R, Bouloumie A. Improvement of postnatal neovascularization by human adipose tissue-derived stem cells. Circulation. 2004;110(3):349-355.

[116] Koh YJ, Koh BI, Kim H, Joo HJ, Jin HK, Jeon J, Choi C, Lee DH, Chung JH, Cho CH, Park WS, Ryu JK, Suh JK, Koh GY. Stromal vascular fraction from adipose tissue forms profound vascular network through the dynamic reassembly of blood endothelial cells. Arterioscler Thromb Vasc Biol. 2011;31(5):1141-1150.

[117] Kang Y, Park C, Kim D, Seong CM, Kwon K, Choi C. Unsorted human adipose tissue-derived stem cells promote angiogenesis and myogenesis in murine ischemic hindlimb model. Microvasc Res. 2010;80(3):310-316.

[118] Bhang SH, Cho SW, La WG, Lee TJ, Yang HS, Sun AY, Baek SH, Rhie JW, Kim BS. Angiogenesis in ischemic tissue produced by spheroid grafting of human adipose-derived stromal cells. Biomaterials. 2011;32(11):2734-2747.

[119] Kim WS, Park BS, Sung JH, Yang JM, Park SB, Kwak SJ, Park JS. Wound healing effect of adipose-derived stem cells: a critical role of secretory factors on human dermal fibroblasts. J Dermatol Sci. 2007;48(1):15-24.

[120] Eltzschig HK, Carmeliet P. Hypoxia and inflammation. N Engl J Med. 2011;364(7): 656-665.

[121] Reichenberger MA, Heimer S, Schaefer A, Lass U, Gebhard MM, Germann G, Leimer U, Kollensperger E, Mueller W. Adipose derived stem cells protect skin flaps against ischemia-reperfusion injury. Stem Cell Rev. 2012;8(3):854-862.

[122] Mazo M, Hernandez S, Gavira JJ, Abizanda G, Arana M, Lopez-Martinez T, Moreno C, Merino J, Martino-Rodriguez A, Uixeira A, de Jalon JA, Pastrana J, Martinez-Caro

D, Prosper F. Treatment of reperfused ischemia with adipose-derived stem cells in a preclinical swine model of myocardial infarction. Cell Transplant. 2011.

[123] Sun CK, Yen CH, Lin YC, Tsai TH, Chang LT, Kao YH, Chua S, Fu M, Ko SF, Leu S, Yip HK. Autologous transplantation of adipose-derived mesenchymal stem cells markedly reduced acute ischemia-reperfusion lung injury in a rodent model. J Transl Med. 2011;9:118.

[124] Froehlich H, Gulati R, Boilson B, Witt T, Harbuzariu A, Kleppe L, Dietz AB, Lerman A, Simari RD. Carotid repair using autologous adipose-derived endothelial cells. Stroke. 2009;40(5):1886-1891.

[125] Malis CD, Bonventre JV. Susceptibility of mitochondrial membranes to calcium and reactive oxygen species: implications for ischemic and toxic tissue damage. Prog Clin Biol Res. 1988;282:235-259.

[126] Clark IA, Cowden WB, Hunt NH. Free radical-induced pathology. Med Res Rev. 1985;5(3):297-332.

[127] Kloner RA, Przyklenk K, Whittaker P. Deleterious effects of oxygen radicals in ischemia/reperfusion. Resolved and unresolved issues. Circulation. 1989;80(5):1115-1127.

[128] Thompson JA, Hess ML. The oxygen free radical system: a fundamental mechanism in the production of myocardial necrosis. Prog Cardiovasc Dis. 1986;28(6):449-462.

[129] Kim WS, Park BS, Kim HK, Park JS, Kim KJ, Choi JS, Chung SJ, Kim DD, Sung JH. Evidence supporting antioxidant action of adipose-derived stem cells: protection of human dermal fibroblasts from oxidative stress. J Dermatol Sci. 2008;49(2):133-142.

[130] Chen YT, Sun CK, Lin YC, Chang LT, Chen YL, Tsai TH, Chung SY, Chua S, Kao YH, Yen CH, Shao PL, Chang KC, Leu S, Yip HK. Adipose-derived mesenchymal stem cell protects kidneys against ischemia-reperfusion injury through suppressing oxidative stress and inflammatory reaction. J Transl Med. 2011;9:51.

[131] Sun CK, Chang CL, Lin YC, Kao YH, Chang LT, Yen CH, Shao PL, Chen CH, Leu S, Yip HK. Systemic administration of autologous adipose-derived mesenchymal stem cells alleviates hepatic ischemia-reperfusion injury in rats. Crit Care Med. 2011;40(4): 1279-1290.

[132] Suga H, Eto H, Aoi N, Kato H, Araki J, Doi K, Higashino T, Yoshimura K. Adipose tissue remodeling under ischemia: death of adipocytes and activation of stem/progenitor cells. Plast Reconstr Surg. 2010;126(6):1911-1923.

[133] Chan RK, Zamora DO, Wrice NL, Baer DG, Renz EM, Christy RJ, Natesan S. Development of a vascularized skin construct using adipose-derived stem cells from debrided burned skin. Stem Cells Int. 2012;2012:841203.

[134]　Zografou A, Tsigris C, Papadopoulos O, Kavantzas N, Patsouris E, Donta I, Perrea D. Improvement of skin-graft survival after autologous transplantation of adipose-derived stem cells in rats. J Plast Reconstr Aesthet Surg. 2011;64(12):1647-1656.

[135]　Lim JS, Yoo G. Effects of adipose-derived stromal cells and of their extract on wound healing in a mouse model. J Korean Med Sci. 2010;25(5):746-751.

[136]　Lee SH, Jin SY, Song JS, Seo KK, Cho KH. Paracrine effects of adipose-derived stem cells on keratinocytes and dermal fibroblasts. Ann Dermatol. 2012;24(2):136-143.

[137]　Song SY, Jung JE, Jeon YR, Tark KC, Lew DH. Determination of adipose-derived stem cell application on photo-aged fibroblasts, based on paracrine function. Cytotherapy. 2012;13(3):378-384.

[138]　Jung H, Kim HH, Lee DH, Hwang YS, Yang HC, Park JC. Transforming growth factor-beta 1 in adipose derived stem cells conditioned medium is a dominant paracrine mediator determines hyaluronic acid and collagen expression profile. Cytotechnology. 2011;63(1):57-66.

[139]　Reichenberger MA, Mueller W, Schafer A, Heimer S, Leimer U, Lass U, Germann G, Kollensperger E. Fibrin-embedded adipose derived stem cells enhance skin flap survival. Stem Cell Rev. 2012;8(3):844-853.

[140]　Song SH, Lee MO, Lee JS, Jeong HC, Kim HG, Kim WS, Hur M, Cha HJ. Genetic modification of human adipose-derived stem cells for promoting wound healing. J Dermatol Sci. 2012;66(2):98-107.

[141]　Altman AM, Yan Y, Matthias N, Bai X, Rios C, Mathur AB, Song YH, Alt EU. IFATS collection: Human adipose-derived stem cells seeded on a silk fibroin-chitosan scaffold enhance wound repair in a murine soft tissue injury model. Stem Cells. 2009;27(1):250-258.

[142]　Fotuhi P, Song YH, Alt E. Electrophysiological consequence of adipose-derived stem cell transplantation in infarcted porcine myocardium. Europace. 2007;9(12):1218-1221.

[143]　Zhang DZ, Gai LY, Liu HW, Jin QH, Huang JH, Zhu XY. Transplantation of autologous adipose-derived stem cells ameliorates cardiac function in rabbits with myocardial infarction. Chin Med J (Engl). 2007;120(4):300-307.

[144]　Kamihata H, Matsubara H, Nishiue T, Fujiyama S, Tsutsumi Y, Ozono R, Masaki H, Mori Y, Iba O, Tateishi E, Kosaki A, Shintani S, Murohara T, Imaizumi T, Iwasaka T. Implantation of bone marrow mononuclear cells into ischemic myocardium enhances collateral perfusion and regional function via side supply of angioblasts, angiogenic ligands, and cytokines. Circulation. 2001;104(9):1046-1052.

[145]　Leobon B, Roncalli J, Joffre C, Mazo M, Boisson M, Barreau C, Calise D, Arnaud E, Andre M, Puceat M, Penicaud L, Prosper F, Planat-Benard V, Casteilla L. Adipose-

derived cardiomyogenic cells: in vitro expansion and functional improvement in a mouse model of myocardial infarction. Cardiovasc Res. 2009;83(4):757-767.

[146] Mazo M, Planat-Benard V, Abizanda G, Pelacho B, Leobon B, Gavira JJ, Penuelas I, Cemborain A, Penicaud L, Laharrague P, Joffre C, Boisson M, Ecay M, Collantes M, Barba J, Casteilla L, Prosper F. Transplantation of adipose derived stromal cells is associated with functional improvement in a rat model of chronic myocardial infarction. Eur J Heart Fail. 2008;10(5):454-462.

[147] Zhang X, Wang H, Ma X, Adila A, Wang B, Liu F, Chen B, Wang C, Ma Y. Preservation of the cardiac function in infarcted rat hearts by the transplantation of adipose-derived stem cells with injectable fibrin scaffolds. Exp Biol Med (Maywood). 2010;235(12):1505-1515.

[148] Cai L, Johnstone BH, Cook TG, Tan J, Fishbein MC, Chen PS, March KL. IFATS collection: Human adipose tissue-derived stem cells induce angiogenesis and nerve sprouting following myocardial infarction, in conjunction with potent preservation of cardiac function. Stem Cells. 2009;27(1):230-237.

[149] Beitnes JO, Oie E, Shahdadfar A, Karlsen T, Muller RM, Aakhus S, Reinholt FP, Brinchmann JE. Intramyocardial injections of human mesenchymal stem cells following acute myocardial infarction modulate scar formation and improve left ventricular function. Cell Transplant. 2012; in press.

[150] Ma T, Liu H, Chen W, Xia X, Bai X, Liang L, Zhang Y, Liang T. Implanted adipose-derived stem cells attenuate small-for-size liver graft injury by secretion of VEGF in rats. Am J Transplant. 2012;12(3):620-629.

[151] Matsumoto D, Sato K, Gonda K, Takaki Y, Shigeura T, Sato T, Aiba-Kojima E, Iizuka F, Inoue K, Suga H, Yoshimura K. Cell-assisted lipotransfer: supportive use of human adipose-derived cells for soft tissue augmentation with lipoinjection. Tissue Eng. 2006;12(12):3375-3382.

[152] Yang YC, Liu BS, Shen CC, Lin CH, Chiao MT, Cheng HC. Transplantation of adipose tissue-derived stem cells for treatment of focal cerebral ischemia. Curr Neurovasc Res. 2011;8(1):1-13.

[153] Kang SK, Lee DH, Bae YC, Kim HK, Baik SY, Jung JS. Improvement of neurological deficits by intracerebral transplantation of human adipose tissue-derived stromal cells after cerebral ischemia in rats. Exp Neurol. 2003;183(2):355-366.

[154] Leu S, Lin YC, Yuen CM, Yen CH, Kao YH, Sun CK, Yip HK. Adipose-derived mesenchymal stem cells markedly attenuate brain infarct size and improve neurological function in rats. J Transl Med. 2010;8:63.

[155] Ryu HH, Lim JH, Byeon YE, Park JR, Seo MS, Lee YW, Kim WH, Kang KS, Kweon OK. Functional recovery and neural differentiation after transplantation of allogenic

adipose-derived stem cells in a canine model of acute spinal cord injury. J Vet Sci. 2009;10(4):273-284.

[156] Wang Y, Zhao Z, Ren Z, Zhao B, Zhang L, Chen J, Xu W, Lu S, Zhao Q, Peng J. Recellularized nerve allografts with differentiated mesenchymal stem cells promote peripheral nerve regeneration. Neurosci Lett. 2012;514(1):96-101.

[157] Santiago LY, Clavijo-Alvarez J, Brayfield C, Rubin JP, Marra KG. Delivery of adipose-derived precursor cells for peripheral nerve repair. Cell Transplant. 2009;18(2): 145-158.

[158] Zhang HT, Cheng HY, Cai YQ, Ma X, Liu WP, Yan ZJ, Jiang XD, Xu RX. Comparison of adult neurospheres derived from different origins for treatment of rat spinal cord injury. Neurosci Lett. 2009;458(3):116-121.

[159] Nakada A, Fukuda S, Ichihara S, Sato T, Itoi S, Inada Y, Endo K, Nakamura T. Regeneration of central nervous tissue using a collagen scaffold and adipose-derived stromal cells. Cells Tissues Organs. 2009;190(6):326-335.

[160] Zhao LR, Duan, W.M., Reyes, M., Keene, C.D., Verfaillie, C.M., Low, W.C. Human bone marrow stem cells exhibit neural phenotypes and ameliorate neurological deficits after grafting into the ischemic brain of rats. Exp. Neurol. 2002;174:11-20.

[161] Croft AP, Przyborski SA. Mesenchymal stem cells expressing neural antigens instruct a neurogenic cell fate on neural stem cells. Exp Neurol. 2009;216(2):329-341.

[162] Wislet-Gendebien S, Bruyere F, Hans G, Leprince P, Moonen G, Rogister B. Nestin-positive mesenchymal stem cells favour the astroglial lineage in neural progenitors and stem cells by releasing active BMP4. BMC Neurosci. 2004;5:33.

[163] Lopatina T, Kalinina N, Karagyaur M, Stambolsky D, Rubina K, Revischin A, Pavlova G, Parfyonova Y, Tkachuk V. Adipose-derived stem cells stimulate regeneration of peripheral nerves: BDNF secreted by these cells promotes nerve healing and axon growth de novo. PLoS One. 2011;6(3):e17899.

[164] Reid AJ, Sun M, Wiberg M, Downes S, Terenghi G, Kingham PJ. Nerve repair with adipose-derived stem cells protects dorsal root ganglia neurons from apoptosis. Neuroscience. 2011;199:515-522.

[165] Wei X, Du Z, Zhao L, Feng D, Wei G, He Y, Tan J, Lee WH, Hampel H, Dodel R, Johnstone BH, March KL, Farlow MR, Du Y. IFATS collection: The conditioned media of adipose stromal cells protect against hypoxia-ischemia-induced brain damage in neonatal rats. Stem Cells. 2009;27(2):478-488.

[166] Cho YJ, Song HS, Bhang S, Lee S, Kang BG, Lee JC, An J, Cha CI, Nam DH, Kim BS, Joo KM. Therapeutic effects of human adipose stem cell-conditioned medium on stroke. J Neurosci Res. 2012;90(9):1794-1802.

[167] Park SS, Lee YJ, Lee SH, Lee D, Choi K, Kim WH, Kweon OK, Han HJ. Functional recovery after spinal cord injury in dogs treated with a combination of Matrigel and

neural-induced adipose-derived mesenchymal Stem cells. Cytotherapy. 2012;14(5): 584-597.

[168] Chung JY, Kim W, Im W, Yoo DY, Choi JH, Hwang IK, Won MH, Chang IB, Cho BM, Hwang HS, Moon SM. Neuroprotective effects of adipose-derived stem cells against ischemic neuronal damage in the rabbit spinal cord. J Neurol Sci. 2012;317(1-2):40-46.

[169] Zhang Y, Luo H, Zhang Z, Lu Y, Huang X, Yang L, Xu J, Yang W, Fan X, Du B, Gao P, Hu G, Jin Y. A nerve graft constructed with xenogeneic acellular nerve matrix and autologous adipose-derived mesenchymal stem cells. Biomaterials. 2010;31(20): 5312-5324.

[170] Hasharoni A, Zilberman Y, Turgeman G, Helm GA, Liebergall M, Gazit D. Murine spinal fusion induced by engineered mesenchymal stem cells that conditionally express bone morphogenetic protein-2. J Neurosurg Spine. 2005;3(1):47-52.

[171] Chang SC, Chuang H, Chen YR, Yang LC, Chen JK, Mardini S, Chung HY, Lu YL, Ma WC, Lou J. Cranial repair using BMP-2 gene engineered bone marrow stromal cells. J Surg Res. 2004;119(1):85-91.

[172] Guo X, Zheng Q, Kulbatski I, Yuan Q, Yang S, Shao Z, Wang H, Xiao B, Pan Z, Tang S. Bone regeneration with active angiogenesis by basic fibroblast growth factor gene transfected mesenchymal stem cells seeded on porous beta-TCP ceramic scaffolds. Biomed Mater. 2006;1(3):93-99.

[173] Studeny M, Marini FC, Champlin RE, Zompetta C, Fidler IJ, Andreeff M. Bone marrow-derived mesenchymal stem cells as vehicles for interferon-beta delivery into tumors. Cancer Res. 2002;62(13):3603-3608.

[174] Chen XC, Wang R, Zhao X, Wei YQ, Hu M, Wang YS, Zhang XW, Zhang R, Zhang L, Yao B, Wang L, Jia YQ, Zeng TT, Yang JL, Tian L, Kan B, Lin XJ, Lei S, Deng HX, Wen YJ, Mao YQ, Li J. Prophylaxis against carcinogenesis in three kinds of unestablished tumor models via IL12-gene-engineered MSCs. Carcinogenesis. 2006;27(12): 2434-2441.

[175] Lin L, Fu X, Zhang X, Chen LX, Zhang JY, Yu CL, Ma KT, Zhou CY. Rat adipose-derived stromal cells expressing BMP4 induce ectopic bone formation in vitro and in vivo. Acta Pharmacol Sin. 2006;27(12):1608-1615.

[176] Dragoo JL, Choi JY, Lieberman JR, Huang J, Zuk PA, Zhang J, Hedrick MH, Benhaim P. Bone induction by BMP-2 transduced stem cells derived from human fat. J Orthop Res. 2003;21(4):622-629.

[177] Hsu WK, Wang JC, Liu NQ, Krenek L, Zuk PA, Hedrick MH, Benhaim P, Lieberman JR. Stem cells from human fat as cellular delivery vehicles in an athymic rat posterolateral spine fusion model. J Bone Joint Surg Am. 2008;90(5):1043-1052.

[178] Diekman BO, Estes BT, Guilak F. The effects of BMP6 overexpression on adipose stem cell chondrogenesis: Interactions with dexamethasone and exogenous growth factors. J Biomed Mater Res A. 2010;93(3):994-1003.

[179] Jin XB, Sun YS, Zhang K, Wang J, Shi TP, Ju XD, Lou SQ. Tissue engineered cartilage from hTGF beta2 transduced human adipose derived stem cells seeded in PLGA/ alginate compound in vitro and in vivo. J Biomed Mater Res A. 2008;86(4):1077-1087.

[180] Jabbarzadeh E, Starnes T, Khan YM, Jiang T, Wirtel AJ, Deng M, Lv Q, Nair LS, Doty SB, Laurencin CT. Induction of angiogenesis in tissue-engineered scaffolds designed for bone repair: a combined gene therapy-cell transplantation approach. Proc Natl Acad Sci U S A. 2008;105(32):11099-11104.

[181] Lu F, Li J, Gao J, Ogawa R, Ou C, Yang B, Fu B. Improvement of the survival of human autologous fat transplantation by using VEGF-transfected adipose-derived stem cells. Plast Reconstr Surg. 2009;124(5):1437-1446.

[182] Kucerova L, Altanerova V, Matuskova M, Tyciakova S, Altaner C. Adipose tissue-derived human mesenchymal stem cells mediated prodrug cancer gene therapy. Cancer Res. 2007;67(13):6304-6313.

[183] Josiah DT, Zhu D, Dreher F, Olson J, McFadden G, Caldas H. Adipose-derived stem cells as therapeutic delivery vehicles of an oncolytic virus for glioblastoma. Mol Ther. 2009;18(2):377-385.

[184] Grisendi G, Bussolari R, Cafarelli L, Petak I, Rasini V, Veronesi E, De Santis G, Spano C, Tagliazzucchi M, Barti-Juhasz H, Scarabelli L, Bambi F, Frassoldati A, Rossi G, Casali C, Morandi U, Horwitz EM, Paolucci P, Conte P, Dominici M. Adipose-derived mesenchymal stem cells as stable source of tumor necrosis factor-related apoptosis-inducing ligand delivery for cancer therapy. Cancer Res. 2010;70(9):3718-3729.

[185] De Ugarte DA, Morizono, K., Elbarbary, A., Alfonso, Z.C., Zuk, P.A., Zhu, M., Dragoo, J.L., Ashjian, P.H., Thomas, B., Benhaim, P., Chen, I., Fraser, J.K., Hedrick, M.H. Comparison of multi-lineage cells from human adipose tissue and bone marrow. Cells Tissues Organs. 2003;174:101-109.

[186] Pittenger MF, Mackay, A. M., Beck, S. C., Jaiswal, R. K., Douglas, R., Mosca, J. D., Moorman, M. A., Simonetti, D. W., Craig, S., and Marshak, D. R. Multilineage potential of adult human mesenchymal stem cells. Science. 1999;284(5411):143-147.

[187] Aust L, Devlin B, Foster SJ, Halvorsen YD, Hicok K, du Laney T, Sen A, Willingmyre GD, Gimble JM. Yield of human adipose-derived adult stem cells from liposuction aspirates. Cytotherapy. 2004;6(1):7-14.

[188] Zhu Y, Liu T, Song K, Fan X, Ma X, Cui Z. Adipose-derived stem cell: a better stem cell than BMSC. Cell Biochem Funct. 2008;26(6):664-675.

[189] Oedayrajsingh-Varma MJ, van Ham SM, Knippenberg M, Helder MN, Klein-Nulend J, Schouten TE, Ritt MJ, van Milligen FJ. Adipose tissue-derived mesenchymal stem

cell yield and growth characteristics are affected by the tissue-harvesting procedure. Cytotherapy. 2006;8(2):166-177.

[190] Lendeckel S, Jodicke A, Christophis P, Heidinger K, Wolff J, Fraser JK, Hedrick MH, Berthold L, Howaldt HP. Autologous stem cells (adipose) and fibrin glue used to treat widespread traumatic calvarial defects: case report. J Craniomaxillofac Surg. 2004;32(6):370-373.

[191] Rigotti G, Marchi A, Galie M, Baroni G, Benati D, Krampera M, Pasini A, Sbarbati A. Clinical treatment of radiotherapy tissue damage by lipoaspirate transplant: a healing process mediated by adipose-derived adult stem cells. Plast Reconstr Surg. 2007;119(5):1409-1422; discussion 1423-1404.

[192] Casteilla L, Planat-Benard V, Laharrague P, Cousin B. Adipose-derived stromal cells: Their identity and uses in clinical trials, an update. World J Stem Cells. 2011;3(4): 25-33.

[193] Yoshimura K, Sato K, Aoi N, Kurita M, Hirohi T, Harii K. Cell-assisted lipotransfer for cosmetic breast augmentation: supportive use of adipose-derived stem/stromal cells. Aesthetic Plast Surg. 2008;32(1):48-55; discussion 56-47.

[194] Lee HC, An SG, Lee HW, Park JS, Cha KS, Hong TJ, Park JH, Lee SY, Kim SP, Kim YD, Chung SW, Bae YC, Shin YB, Kim JI, Jung JS. Safety and effect of adipose tissue-derived stem cell implantation in patients with critical limb ischemia. Circ J. 2012;76(7):1750-1760.

[195] Akita S, Akino K, Hirano A, Ohtsuru A, Yamashita S. Mesenchymal stem cell therapy for cutaneous radiation syndrome. Health Phys. 2010;98(6):858-862.

[196] Mesimaki K, Lindroos B, Tornwall J, Mauno J, Lindqvist C, Kontio R, Miettinen S, Suuronen R. Novel maxillary reconstruction with ectopic bone formation by GMP adipose stem cells. Int J Oral Maxillofac Surg. 2009;38(3):201-209.

[197] Peterson B, Zhang J, Iglesias R, Kabo M, Hedrick M, Benhaim P, Lieberman JR. Healing of critically sized femoral defects, using genetically modified mesenchymal stem cells from human adipose tissue. Tissue Eng. 2005;11(1-2):120-129.

[198] Dudas JR, Marra KG, Cooper GM, Penascino VM, Mooney MP, Jiang S, Rubin JP, Losee JE. The osteogenic potential of adipose-derived stem cells for the repair of rabbit calvarial defects. Ann Plast Surg. 2006;56(5):543-548.

[199] Chen Q, Yang Z, Sun S, Huang H, Sun X, Wang Z, Zhang Y, Zhang B. Adipose-derived stem cells modified genetically in vivo promote reconstruction of bone defects. Cytotherapy. 2010;12(6):831-840.

[200] Sheyn D, Kallai I, Tawackoli W, Cohn Yakubovich D, Oh A, Su S, Da X, Lavi A, Kimelman-Bleich N, Zilberman Y, Li N, Bae H, Gazit Z, Pelled G, Gazit D. Gene-modified adult stem cells regenerate vertebral bone defect in a rat model. Mol Pharm. 2011;8(5):1592-1601.

[201] Yang M, Ma QJ, Dang GT, Ma K, Chen P, Zhou CY. In vitro and in vivo induction of bone formation based on ex vivo gene therapy using rat adipose-derived adult stem cells expressing BMP-7. Cytotherapy. 2005;7(3):273-281.

[202] Chou Y-F, Zuk PA, Chang T-L, Benhaim P, Wu BM. Adipose-Derived Stem Cells and BMP2: Part 1 eated Adipose-Derived Stem Cells Do Not Improve Repair of Segmental Femoral Defects. Conn. Tiss. Res. 2011; 52(2):119-132

[203] Keibl C, Fugl A, Zanoni G, Tangl S, Wolbank S, Redl H, van Griensven M. Human adipose derived stem cells reduce callus volume upon BMP-2 administration in bone regeneration. Injury. 2011;42(8):814-820.

[204] Ra JC, Shin IS, Kim SH, Kang SK, Kang BC, Lee HY, Kim YJ, Jo JY, Yoon EJ, Choi HJ, Kwon E. Safety of intravenous infusion of human adipose tissue-derived mesenchymal stem cells in animals and humans. Stem Cells Dev. 2011;20(8):1297-1308.

[205] Garcia-Olmo D, Garcia-Arranz M, Garcia LG, Cuellar ES, Blanco IF, Prianes LA, Montes JA, Pinto FL, Marcos DH, Garcia-Sancho L. Autologous stem cell transplantation for treatment of rectovaginal fistula in perianal Crohn's disease: a new cell-based therapy. Int J Colorectal Dis. 2003;18(5):451-454.

[206] Garcia-Olmo D, Garcia-Arranz M, Herreros D, Pascual I, Peiro C, Rodriguez-Montes JA. A phase I clinical trial of the treatment of Crohn's fistula by adipose mesenchymal stem cell transplantation. Dis Colon Rectum. 2005;48(7):1416-1423.

[207] Garcia-Olmo D, Herreros D, De-La-Quintana P, Guadalajara H, Trebol J, Georgiev-Hristov T, Garcia-Arranz M. Adipose-derived stem cells in Crohn's rectovaginal fistula. Case Report Med. 2010;2010:961758.

[208] Garcia-Olmo D, Herreros D, Pascual M, Pascual I, De-La-Quintana P, Trebol J, Garcia-Arranz M. Treatment of enterocutaneous fistula in Crohn's Disease with adipose-derived stem cells: a comparison of protocols with and without cell expansion. Int J Colorectal Dis. 2009;24(1):27-30.

[209] Guadalajara H, Herreros D, De-La-Quintana P, Trebol J, Garcia-Arranz M, Garcia-Olmo D. Long-term follow-up of patients undergoing adipose-derived adult stem cell administration to treat complex perianal fistulas. Int J Colorectal Dis. 2012;27(5):595-600.

[210] Song KH. New techniques for treating an anal fistula. J Korean Soc Coloproctol. 2012;28(1):7-12.

[211] Garcia-Olmo D, Herreros D, Pascual I, Pascual JA, Del-Valle E, Zorrilla J, De-La-Quintana P, Garcia-Arranz M, Pascual M. Expanded adipose-derived stem cells for the treatment of complex perianal fistula: a phase II clinical trial. Dis Colon Rectum. 2009;52(1):79-86.

[212] Herreros MD, Garcia-Arranz M, Guadalajara H, De-La-Quintana P, Garcia-Olmo D. Autologous expanded adipose-derived stem cells for the treatment of complex cryptoglandular perianal fistulas: a phase III randomized clinical trial (FATT 1: fistula

Advanced Therapy Trial 1) and long-term evaluation. Dis Colon Rectum. 2012;55(7): 762-772.

[213] Riordan NH, Ichim TE, Min WP, Wang H, Solano F, Lara F, Alfaro M, Rodriguez JP, Harman RJ, Patel AN, Murphy MP, Lee RR, Minev B. Non-expanded adipose stromal vascular fraction cell therapy for multiple sclerosis. J Transl Med. 2009;7:29.

[214] Ra JC, Kang SK, Shin IS, Park HG, Joo SA, Kim JG, Kang BC, Lee YS, Nakama K, Piao M, Sohl B, Kurtz A. Stem cell treatment for patients with autoimmune disease by systemic infusion of culture-expanded autologous adipose tissue derived mesenchymal stem cells. J Transl Med. 2011;9:181.

[215] Fang B, Song Y, Liao L, Zhang Y, Zhao RC. Favorable response to human adipose tissue-derived mesenchymal stem cells in steroid-refractory acute graft-versus-host disease. Transplant Proc. 2007;39(10):3358-3362.

[216] Fang B, Song Y, Lin Q, Zhang Y, Cao Y, Zhao RC, Ma Y. Human adipose tissue-derived mesenchymal stromal cells as salvage therapy for treatment of severe refractory acute graft-vs.-host disease in two children. Pediatr Transplant. 2007;11(7):814-817.

[217] Fang B, Song YP, Liao LM, Han Q, Zhao RC. Treatment of severe therapy-resistant acute graft-versus-host disease with human adipose tissue-derived mesenchymal stem cells. Bone Marrow Transplant. 2006;38(5):389-390.

[218] Yanez R, Lamana ML, Garcia-Castro J, Colmenero I, Ramirez M, Bueren JA. Adipose tissue-derived mesenchymal stem cells have in vivo immunosuppressive properties applicable for the control of the graft-versus-host disease. Stem Cells. 2006;24(11): 2582-2591.

[219] Yoshimura K, Sato K, Aoi N, Kurita M, Inoue K, Suga H, Eto H, Kato H, Hirohi T, Harii K. Cell-assisted lipotransfer for facial lipoatrophy: efficacy of clinical use of adipose-derived stem cells. Dermatol Surg. 2008;34(9):1178-1185.

[220] Wang L, Lu Y, Luo X, Fu MG, Hu X, Dong H, Fan ZH. [Cell-assissted lipotransfer for breast augmentation: a report of 18 patients]. Zhonghua Zheng Xing Wai Ke Za Zhi. 2012;28(1):1-6.

[221] Fierro FA, Sierralta WD, Epunan MJ, Minguell JJ. Marrow-derived mesenchymal stem cells: role in epithelial tumor cell determination. Clin Exp Metastasis. 2004;21(4): 313-319.

[222] Zhu W, Xu W, Jiang R, Qian H, Chen M, Hu J, Cao W, Han C, Chen Y. Mesenchymal stem cells derived from bone marrow favor tumor cell growth in vivo. Exp Mol Pathol. 2006;80(3):267-274.

[223] Zimmerlin L, Donnenberg AD, Rubin JP, Basse P, Landreneau RJ, Donnenberg VS. Regenerative therapy and cancer: in vitro and in vivo studies of the interaction between adipose-derived stem cells and breast cancer cells from clinical isolates. Tissue Eng Part A. 2011;17(1-2):93-106.

[224] Vona-Davis L, Rose DP. Adipokines as endocrine, paracrine, and autocrine factors in breast cancer risk and progression. Endocr Relat Cancer. 2007;14(2):189-206.

[225] Sasser AK, Sullivan NJ, Studebaker AW, Hendey LF, Axel AE, Hall BM. Interleukin-6 is a potent growth factor for ER-alpha-positive human breast cancer. FASEB J. 2007;21(13):3763-3770.

[226] Razmkhah M, Jaberipour M, Erfani N, Habibagahi M, Talei AR, Ghaderi A. Adipose derived stem cells (ASCs) isolated from breast cancer tissue express IL-4, IL-10 and TGF-beta1 and upregulate expression of regulatory molecules on T cells: do they protect breast cancer cells from the immune response? Cell Immunol. 2011;266(2):116-122.

[227] Liang W, Xia H, Li J, Zhao RC. Human adipose tissue derived mesenchymal stem cells are resistant to several chemotherapeutic agents. Cytotechnology. 2011;63(5): 523-530.

[228] Fantuzzi G. Adiponectin and inflammation: consensus and controversy. J Allergy Clin Immunol. 2008;121(2):326-330.

[229] Lago F, Gomez R, Gomez-Reino JJ, Dieguez C, Gualillo O. Adipokines as novel modulators of lipid metabolism. Trends Biochem Sci. 2009;34(10):500-510.

[230] Zeyda M, Farmer D, Todoric J, Aszmann O, Speiser M, Gyori G, Zlabinger GJ, Stulnig TM. Human adipose tissue macrophages are of an anti-inflammatory phenotype but capable of excessive pro-inflammatory mediator production. Int J Obes (Lond). 2007;31(9):1420-1428.

[231] Deng Y, Scherer PE. Adipokines as novel biomarkers and regulators of the metabolic syndrome. Ann N Y Acad Sci. 2010;1212:E1-E19.

[232] Maury E, Ehala-Aleksejev K, Guiot Y, Detry R, Vandenhooft A, Brichard SM. Adipokines oversecreted by omental adipose tissue in human obesity. Am J Physiol Endocrinol Metab. 2007;293(3):E656-665.

[233] Cancello R, Clement K. Is obesity an inflammatory illness? Role of low-grade inflammation and macrophage infiltration in human white adipose tissue. BJOG. 2006;113(10):1141-1147.

[234] Balistreri CR, Caruso C, Candore G. The role of adipose tissue and adipokines in obesity-related inflammatory diseases. Mediators Inflamm. 2010;2010:802078.

[235] Fain JN. Release of inflammatory mediators by human adipose tissue is enhanced in obesity and primarily by the nonfat cells: a review. Mediators Inflamm. 2010;2010:513948.

[236] Codoner-Franch P, Valls-Belles V, Arilla-Codoner A, Alonso-Iglesias E. Oxidant mechanisms in childhood obesity: the link between inflammation and oxidative stress. Transl Res. 2011;158(6):369-384.

[237] Zhang K, Kaufman RJ. Identification and characterization of endoplasmic reticulum stress-induced apoptosis in vivo. Methods Enzymol. 2008;442(395-419.

[238] Gao CL, Zhu C, Zhao YP, Chen XH, Ji CB, Zhang CM, Zhu JG, Xia ZK, Tong ML, Guo XR. Mitochondrial dysfunction is induced by high levels of glucose and free fatty acids in 3T3-L1 adipocytes. Mol Cell Endocrinol. 2010;320(1-2):25-33.

[239] Malhotra JD, Kaufman RJ. Endoplasmic reticulum stress and oxidative stress: a vicious cycle or a double-edged sword? Antioxid Redox Signal. 2007;9(12):2277-2293.

[240] Bulua AC, Simon A, Maddipati R, Pelletier M, Park H, Kim KY, Sack MN, Kastner DL, Siegel RM. Mitochondrial reactive oxygen species promote production of proinflammatory cytokines and are elevated in TNFR1-associated periodic syndrome (TRAPS). J Exp Med. 2011;208(3):519-533.

[241] Lumeng CN, Bodzin JL, Saltiel AR. Obesity induces a phenotypic switch in adipose tissue macrophage polarization. J Clin Invest. 2007;117(1):175-184.

[242] Weisberg SP, McCann D, Desai M, Rosenbaum M, Leibel RL, Ferrante AW, Jr. Obesity is associated with macrophage accumulation in adipose tissue. J Clin Invest. 2003;112(12):1796-1808.

[243] Harman-Boehm I, Bluher M, Redel H, Sion-Vardy N, Ovadia S, Avinoach E, Shai I, Kloting N, Stumvoll M, Bashan N, Rudich A. Macrophage infiltration into omental versus subcutaneous fat across different populations: effect of regional adiposity and the comorbidities of obesity. J Clin Endocrinol Metab. 2007;92(6):2240-2247.

[244] Cinti S, Mitchell G, Barbatelli G, Murano I, Ceresi E, Faloia E, Wang S, Fortier M, Greenberg AS, Obin MS. Adipocyte death defines macrophage localization and function in adipose tissue of obese mice and humans. J Lipid Res. 2005;46(11):2347-2355.

[245] Lumeng CN, Deyoung SM, Bodzin JL, Saltiel AR. Increased inflammatory properties of adipose tissue macrophages recruited during diet-induced obesity. Diabetes. 2007;56(1):16-23.

[246] Subramanian V, Ferrante AW, Jr. Obesity, inflammation, and macrophages. Nestle Nutr Workshop Ser Pediatr Program. 2009;63:151-159; discussion 159-162, 259-168.

[247] Wozniak SE, Gee LL, Wachtel MS, Frezza EE. Adipose tissue: the new endocrine organ? A review article. Dig Dis Sci. 2009;54(9):1847-1856.

[248] Ye J, Gimble JM. Regulation of stem cell differentiation in adipose tissue by chronic inflammation. Clin Exp Pharmacol Physiol. 2011;38(12):872-878.

[249] Dercum FX. Three cases of a hitherto unclassified affection resembling in its grosser aspects obesity, but associated with special nervous symptoms - adiposis dolorosa. Am J Med Sci. 1892;civ:521.

[250] Madelung O. Uber den Fetthals. Langenbecks Arch Chir. 1888;37:106.

[251] Fife CE, Maus EA, Carter MJ. Lipedema: a frequently misdiagnosed and misunderstood fatty deposition syndrome. Adv Skin Wound Care. 2010;23(2):81-92; quiz 93-84.

[252] Herbst KL. Rare adipose disorders (RADs) masquerading as obesity. Acta Pharmacol Sin. 2012;33(2):155-172.

[253] Langendoen SI, Habbema L, Nijsten TE, Neumann HA. Lipoedema: from clinical presentation to therapy. A review of the literature. Br J Dermatol. 2009;161(5): 980-986.

[254] Curri SB, Merlen JF. [Microvascular disorders of adipose tissue]. J Mal Vasc. 1986;11(3):303-309.

[255] Foldi E, Foldi M. Foldi's Textbook of Lymphology. Munich: Elsevier; 2006.

[256] Kim JH, Lee YM, Ahn EM, Kim KW, Yu YS. Decursin inhibits retinal neovascularization via suppression of VEGFR-2 activation. Mol Vis. 2009;15:1868-1875.

[257] Frank RN. Vascular endothelial growth factor--its role in retinal vascular proliferation. N Engl J Med. 1994;331(22):1519-1520.

[258] Cao R, Brakenhielm E, Wahlestedt C, Thyberg J, Cao Y. Leptin induces vascular permeability and synergistically stimulates angiogenesis with FGF-2 and VEGF. Proc Natl Acad Sci U S A. 2001;98(11):6390-6395.

[259] Siems W, Grune T, Voss P, Brenke R. Anti-fibrosclerotic effects of shock wave therapy in lipedema and cellulite. Biofactors. 2005;24(1-4):275-282.

[260] Partsch H, Stoberl C, Urbanek A, Wenzel-Hora BI. Clinical use of indirect lymphography in different forms of leg edema. Lymphology. 1988;21(3):152-160.

[261] Schneider M, Conway EM, Carmeliet P. Lymph makes you fat. Nat Genet. 2005;37(10):1023-1024.

[262] Nougues J, Reyne Y, Dulor JP. Differentiation of rabbit adipocyte precursors in primary culture. Int J Obes. 1988;12(4):321-333.

[263] Bagheri S, Ohlin K, Olsson G, Brorson H. Tissue tonometry before and after liposuction of arm lymphedema following breast cancer. Lymphat Res Biol. 2005;3(2):66-80.

[264] Wigle JT, Harvey N, Detmar M, Lagutina I, Grosveld G, Gunn MD, Jackson DG, Oliver G. An essential role for Prox1 in the induction of the lymphatic endothelial cell phenotype. EMBO J. 2002;21(7):1505-1513.

[265] Harvey NL, Srinivasan RS, Dillard ME, Johnson NC, Witte MH, Boyd K, Sleeman MW, Oliver G. Lymphatic vascular defects promoted by Prox1 haploinsufficiency cause adult-onset obesity. Nat Genet. 2005;37(10):1072-1081.

[266] Wigle JT, Oliver G. Prox1 function is required for the development of the murine lymphatic system. Cell. 1999;98(6):769-778.

[267] Blaber SP, Webster RA, Hill CJ, Breen EJ, Kuah D, Vesey G, Herbert BR. Analysis of in vitro secretion profiles from adipose-derived cell populations. J Transl Med. 2012;10(1):172.

[268] Hsiao ST, Asgari A, Lokmic Z, Sinclair R, Dusting GJ, Lim SY, Dilley RJ. Comparative analysis of paracrine factor expression in human adult mesenchymal stem cells derived from bone marrow, adipose, and dermal tissue. Stem Cells Dev. 2012;21(12): 2189-2203.

[269] Banas A, Teratani T, Yamamoto Y, Tokuhara M, Takeshita F, Osaki M, Kawamata M, Kato T, Okochi H, Ochiya T. IFATS collection: in vivo therapeutic potential of human adipose tissue mesenchymal stem cells after transplantation into mice with liver injury. Stem Cells. 2008;26(10):2705-2712.

Chapter 2

Placenta-Derived Stem Cells as a Source for Treatment of Lung and Liver Disease in Cystic Fibrosis

Annalucia Carbone, Stefano Castellani,
Valentina Paracchini, Sante Di Gioia,
Carla Colombo and Massimo Conese

Additional information is available at the end of the chapter

1. Introduction

In the first part of this chapter we will summarize the main clinical aspects of cystic fibrosis as well as the pathophysiology of lung and liver diseases, with particular reference to the role of airway and biliary duct epithelia, where the cystic fibrosis gene is expressed. In the second part we will describe the main features of placenta-derived stem cells and their potential use for the treatment of lung and liver diseases in cystic fibrosis.

1.1. Cystic fibrosis

Cystic fibrosis (CF) is an autosomal recessive disease of epithelia in the lung, liver, pancreas, small intestine, reproductive organs, sweat glands and other fluid-transporting tissues [1, 2]. In Caucasians the disease affects about 1 in 2500 live births and is the most common eventually lethal genetic disease [3]. The cause of CF is different mutations in the *CFTR* (cystic fibrosis transmembrane conductance regulator) gene, the product of which is a protein expressed in the apical membrane of most epithelia. This membrane protein is a cyclic AMP (cAMP) regulated chloride (Cl⁻)-channel involved in different regulatory processes of the cell, *e.g.* both transcellular and paracellular ion and water transport [1, 4].

Chronic progressive obstructive lung disease and pancreatic insufficiency are the main clinical symptoms of CF, where pulmonary disease is the major cause (95%) of morbidity and mortality [5]. However, liver disease is also increasing as the life span of these individuals becomes longer.

The succession of events leading from the defective CFTR to the clinical symptoms is not completely understood. However, it is obvious that the abnormal ion transport with hyper-absorption of Na^+ and impaired Cl^- and $HCO3^-$ secretion in airway epithelial cells and cholangiocytes leads to a disturbance of the fluid lining the airways and the bile ducts [6-10].

1.1.1. The CFTR gene

The CFTR gene was identified in 1989 and this has sharply accelerated the research on CF. The gene, which is situated on the long arm of human chromosome 7 (7q31.2), spans approximately 250 kilobases (kb) of nucleotide sequences together with its promoter and regulatory regions. The 27 exons form a 6.5 kb long coding sequence, which is capable of encoding a protein of 1480 amino acids [11].

The CFTR gene product is not limited to the cells of epithelial origin. In fact, CFTR mRNA transcripts and/or CFTR protein have been demonstrated in lung fibroblasts, blood cells, hematopoietic stem/progenitor stem cells (HSPC), alveolar macrophages, and smooth muscle cells [12-14]. In addition to its typical plasma membrane location, CFTR was also found in membranous organelles such as lysosomes of alveolar macrophages [15] and in both apical and basolateral membrane of the sweat duct [16].

Although over 1,900 different mutations in the CFTR gene are known (Cystic Fibrosis Mutation Database, http://www.genet.sickkids.on.ca/cftr/Home.html), approximately 66% of the patients worldwide carry the F508del mutation (a deletion of three nucleotides that results in a loss of phenylalanine at position 508 of the CFTR protein) with somewhat higher prevalence in Western Europe and USA [17]. This type of mutation causes an incorrectly assembled CFTR protein resulting in endoplasmatic reticulum (ER) retention and degradation of the protein [18] as well as defective regulation [19]. Patients homozygous for F508del usually have more pronounced clinical manifestations compared to heterozygotes and genotypes without F508del [20-22] although these differences are highly variable [23].

1.1.2. The CFTR protein

Based on the amino-acid sequence and its structure, CFTR is identified as a member of the superfamily of ATP-binding cassette (ABC) transporters. However, among the thousands of ABC family members, only CFTR is an ion channel [24, 25]. ABC transporters are ubiquitous in the entire animal kingdom due to their role in coupling transport to ATP hydrolysis. They also are involved in many genetic diseases [26]. Like other ABC transporters CFTR contains two membrane-spanning domains (MSDs), two hydrophilic nucleotide-binding domains (NBDs) located at the cytoplasmic site of the protein, and, as a unique feature among ABC transporters, a regulatory domain (R domain) located between NBD1 and MSD2. The R domain contains several consensus phosphorylation sites for protein kinases A (PKA) and C (PKC) [27]. The opening and closing of the CFTR Cl^- channel is tightly controlled by the balance of kinase and phosphatase activity within the cell and by cellular ATP levels [28]. Activation of PKA causes the phosphorylation of multiple serine residues within the R domain leading to conformational changes in this domain [29] relieving its inhibitory functions on CFTR channel gating [30]. Once the R domain is phosphorylated, channel opening requires binding of cytosolic ATP. NBD1-NBD2 dimerization induces channel opening, whereas ATP hydrolysis at the NBD2 induces dimer disruption and channel closure [24, 31, 32]. Finally, channel activity is terminated by protein phosphatases that dephosphorylate the R domain and return CFTR to its quiescent state [28].

Besides its cAMP-induced chloride channel function, CFTR is reported to have important regulatory functions on other ion channels and transporters. Below some of these interactions are presented: $HCO3^-$ is conducted from the cell into the lumen [33] through reciprocal regulatory interactions between CFTR and the SLC26 chloride/bicarbonate exchanger [34] and loss of this mechanism contributes to both airway and pancreatic-duct disease in CF [33, 35]. CFTR enhances ATP release by a separate channel [36], not yet identified [37]. This CFTR mediated release, although debated, is thought to be stimulated by hypotonic challenge to strengthen autocrine control of cell volume regulation through a purinergic receptor-dependent signalling mechanism [36, 37]. Furthermore, transport of glutathione is directly mediated by CFTR, which is essential for control of oxidative stress [38]. The interaction between CFTR and epithelial sodium channel (ENaC) is of crucial importance for lung disease development (see below). CFTR downregulates calcium-activated chloride channels (CaCC) [39], and stimulates outwardly rectifying chloride channels [40]. Other channels regulated are the volume-regulated anion channel [41] and ATP-sensitive K_{ATP} channels such as inwardly rectifying outer medullary potassium channels [42].

Regulatory sites on NBD1 interact with several of the above processes. For example, NBD1 contains a CFTR-specific regulatory site that downregulates ENaC. This regulatory site is also needed for CFTR-mediated interactions with other transporting membrane proteins [1, 43]. Several studies also have identified a short stretch of amino acids (-DTRL-) at the COOH terminal end, forming a PDZ binding domain [1, 44]. This PDZ binding domain interacts with different PDZ-domain-containing proteins, anchors CFTR to the cytoskeleton and stimulates the channel activities through downstream signaling elements [44, 45].

2. The airway epithelium

The airway epithelium is a target for potentially noxious substances and pathogens. It plays a critical role in maintaining a sterile undamaged airway and also separates the connective tissue as well as the smooth muscle from the airway luminal contents. In addition to its barrier function, the airway epithelium has a regulated fluid and ion transport together with a secretory function, although its function is mainly absorptive [46]. It can produce mucus, and can release mediators of the immune system such as lysozyme, lactoferrin, mucous glycoprotein, immunoglobulins, chemokines, cytokines, lectins and β-defensin (cationic antimicrobial peptides) [47, 48].

Furthermore, the airway epithelium produces antioxidants such as glutathione and ascorbic acid [49]. Aside from these protective functions it also regulates the airway physiology via production of smooth muscle relaxant factors such as prostaglandin E_2, nitric oxide and enzymes, which catabolize smooth muscle contractile agonists [50, 51].

In normal human airways the surface epithelium is on average 50 μm thick and rests on a basement membrane. The epithelium in the major bronchi and proximal bronchioles is ciliated pseudostratified with the main cell types: ciliated and secretory columnar cells, and underlying basal cells. In addition, immune cells, inflammatory cells and phagocytic cells migrate to and remain within the epithelium [52].

More distally, in the terminal bronchioles, the epithelium changes towards a simple ciliated columnar and, finally, to simple cuboidal epithelium with ciliated and non-ciliated cells (Clara cells) [53]. In addition brush cells (columnar with microvilli only) have been identified in the respiratory tract from nose to alveoli [54]. Scattered along the respiratory tree, various progenitor niches are present in the airway epithelium [55].

It has been widely accepted that acinar gland serous cells are the predominant site for CFTR expression in the human large airways, arguing for a dominant role of submucosal glands in the volume regulation of airway surface liquid (ASL) and CF [56-59]. However, these findings have later been debated. It has been demonstrated that normal (but not the F508del) surface airway epithelia express CFTR in every ciliated cell, also in glandular ducts, with decreased expression towards the distal airways. This suggests a key role for the superficial epithelium in the initiation of ASL volume depletion and as the site for early disease [60]. It also supports a role for CFTR in regulating glandular secretion homeostasis, but predominantly in the submucosal ducts rather than in the serous acini as was earlier proposed.

2.1. Ion and water transport in airway epithelium

Net vectorial fluid transport depends critically on ENaC and CFTR operating in concert with the paracellular and transcellular pathways [61].

Fluid absorption is mainly controlled by the transport of Na^+ through apical ENaC, which is also the dominant basal ion transport process. *Fluid secretion* is regulated by cell-to-lumen movement of Cl^-, via CFTR, CaCC and volume regulated chloride channel, and/or $HCO3^-$ via the interactions between CFTR and the SLC26 channel. In both cases the transport occurs along the electrochemical gradient and the movement of counterions likely takes place predominantly through leaky tight junctions [61].

Over the basolateral membrane a Na^+ gradient is maintained by the Na^+-K^+-ATPase, which pumps 3 Na^+ ions out of the cell for every 2 K^+ ions coming in. As a result the intracellular concentration of Na^+ is low (20 mM), whereas the K^+ concentration is high (150 mM) [62]. In addition, the Na^+-K^+-2Cl^- co-transporter moves Cl^- against its electrochemical gradient and accumulates Cl^- inside the cell to be released via apical channels. Secretion of Cl^- is electrically coupled to efflux of K^+ through basolateral K^+ conductance channels [63]. Through the paracellular pathway, Cl^- is absorbed or Na^+ secreted and the water-flow is regulated by diffusion following osmotic gradients.

The maintenance of the electro-osmotic gradients is dependent on limiting back diffusion. The tightness of the paracellular barrier and the molecular selectivity together contribute to the overall epithelial transport characteristics [64]. In many epithelia the transport of different ions is performed by different cell types, however, in airway epithelia the ciliated cell is responsible for both secreting Cl⁻ and absorbing Na⁺ [65].

2.2. The airway surface liquid

ASL, the fluid covering the airway epithelium, consists of a periciliary layer (PCL), which is a watery layer surrounding the cilia, and of mucus on top of the cilia. Mucus is produced mainly by the submucosal glands, while a small amount is produced by the goblet cells. In normal airways PCL height is defined as the length of an outstretched cilium (~6 μm) [66], whereas the ASL layer (mucus plus PCL) varies in thickness of 20-150 μm for different species (20-58 μm in humans) [67]. ASL is the first line of defense against inhaled pathogens and is important for mucociliary clearance. It contains *e.g.*, mucins, phospholipids, albumin, lactoferrin, lysozyme, proteases, defensins and other peptides, ions and water [68], see also paragraph 2.1. The composition, volume and physical properties of the ASL depend manly on secretions of the airway submucosal glands and the absorptive properties of the surface epithelial cells. Regulation of the balance between absorption and secretion determines the net transport of ions across the epithelium through transcellular and paracellular pathways and, thus the mass of salt on an epithelial surface [69].

2.3. Pathogenesis of CF lung disease

The lung of CF patients is normal at birth, but soon after birth an endobronchiolitis ensues with surprisingly few pathogenic bacterial species (*Pseudomonas aeruginosa* in most cases), and which is associated with an intense neutrophilic response localized to the peribronchial and endobronchial spaces [70-72]. The neutrophil-dominated inflammatory response is harmful for the host by causing exaggerated production of inflammatory cytokines and proteases which may sustain infection [73]. CF primarily affects the airways and submucosal glands with sparing of the interstitium and alveolar spaces until late in the disease [74, 75]. The CF lung disease is characterized by a picture of airway epithelial injury [76] and remodeling, such as squamous metaplasia [77], cell hyperproliferation [78], basal and goblet cell hyperplasia, and hypersecretion of mucus due to the inflammatory profile [79-81]. The epithelial regeneration characterized by successive steps of cell adhesion and migration, proliferation, pseudostratification, and terminal differentiation is disturbed and characterized by delayed differentiation, increased proliferation, and altered pro-inflammatory responses [82].

There are several hypotheses about the early pathogenetic steps in the CF lung disease and how defective CFTR leads to the airway disease:

- *The low ASL volume hypothesis* claims that the ASL is isotonic both normally and in CF. CFTR functions both as a Cl⁻ channel and as an inhibitor of the ENaC. In CF airway epithelia, with an absence of either molecular or functional CFTR, there will be unregulated Na⁺ absorption and a decreased capacity to secrete Cl⁻. This leads to dehydration of the airway surface, with a collapsed PCL, concentration of mucins within the mucus layer, and adhesion of mucus to the airway surface [83].

- *The high salt hypothesis* suggests that the ASL normally is hypotonic [84] and provides an optimal environment for defensins. According to this view the ASL in CF patients would have a higher salt concentration than normal because the absorbing function of ENaC depends on the state of CFTR and cannot be activated when CFTR is defective or absent [84].

- *The low pH hypothesis* focuses on the interactions between CFTR and the SLC26 and proposes an acidic ASL. This may compromise the function of airway immune cells and increase toxic oxidant species. Lowering the pH may also eliminate electrostatic repulsive charges between organisms and facilitate "tighter" biofilm formation as well as reduce electrorepulsive forces between bacteria and negatively charged mucins. Furthermore, ciliary beat frequency in bronchial epithelium is reduced when external pH falls [85]. All the above factors may inhibit mucociliary clearance (MCC) and thus elimination of bacteria from the airways [86].

- *The low oxygenation hypothesis* postulates that the oxygen content of the ASL is low, due to build-up of mucus plugs, resulting in enhanced growth of the facultative anaerobic *P.aeruginosa* [87].

- *The defect gland function hypothesis* suggests that the primary defect in CF is reduced fluid secretion by airway submucosal glands and possibly altered secretion of mucous glycoproteins [88].

- *The soluble mediator hypothesis* proposes that signalling molecules within the ASL itself are controlling ASL volume [89]. These molecules are ATP, which is breathing- or shear-stress induced [90], and adenosine. ATP interacts with receptors such as the purinergic P2Y2 receptors and adenosine reacts with the adenosine A2b receptors, that mediate inhibition of ENaC and activation of both CFTR and CaCC [91, 92]. This mechanism is also supposed to include PDZ interactions and cytoskeletal elements [1].

An interesting question is what the role of aquaporins (AQP) is in the production of ASL, compared to paracellular water flow and CFTR. In the epididymis, CFTR appears to regulate AQP-mediated water permeability [93]. In this tissue, CFTR is co-localized with AQP9 in the apical membrane, and this association promotes the activation of AQP9 by cAMP [94]. In a heavily debated study, concerning the clinical benefit of nebulized hypertonic saline in cystic fibrosis, an important role of amiloride-inhibitable AQP water channels in the generation of ASL was proposed [95]. However, although the positive effect of hypertonic saline as such is not disputed, the question whether this effect is mediated by AQP has received conflicting answers [96, 97] and is still open. Recently, it has been found that interleukin (IL)-13 enhances the expression of CFTR but abolishes the expression of AQP in airway epithelial cells [98]. In conclusion, the relation between CFTR and AQP needs further study.

The differences in the proposed hypotheses are due to difficulties in determining the accurate composition of the ASL because of the very small depth of the layer. Among the problems encountered there are difficulties to collect an adequate amount of ASL without disturbing the epithelium and inducing secretion from submucosal glands or leakage of interstitial fluid into the lumen, which may modify the composition of the ASL [99].

Furthermore, fluid secretion by submucosal glands differs markedly between mammalian species. For example, in transgenic mice that serve as animal models for CF, the fluid transport in the airways is much less affected than in CF patients [100]. It is also possible that variant forms of ENaC or different regulatory components operate in different systems [101].

3. The biliary duct epithelium

The biliary tree is a complex network of conduits within the liver that begins with the canals of Hering and progressively merges into a system of ducts, which finally deliver bile to the gallbladder and to the intestine. Cholangiocytes are the epithelial cells forming the biliary epithelium which shows a morphological heterogeneity that is strictly associated with a variety of functions performed at the different levels of the biliary tree [102]. Thus, the canals of Hering, located at the ductular-hepatocellular junction, constitute the physiologic link of the biliary tree with the hepatocyte canalicular system and they are the site where a facultative progenitor cell compartment resides; these liver progenitor cells are variably elicited only after liver injury. Given the strong capacity of mature hepatocytes to proliferate, cholangiocyte ability to behave as liver progenitor cells becomes evident only when hepatocellular proliferation is hampered as a result of severe liver damage, as that induced by several toxins or drugs, or occurring under certain conditions, *i.e.* viral hepatitis or non alcoholic steatohepatitis [103]. Cells lining the intrahepatic biliary tree have different functional and morphological specializations: the terminal cholangioles (size <15 μm) have some biological properties such as plasticity (i.e., the ability to undergo limited phenotypic changes) and reactivity (*i.e.*, the ability to participate in the inflammatory reaction to liver damage); interlobular (15-100 μm) and large ducts (100 μm to 800 μm) modulates fluidity and alkalinity of the primary hepatocellular bile.

3.1. Ion and water transport in cholangiocytes

In addition to funnelling bile into the intestine, cholangiocytes are actively involved in bile production. In humans, around 40% of the total bile production is of ductal origin. Cholangiocytes exert a series of reabsorptive and secretory process which dilute and alkalinize the bile during its passage along the biliary tract. Modifications of ductal bile appear to be tightly regulated by the actions of nerves, biliary constituents, and some peptide hormones like secretin [104]. Accordingly to *in vivo* and *in vitro* models, it is possible to distinguish between three different bile flow fractions: 1) the canalicular bile salt-dependent flow that is driven by concentrative secretion of bile acids by the hepatocytes followed by a facilitated efflux of water; 2) the canalicular bile salt-independent flow, which is also created by hepatocytes but through active secretion of both inorganic (bicarbonate) and organic (glutathione) compounds; and 3) the ductal bile flow, that is the bile salt-independent flow contributed by cholangiocytes, mainly through production of a bicarbonate-rich fluid in response to secretin and other regulatory factors. Cl⁻ secretion into the ductal lumen is the driving force of a chloride/

bicarbonate exchanger that exports HCO_3^- into the bile flowing into the biliary tree. Indeed, this AE (anion exchanger) activity is facilitated by the outside to inside transmembrane gradient of Cl^- at relatively high intracellular concentrations of $HCO3^-$, specially upon secretin stimulation. The AE activity in the liver is operated by AE2/SLC4A2 which is localized not only in the canaliculi but also in the luminal membrane of bile duct cells [105]. Experiments of RNA interference with recombinant adenovirus expressing short/small hairpin RNA have confirmed that AE2/SL4A2 is indeed the main effector of both basal and stimulated Na^+-independent Cl^-/HCO_3^- exchange in rat cholangiocytes [106]. Besides acid/base transporters cholangiocytes possess other ion carriers like those for Cl^-, Na^+, and K^+, which greatly contribute to intracellular pH regulation and bicarbonate secretion. Thus, CFTR had been localized at the apical side, where it plays a role in biliary excretion of bicarbonate [107, 108]. Although bicarbonate permeability through activated CFTR has been shown in several epithelia [109], its main contribution to biliary bicarbonate secretion appears to occur through a coordinated action with AE2/SL4A2 [106, 110, 111]. In addition to CFTR, cholangiocytes possess a dense population of Ca^{2+}-activated Cl^- channels. These channels are responsive to interaction of the purinergic-2 (P2) receptors with nucleotides (mainly ATP or UTP) [112, 113]. The apical fluxes of anions results in increased osmotic forces in the bile duct lumen which in the presence of AQPs contributes to water flux. AE2/SLC4A2 and CFTR colocalize with AQP1 in cholangiocyte intracellular vesicles wich coredistribute to the apical cholangiocyte membrane upon both cAMP and secretin stimulations [114].

3.2. The pathogenesis of CF liver disease

CF is associated with liver disease in almost 30% of all patients. In general, CF-associated liver disease develops during the first decades of life and does not progress rapidly. The diagnostic criteria were initially established by Colombo et al. [115]. Hepatobiliary disease in CF encompass a wide variety of complications, including steatosis, focal biliary cirrhosis (FBC), multilobular biliary cirrhosis (MBC), microgallbladder, distended gallbladder, cholelithiasis, intraheapatic sludge or stones, and cholangiocarcinoma [116]. The pathogenesis of steatosis (fatty liver) is not directly ascribed to the CFTR gene defect but has been attributed to malnutrition, essentially fatty acid deficiency, carnitine or choline deficiency, or insulin resistance [117].

With regarding to the pathogenesis of FBC and MBC, various hypotheses have been proposed [118, 119]:

- *The low chloride secretion hypothesis* proposes that loss of CFTR function leads to blocked biliary ductules with thick periodic acid-Schiff positive material leading to acute and chronic periductal inflammation, bile duct proliferation and increased fibrosis in scattered portal tracts. Hepatic stellate cells (important drivers of hepatic fibrosis) become activated to produce collagen and stimulate the bile duct epithelium to produce the profibrogenic cytokine TGF-β. The progression of FBC to MBC and portal hypertension, which occurs in up to 8% of patients, may take years to decades, and should be viewed as a continuum [120]. Considering CFTR as a driving force for Cl^-/HCO_3^- exchange, the postulated sequence of CF-associated hepatobiliary complications is that loss of functional CFTR protein in the apical membrane of cholangiocytes presumably initiates a cascade of abnormal Cl^- and HCO_3^- secretion, decreased bile flow, bile duct plugging by thickened secretions, and cholangiocyte/hepatocyte injury [10].

- *The cholangiocyte damage hypothesis* has been put forward by the studies of Freudenberg et al. in the F508del mouse model for CF [121]. These mice present with increased fecal loss of bile acids and a higher bile salt-to-phospholipid ratio in cell membranes, which was found to be associated with damage to intrahepatic bile ducts determining increased permeability of unconjugated bilirubin into cholangiocytes. They suggest that cholangiocytes injury is caused by a more hydrophobic bile acid pattern and an increased detergency from augmented bile salt-to-phospholipid ratio caused by hyperbilirubinbilia. In addition, lower gallbladder pH values and elevated calcium bilirubinate ion products in bile of CF mice raise the likelihood of supersaturating bile and forming black pigment gallstones [122].

- *The purinergic hypothesis* suggests that CFTR regulates the release of ATP into the bile duct lumen which regulates cholangiocyte secretion via the activation of the purinergic P2Y receptors [123]. Accordingly, Fiorotto et al. [124] have demonstrated that the choleretic effect of ursodeoxycholic acid (UDCA) is mediated via CFTR-dependent ATP secretion.

- *The mechanosensitive pathway hypothesis* indicates that the mechanical effects of fluid flow or shear stress at the apical membrane of biliary epithelial cells results in stimulation of ATP release and Cl^- secretion [123, 125]. The decreased bile flow due to CFTR dysfunction may be associated with alterations in mechanosensitive pathways which exacerbate abnormalities in Cl^- secretion and bile formation [123, 125].

- Finally, *the biliary HCO_3^- umbrella hypothesis* postulates that adequate apical biliary HCO_3^- secretion would appear crucial for protection of cholangiocytes against uncontrolled invasion of protonated bile acid monomers from bile via apical membranes into the cholangiocyte interior, inducing damage and apoptosis [126]. The Cl^-/HCO_3^- exchanger AE2/SLC4A2 and an intact glycocalyx appear to be crucial for the biliary HCO_3^- umbrella [127].

4. Placenta-derived stem cells

The placenta is a highly specialised organ, about 15 to 25 centimetres in diameter, that plays an important role in maintaining normal pregnancy and supporting the normal growth and development of the fetus. It is made up of a fetal and a maternal component: the fetal component include amnion and chorion as well as the chorionic plate, from which chorionic villi extend and make intimate contact with the uterine decidua during pregnancy; the maternal part of the placenta is the decidua basalis and it derived from endometrium.

As reported by Parolini et al. [128], different cell types can be isolated from the regions of the placenta:

- human amniotic epithelial cells (hAEC),

- human amniotic mesenchymal stromal cells (hAMSC),

- human chorionic mesenchymal stromal cells (hCMSC),

- human chorionic trophoblastic cells (hCTC).

In several studies hAEC, hAMSC, and hCMSC have been isolated and characterized for phenotypic and pluripotency molecular markers; moreover, has been demonstrated that these cells display differentiation potential and immunomodulatory effects [129].

hAEC express a pattern of mesenchymal markers while are negative for those of hematopoietic origin (CD90+, CD73+, CD105+, CD44+, CD29+, CD45-, CD34-, CD14-, HLA-DR-), and these cells are capable to differentiate in vitro into cell types of all 3 germ layers [128]. Like the amniotic epithelial fraction, the human amniotic and chorionic mesenchymal regions display the same pattern of phenotypic markers of bone marrow (BM) MSC, also displaying the expression of pluripotency markers (such as *Oct*-4) and the capability to differentiate toward different lineages including osteogenic, adipogenic, chondrogenic, and vascular/endothelial [128].

Placenta-derived stem cells seems to have a multipotent potential towards other cell types different from mesenchyme cells. hAMSC and hCMSC were shown to differentiate in vitro into a range of neuronal, oligodendrocyte and astrocyte precursors [130-132]. In addition, the use of amniochorionic membrane as a scaffold has been proposed for improving osteogenic differentiation of chorionic membrane-derived cells [133]. Alviano and colleagues reported that hAMSC display the ability to differentiate into endothelial cells in vitro [134]. Recently it has been shown that hAEC can differentiate in vitro in cells with hepatic characteristics, in particular in cells with the ability to differentiate into parenchymal hepatocytes as well as biliary cells that form duct-like three-dimensional structures when cultured on extracellular matrix [135]. hAMSC were demonstrated to differentiate into hepatocyte-like cells as judged by functional and phenotypic markers [136].

As regard the osteogenic and adipogenic differentiation of hAEC and hAMSC, discrepant results have been reported [137, 138], most likely due to the heterogeneous nature of these cell populations and due to the need to isolate the right population of progenitor cells from placental tissues. In this respect, recent efforts have been dedicated to optimizing isolation, culture, and preservation methods for placenta-derived cells; these include a study to determine the quantity and quality of amnion cells after isolation and culture [138], while other studies aimed to define long-term expansion methods to obtain a large cell population for analysis before use in cell-based therapies.

Sources such as amnion tissue offer outstanding possibilities for allogeneic transplantation due to their high differentiation potential and their ability to modulate immune reaction. Limitations, however, concern the reduced replicative potential as a result of progressive telomere erosion, which hampers scalable production and long-term analysis of these cells. The establishment and characterization of human amnion-derived stem cells lines immortalized by ectopic expression of the catalytic subunit of human telomerase (hTERT) resulted in continuously growing stem cells lines that were unaltered concerning surface marker profile, morphology, karyotype, and immunosuppressive capacity with similar or enhanced differentiation potential for up to 87 population doublings [139].

Interestingly, two groups found a more reliable and unlimited non-animal source for large-scale expansion of hMSC for future allogeneic clinical use: they cultured MSC with animal-free culture supplements such as human platelet lysate (PL), a suitable alternative to fetal calf serum (FCS) showing that these cells exhibit an increased proliferation potential and in vitro life span compared to cells cultured with FCS [140, 141]. On the other hand, it has been demonstrated that phenotypic shift of hAEC in culture is associated with reduced osteogenic differentiation in vitro, therefore different culturing methods may influence cell behavior [137].

In a recent comparative phenotypical study, BM- and placenta-derived mesenchymal cells has been shown that have a very similar morphology, size and cell surface phenotype for characteristics MSC markers [142]; in contrast, differences in proliferation potential have been observed between these two cell types [142]. Another study found different expressions of the chemokine receptors CCR1 and CCR3, which are only present on placenta-derived cells, while the adhesion molecules such as CD56, CD10, and CD49d have been shown to be more highly expressed on placenta-derived mesenchymal cells [143]. On the basis of numerous studies in the literature which clearly show the lack of significant differences between BM- and placenta-derived mesenchymal cells types, and on the basis of the fact that placenta is readily and widely available, a good manufacturing practice-compliant (GMP) reagents and protocols has been established for isolating and expanding human placenta-derived MSC that can be directly translated to the clinical trial setup [144].

4.1. Immunomodulatory features of placenta-derived stem cells

Since the placenta is fundamental for maintaining fetomaternal tolerance during pregnancy, the cells present in placental tissue may have immunomodulatory characteristics; this aspect contributes to make cells from placenta good candidates for possible use in cell therapy approaches, with the possibility of providing cells that display immunological properties that would allow their use in an all-transplantation setting.

It has been demonstrated that cells derived from placenta are negative for the expression of major histocompatibility complex (MHC) class II and for co-stimulatory molecules; all this is reflected as immune tolerance [128, 145]. Furthermore, these cells possess remarkable immunosuppressive properties and can inhibit the proliferation and function of the major immune cell populations, including dendritic cells (DCs), T cells, B cells and natural killer (NK) cells. Most of these studies have been recently summarized in up-to-date reviews [146-148]. Here, we give a brief account of the major findings concerning hAMSC.

Numerous studies showed that amniotic and chorionic membrane-derived cells can suppress the T lymphocyte proliferation induced by alloantigens, mitogens, anti-CD3 and anti-CD28 antibodies in *in vitro* and *in vivo* models [149-152]. The suppression of lymphocyte population was shown to be not dependent on cell death but on decreased proliferation and increased numbers of regulatory T cells [145]. Inhibition of T cell proliferation by placenta-derived stem cells appears to be mediated by both cell–cell interaction [153] and release of soluble factors such as indoleamine 2,3-dioxygenase (IDO), transforming growth factor β (TGF-β), and IL-10 [145, 154, 155]. The immunosuppressive activity of hAMSC on T cells seems to be not only direct but involves also DCs. Indeed, cells derived from the mesenchymal region of human amnion impaired the differentiation of monocytes into DCs by inhibiting the response of the former to maturation signals, reducing the expression of co-stimulatory molecules and hampering the ability of monocytes to stimulate naive T cell proliferation [156]. The mechanism involved is not known, however, this inhibitory effect might be mediated via soluble factors, like IL-6, and may be dose-dependent, as it has been shown for BM-derived MSCs [157] (Figure 1).

This immune-privileged status of placenta-derived stem cells has been indicated as the cause of lack of rejection in allo- and xeno-transplantation settings. In this regard, several studies examined the fate of amniotic membrane derived stem cells grafts. Wang et al. [158] studied allogeneic GFP+ mouse intact amniotic epithelium grafts heterotopically transplanted in the eye. Kubo et al. [159] studied xenotransplanted human amniotic membrane in the eye of rats. Several preclinical studies have already reported prolonged survival of human placenta-derived cells after xenogeneic transplantation into immunocompetent animals including swine [152] and bonnet monkeys [128], with no evidence of immunological rejection.

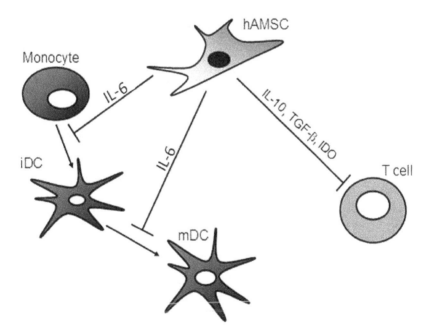

Figure 1. Effects of placenta-derived stem cells on immunocytes. Placenta-derived cells exert immunomodulatory effects both on dendritic cells and T cells. Their inhibitory role is dependent on cell–cell contact and secreted soluble factors. Since most of the studies have focused on hAMSC, this cell type is represented in the scheme. iDC: immature dendritic cell; IDO: indoleamine 2, 3-dioxygenase; IL-6: interleukin-6; IL-10: interleukin-10; mDC: mature dendritic cell; TGF-β: transforming growth factor β.

4.2. Clinical application of placenta-derived stem cells

More than once century ago, Davis was the first to report the use of the amniotic membrane (AM) to heal skin wounds [160], prompting subsequent applications in the treatment of leg ulcers [161, 162] and burns [163], as well as for applications in ophthalmology [164]. These studies have suggested that placenta-derived stem cells may be useful for treating a range of pathologic conditions, including neurological disorders [165-167], spinal cord injury [128, 168], critical limb ischemia [169], inflammatory bowel diseases [170], and myocardial infarction [171]. Here, we will focus on the potential application of placenta-derived stem cells to lung and liver, the major organs interested by CF.

5. Potential application of placenta-derived stem cells to CF

5.1. Placenta-derived stem cells for lung diseases

The first report demonstrating a therapeutic effect of placenta-derived stem cells in lung diseases is that by Cargnoni and colleagues [172]. In a mouse model of bleomycin-induced lung injury, transplantation of fetal membrane-derived cells resulted in a reduction in the severity of pulmonary fibrosis. This result was obtained when cells were administered either systemically (intravenous or intraperitoneal) or locally (intratracheal) 15 min after intratracheal bleomycin instillation and in two different settings, *i.e.* either using allogeneic or xenogeneic (a mixture of 50% human amnion/chorion mensenchymal stem cells and 50% hAEC) cells. Although the inflammatory score was not decreased, a reduction in the number of infiltrating neutrophils was observed. It is worth noting that that the presence of neutrophils is known to be associated with poor prognosis in idiopathic pulmonary fibrosis in humans [173]. The question arises whether these anti-inflammatory and anti-fibrotic effects may be due to the engraftment of placenta-derived stem cells or to the secretion of soluble factors. In this study allogeneic or xenogeneic cells were detected in the injured lung of transplanted mice, although not in a quantitatively fashion, by means of PCR analysis, and these results are in accordance with those obtained by Bailo and colleagues, who demonstrated microchimerism upon transplantation of human amnion and chorionic cells in neonatal swine and rats [152]. The release of soluble factors has been addressed in a further study. The administration of conditioned medium generated from hAMSC to bleomycin-treated mice determined a reduction in lung fibrosis scores in terms of fibrosis distribution, fibroblast proliferation, collagen deposition and alveolar obliteration [174]. This study support the increasing evidence that MSC isolated from various sources produce bioactive molecules, so that injection of conditioned medium obtained from MSC could be an effective experimental treatment for different tissue injuries [175, 176]. Further studies are therefore warranted to elucidate the mechanisms of action of placenta-derived cells in this model, in particular paracrine factors that act to down-regulate neutrophil recruitment.

It has to be said that the role of exogenous stem cells in pulmonary fibrosis is controversial, meaning that some studies have demonstrated that these cells can act as a potential source of fibroblast, which may accentuate the fibrotic process [177]. Since these findings were obtained with BM-derived stem cells, it should be further assessed if a similar behaviour is presented by amniotic-derived stem cells. Of note, placenta-derived cells did not exert any profibrotic effect after their transplantation [172].

In vitro studies have so far demonstrated that co-cultures of hAMSC and CF epithelial cells originated from bronchi can elicit CFTR protein expression in 33-50% hAMSC, in front of 6% prior to the co-cultures, and the lower the hAMSC:CFBE41o- ratios the lower the CFTR expression in hAMSC [136]. Indirect co-cultures data indicate that this effect is primarily due to the contact between hAMSC and epithelial cells, and not due to factors acting by a paracrine manner. BM-MSC acquired an airway epithelium phenotype when co-cultured with respiratory epithelial cells and determined a partial resumption of the chloride secretion defect in CF epithelia [178]. Preliminary analysis of the chloride transport defect in co-cultures between CF cells and hAMSC showed a partial correction of the chloride efflux (Carbone et al., unpublished results). Furthermore, since only 6-20% of corrected cells is needed to revert the basic defect in chloride secretion [179], our data showing that 33-50% of hAMSC acquired CFTR expression shed a positive light on the use of amnion MSCs in the CF treatment. Overall, these data point out to a cross talk between amniotic and epithelial cells, for which a critical number of hAMSC is needed. Indeed, in other co-culture systems, developed with MSC and chondrocytes, it has been shown universally that the more chondrocytes the lower the expression of extracellular matrix genes and functional properties of engineered cartilage [180, 181]. Since the cellular interactions between epithelial and mesenchymal cells in monolayer co-culture are likely to be bi-directional, a possible mode of action could be cross talk between cells via gap junctions, which has been observed *in vivo* in the lung between transplanted MSC and resident epithelial cells [182].

Overall, the potential usefulness of placenta-derived stem cells in CF lung disease might be either in the correction of the early basic defect (chloride transport) or in late remodelling events (pulmonary fibrosis).

5.2. Placenta-derived stem cells for liver diseases

Several preclinical studies have reported to date that placenta-derived stem cells can engraft into the liver and perform hepatic functions *in vivo*. Takashima and colleagues [183] showed that after transplantation of human amniotic membrane into the peritoneum of SCID mice, human albumin could be detected in the sera and peritoneal fluid of these animals from day 1 until day 7. Sakuragawa and colleagues [184] showed that the transplantation of hAEC transduced with the β-galactosidase gene into the livers of SCID mice resulted in detection of β-galactosidase-positive cells at 1 week after transplantation, indicating that the transplanted cells had been integrated into the hepatic parenchyma within a few days [184]. More recently, it has been shown that six months after transplantation of hAEC into the livers of SCID/beige mice that had been pretreated with retrorsine, most mature liver genes were expressed at levels comparable to those of authentic human adult livers, including the major CYP genes, other metabolic enzymes, plasma proteins, and hepatocyte-enriched transcription factors and genes encoding hepatic-transporter proteins [185].

These studies provide compelling evidence in support of the functional hepatic potential of hAEC *in vivo*, thereby supporting the potential of hAEC as a useful tool for liver regeneration in the future.

MSC represent an alternative tool for the establishment of a successful stem-cell-based therapy of liver diseases [186] with preliminary clinical improvements in acute and chronic hepatic diseases [187, 188]. To date, several studies on animal models reported the beneficial effects of MSC in promoting hepatic tissue regeneration [189]. Overall, a number of different mechanisms contribute to the therapeutic effects exerted by MSC, among which their differentiation into functional hepatic cells. However, these studies have not provided definitive evidence that MSC have a capability to differentiate into functional hepatocytes *in vivo* [190]. Rather, the observed improvements could be attributed to the known property of MSC to produce a series of growth factors and cytokines that could suppress inflammatory response, reduce hepatocytes apoptosis, regress liver fibrosis, and enhance hepatocytes functionality [191, 192].

Although numerous studies have reported that BM-derived MSC can reduce carbon tetrachloride (CCl_4)-induced liver fibrosis in mice, the mechanism by which MSC repair the fibrosis is unclear, and the results are controversial [190, 193-197]. One possibility is that MSC differentiate into hepatocytes, because of the *in vivo* niche, and secrete growth factors that promote liver regeneration. Another possibility is that MSC suppress hepatic stellate cells activity and secrete metalloproteinases (MMPs), thereby eliminating deposition of extracellular matrix [198]. It has been demonstrated that fibrosis, infiltration of neutrophils, synthesis of collagen I and α-smooth muscle actin (α-SMA), and expression of inflammatory were all reduced by infusion of isogenic MSC [199]. It is possible that these responses were partly due to the upregulation of cytoglobin expression by hepatic stellate cells, which protect against oxidative stress and controls tissue fibrosis and at the same time inhibits the activation of those cells to become myofibroblasts [200]. Finally, it has been demonstrated that intravenous administration of MSC caused an increase in IL-10 mRNA in the liver and protein in the blood in a CCl_4-induced liver fibrosis rat model [201]. IL-10 is an inhibitor of many cytokines that stimulate liver fibrosis, such as IL-6, TNF-α and TGF-β, all downregulated by the MSC infusion. In addition, IL-10 can suppress tissue inhibitor of metalloproteinase (TIMP)-1 expression and thereby relieve MMP-1 to degrade liver collagen deposits [202, 203].

In a recent study, hAMSC were infused in mice with CCl_4-induced hepatic cirrhosis and exerted various beneficial effects such as reduction of hepatic stellate cell activation, decrease of hepatocyte apoptosis, and reduction of hepatic fibrosis [204]. Infusion of hAMSC also depressed hepatocyte senescence and resulted in engraftment of hAMSC into the host liver as judged by the expression of the hepatocyte-specific markers, human albumin and α-fetoprotein. Finally, a study demonstrated that human AM, when applied as a patch onto the liver surface, reduced progression of experimental biliary fibrosis induced in rats by the biliary duct ligation procedure [205]. Again, a beneficial effect related to the release of soluble factors by the human AM patch has been invoked, since no massive (or at least very low/undetectable) engraftment of AM-derived cells occurred in the host liver.

6. Conclusion

Placenta-derived stem cells are endowed with interesting features that are important for choosing them as a source for approaches aimed to regenerative medicine: immune-privileged status, secretion of biomolecules with anti-scarring and anti-inflammatory properties, and, least but not last, no ethical concerns. Although the AM and AM-derived stem cells have been used in the clinics for over one hundred years, their employment in lung and liver diseases is coming on the stage only in the last few years. Placenta-derived stem cells have been recently more thoroughly characterized for their phenotype, multipotency and expression of pluripotency genes.

In CF, lung disease has been the target first of gene therapy approaches brought to the clinical stage [206, 207], hesitated in a slow progression due to limited efficiency of gene transfer vectors and pathophysiological barriers, and then of stem cell-based experimental treatments in mice [208]. Despite a very low level of engraftment of donor HSPC into the nose and the gut, significant CFTR mRNA expression and a measurable level of correction of the electro-physiological defect were observed after transplantation of wild-type marrow cells into CF mice [209]. It is uncertain whether this effect is due to the presence of CFTR-expressing epithelial cells derived from donor cells or to the paracrine effects of transplanted cells. Other sources, such as umbilical cord blood, embryonic stem cells, and induced pluripotent stem cells are being evaluated [210, 211]. Recent *in vitro* data on the acquisition of CFTR expression by hAMSC indicate placenta-derived stem cells as a possible source for treating the early phases of CF lung disease. Anyhow, caution should be taken when stem cell-based therapies are proposed for an inflammatory disease like that of CF lung, in view of the fact that these cells could be immunosuppressive and/or contribute to the inflammatory process. There is no available information concerning the immunomodulatory effects of placenta-derived stem cells in CF lungs.

Liver fibrosis is a common outcome of a variety of chronic liver diseases following different insults, including the biliary disorder occurring in CF. Orthotopic liver transplantation remains the only viable therapeutic option to treat CF patients with hepatic cirrhosis, and hepatocyte transplantation has never been attempted in this disease. The use of progenitor cell transplantation is emerging as a potential alternative, and several potential sources have been identified for the isolation of these cells [212]. For the treatment of liver cirrhosis, this approach has been performed mainly with BM-derived MSC [213, 214]. Given the drawbacks related to the use of BM-derived MSC (limited frequency, invasive procedure, age and disease state affecting the collection of healthy autologous BM), placenta-derived stem cells could represent a prime candidate for the treatment of liver fibrosis, since they are immunotolerated, can be isolated and produced at high yield, and do not provoke ethical debate. AM and AM-derived stem cells have been demonstrated to halt the progression of liver fibrosis and its evolution towards cirrhosis, but the long-term safety and therapeutic efficacy are not known yet, which warrant further studies. Moreover, optimal therapeutic regimens for clinical application of placenta-derived stem cells, such as optimal doses, transplantation route and interval period for transplantation should be evaluated in detail [215].

Acknowledgements

This work was supported by the Italian Ministry of Health (Ricerca Corrente and Law 548/93).

Author details

Annalucia Carbone[1,2*], Stefano Castellani[2], Valentina Paracchini[1], Sante Di Gioia[2], Carla Colombo[1] and Massimo Conese[2]

*Address all correspondence to: annalucia.carbone@gmail.com

1 Fondazione IRCCS Ca' GrandaOspedale Maggiore Policlinico, Cystic Fibrosis Center, Milan, Italy

2 Department of Medical and Surgical Sciences, University of Foggia, Foggia, Italy

References

[1] Kunzelmann K. CFTR: interacting with everything? News Physiol Sci 2001;16: 167-70

[2] Amaral MD, Kunzelmann K. Molecular targeting of CFTR as a therapeutic approach to cystic fibrosis. Trends Pharmacol Sci 2007;28: 334-41

[3] Zielenski J. Genotype and phenotype in cystic fibrosis. Respiration 2000;67: 117-33

[4] Blaug S, Hybiske K, Cohn J, Firestone GL, Machen TE, Miller SS. ENaC- and CFTR-dependent ion and fluid transport in mammary epithelia. Am J Physiol Cell Physiol 2001;281: C633-48

[5] Gibson RL, Burns JL, Ramsey BW. Pathophysiology and management of pulmonary infections in cystic fibrosis. Am J Respir Crit Care Med 2003;168: 918-51

[6] Knowles MR, Stutts MJ, Spock A, Fischer N, Gatzy JT, Boucher RC. Abnormal ion permeation through cystic fibrosis respiratory epithelium. Science 1983;221: 1067-70

[7] Boucher RC, Stutts MJ, Knowels MR, Cantley L, Gatzy JT. Na+ transport in cystic fibrosis respiratory epithelia. J Clin Invest 1986;78: 1245-52

[8] Boucher RC. Cystic fibrosis: a disease of vulnerability to airway surface dehydration. Trends Mol Med 2007;13: 231-40

[9] Fischer H, Widdicombe JH. Mechanisms of acid and base secretion by the airway epithelium. J Membr Biol 2006;211: 139-50

[10] Quinton PM. Cystic fibrosis: impaired bicarbonate secretion and mucoviscidosis. Lancet 2008;372: 415-7

[11] Rommens JM, Iannuzzi MC, Kerem B, Drumm ML, Melmer G. Identification of the cystic fibrosis gene: chromosome walking and jumping. Science 1989;245: 1059-65

[12] Yoshimura K, Nakamura H, Trapnell BC, Chu C-S, Dalemans W, Pavirani A, et al. Expression of the cystic fibrosis transmembrane conductance regulator gene in cells of non-epithelial origin. Nucleic Acids Research 1991;19: 5417-23

[13] Vandebrouck C, Melin P, Norez C, Robert R, Guibert C, Mettey Y, et al. Evidence that CFTR is expressed in rat tracheal smooth muscle cells and contributes to bron-chodilation. Respir Res 2006;7: 113

[14] Piro D, Piccoli C, Guerra L, Sassone F, D'Aprile A, Favia M, et al. Hematopoietic stem/progenitor cells express functional mitochondrial energy-dependent cystic fib-rosis transmembrane conductance regulator. Stem Cells Dev 2012;21: 634-46

[15] Di A, Brown ME, Deriy LV, Li C, Szeto FL, Chen Y, et al. CFTR regulates phagosome acidification in macrophages and alters bactericidal activity. Nat Cell Biol 2006;8: 933-44

[16] Reddy MM, Quinton PM. cAMP activation of CF-affected Cl- conductance in both cell membranes of an absorptive epithelium. J Membr Biol 1992;130: 49-62

[17] Bobadilla JL, Macek M, Jr., Fine JP, Farrell PM. Cystic fibrosis: a worldwide analysis of CFTR mutations--correlation with incidence data and application to screening. Hum Mutat 2002;19: 575-606

[18] Gelman MS, Kopito RR. Rescuing protein conformation: prospects for pharmacologi-cal therapy in cystic fibrosis. J Clin Invest 2002;110: 1591-7

[19] Vankeerberghen A, Cuppens H, Cassiman JJ. The cystic fibrosis transmembrane con-ductance regulator: an intriguing protein with pleiotropic functions. J Cyst Fibros 2002;1: 13-29

[20] McKone EF, Emerson SS, Edwards KL, Aitken ML. Effect of genotype on phenotype and mortality in cystic fibrosis: a retrospective cohort study. Lancet 2003;361: 1671-6

[21] Kerem E, Corey M, Kerem BS, Rommens J, Markiewicz D, Levison H, et al. The rela-tion between genotype and phenotype in cystic fibrosis--analysis of the most com-mon mutation (delta F508). N Engl J Med 1990;323: 1517-22

[22] Santis G, Osborne L, Knight RA, Hodson ME. Independent genetic determinants of pancreatic and pulmonary status in cystic fibrosis. Lancet 1990;336: 1081-4

[23] Burke DT, Carle GF, Olson MV. Cloning of large segments of exogenous DNA into yeast by means of artificial chromosome vectors. Science 1992;236: 806-12

[24] Gadsby DC, Vergani P, Csanady L. The ABC protein turned chloride channel whose failure causes cystic fibrosis. Nature 2006;440: 477-83

[25] Bear CE, Li C, Kartner N, Bridges RD, Jensen TJ, Ramjeesingh M, et al. Purification and functional reconstitution of the cystic fibrosis transmembrane conductance regulator (CFTR). Cell 1992;68: 809-18

[26] Jones PM, George AM. The ABC transporter structure and mechanism: perspectives on recent research. Cell Mol Life Sci 2004;61: 682-99

[27] Riordan JR, Rommens JM, Kerem B, Alon N, Rozmahel R, Grzelczak Z, et al. Identification of the cystic fibrosis gene: cloning and characterization of complementary DNA. Science 1989;245: 1066-73 [Erratum, Science 989;245:437.]

[28] Sheppard DN, Welsh MJ. Structure and function of the CFTR chloride channel. Physiol Rev 1999;79: S23-45

[29] Dulhanty AM, Riordan JR. Phosphorylation by cAMP-dependent protein kinase causes a conformational change in the R domain of the cystic fibrosis transmembrane conductance regulator. Biochemistry 1994;33: 4072-9

[30] Ma J, Tasch JE, Tao T, Zhao J, Xie J, Drumm ML, et al. Phosphorylation-dependent block of cystic fibrosis transmembrane conductance regulator chloride channel by exogenous R domain protein. J Biol Chem 1996;271: 7351-6

[31] Hopfner KP, Karcher A, Shin DS, Craig L, Arthur LM, Carney JP, et al. Structural biology of Rad50 ATPase: ATP-driven conformational control in DNA double-strand break repair and the ABC-ATPase superfamily. Cell 2000;101: 789-800

[32] Vergani P, Nairn AC, Gadsby DC. On the mechanism of MgATP-dependent gating of CFTR Cl- channels. J Gen Physiol 2003;121: 17-36

[33] Quinton PM. The neglected ion: HCO3. Nat Med 2001;7: 292-3

[34] Ko SB, Zeng W, Dorwart MR, Luo X, Kim KH, Millen L, et al. Gating of CFTR by the STAS domain of SLC26 transporters. Nat Cell Biol 2004;6: 343-50

[35] Wine JJ. Acid in the airways. Focus on "Hyperacidity of secreted fluid from submucosal glands in early cystic fibrosis". Am J Physiol Cell Physiol 2006;290: C669-71

[36] Braunstein GM, Roman RM, Clancy JP, Kudlow BA, Taylor AL, Shylonsky VG, et al. Cystic fibrosis transmembrane conductance regulator facilitates ATP release by stimulating a separate ATP release channel for autocrine control of cell volume regulation. J Biol Chem 2001;276: 6621-30

[37] Sabirov RZ, Okada Y. ATP release via anion channels. Purinergic Signal 2005;1: 311-28

[38] Kogan I, Ramjeesingh M, Li C, Kidd JF, Wang Y, Leslie EM, et al. CFTR directly mediates nucleotide-regulated glutathione flux. EMBO J 2003;22: 1981-9

[39] Wei L, Vankeerberghen A, Cuppens H, Eggermont J, Cassiman JJ, Droogmans G, et al. Interaction between calcium-activated chloride channels and the cystic fibrosis transmembrane conductance regulator. Pflugers Arch 1999;438: 635-41

[40] Schwiebert EM, Egan ME, Hwang TH, Fulmer SB, Allen SS, Cutting GR, et al. CFTR regulates outwardly rectifying chloride channels through an autocrine mechanism involving ATP. Cell 1995;81: 1063-73.

[41] Vennekens R, Trouet D, Vankeerberghen A, Voets T, Cuppens H, Eggermont J, et al. Inhibition of volume-regulated anion channels by expression of the cystic fibrosis transmembrane conductance regulator. J Physiol 1999;515 (Pt 1): 75-85

[42] McNicholas CM, Nason MW, Guggino WB, Schwiebert EM, Hebert SC, Giebisch G, et al. A funtional CFTR-NBF1 is required for ROMK2-CFTR interaction. Am J Physiol 1997;273: F843-F8

[43] Schreiber R, Hopf A, Mall M, Greger R, Kunzelmann K. The first-nucleotide binding domain of the cystic-fibrosis transmembrane conductance regulator is important for inhibition of the epithelial Na+ channel. Proc Natl Acad Sci U S A 1999;96: 5310-5

[44] Short DB, Trotter KW, Reczek D, Kreda SM, Bretscher A, Boucher RC, et al. An apical PDZ protein anchors the cystic fibrosis transmembrane conductance regulator to the cytoskeleton. J Biol Chem 1998;273: 19797-801

[45] Guggino WB, Stanton BA. New insights into cystic fibrosis: molecular switches that regulate CFTR. Nat Rev Mol Cell Biol 2006;7: 426-36

[46] Kunzelmann K. ENaC is inhibited by an increase in the intracellular Cl(-) concentration mediated through activation of Cl(-) channels. Pflugers Arch 2003;445: 504-12

[47] Bals R, Hiemstra PS. Innate immunity in the lung: how epithelial cells fight against respiratory pathogens. Eur Respir J 2004;23: 327-33

[48] Parker D, Prince A. Innate immunity in the respiratory epithelium. Am J Respir Cell Mol Biol 2011;45: 189-201

[49] Yadav AK, Bracher A, Doran SF, Leustik M, Squadrito GL, Postlethwait EM, et al. Mechanisms and modification of chlorine-induced lung injury in animals. Proc Am Thorac Soc 2010;7: 278-83

[50] Folkerts G, van der Linde H, Verheyen AK, Nijkamp FP. Endogenous nitric oxide modulation of potassium-induced changes in guinea-pig airway tone. Br J Pharmacol 1995;115: 1194-8

[51] Zalewski PD, Truong-Tran AQ, Grosser D, Jayaram L, Murgia C, Ruffin RE. Zinc metabolism in airway epithelium and airway inflammation: basic mechanisms and clinical targets. A review. Pharmacol Ther 2005;105: 127-49

[52] Knight DA, Holgate ST. The airway epithelium: structural and functional properties in health and disease. Respirology 2003;8: 432-46

[53] Engelhardt JF, Zepeda M, Cohn JA, Yankaskas JR, Wilson JM. Expression of the cystic fibrosis gene in adult human lung. J Clin Invest 1994;93: 737-49

[54] Reid L, Meyrick B, Antony VB, Chang LY, Crapo JD, Reynolds HY. The mysterious pulmonary brush cell: a cell in search of a function. Am J Respir Crit Care Med 2005;172: 136-9

[55] Weiss DJ, Kolls JK, Ortiz LA, Panoskaltsis-Mortari A, Prockop DJ. Stem cells and cell therapies in lung biology and lung diseases. Proc Am Thorac Soc 2008;5: 637-67

[56] Joo NS, Irokawa T, Wu JV, Robbins RC, Whyte RI, Wine JJ. Absent secretion to vasoactive intestinal peptide in cystic fibrosis airway glands. J Biol Chem 2002;277: 50710-5

[57] Engelhardt JF, Yankaskas JR, Ernst SA, Yang Y, Marino CR, Boucher RC, et al. Submucosal glands are the predominant site of CFTR expression in the human bronchus. Nat Genet 1992;2: 240-7

[58] Ballard ST, Inglis SK. Liquid secretion properties of airway submucosal glands. J Physiol 2004;556: 1-10

[59] Verkman AS, Song Y, Thiagarajah JR. Role of airway surface liquid and submucosal glands in cystic fibrosis lung disease. Am J Physiol Cell Physiol 2003;284: C2-15

[60] Kreda S, Mall M, Mengos A, Rochelle L, Yankaskas J, Riordan JR, et al. Characterization of wild-type and deltaF508 cystic fibrosis transmembrane regulator in human respiratory epithelia. Mol Biol Cell 2005;16: 2154-67

[61] Hollenhorst MI, Richter K, Fronius M. Ion transport by pulmonary epithelia. J Biomed Biotechnol 2011;2011: 174306

[62] Widdicombe JH, Basbaum CB, Highland E. Ion contents and other properties of isolated cells from dog tracheal epithelium. Am J Physiol 1981;241: C184-92

[63] McCann JD, Welsh MJ. Regulation of Cl- and K+ channels in airway epithelium. Annu Rev Physiol 1990;52: 115-35

[64] Mitic LL, Van Itallie CM, Anderson JM. Molecular physiology and pathophysiology of tight junctions I. Tight junction structure and function: lessons from mutant animals and proteins. Am J Physiol Gastrointest Liver Physiol 2000;279: G250-4

[65] Welsh MJ. Electrolyte transport by airway epithelia. Physiol Rev 1987;67: 1143-84

[66] Sleigh MA, Blake JR, Liron N. The propulsion of mucus by cilia. Am Rev Respir Dis 1988;137: 726-41

[67] Widdicombe JH, Bastacky SJ, Wu DX, Lee CY. Regulation of depth and composition of airway surface liquid. Eur Respir J 1997;10: 2892-7

[68] Widdicombe JH, Widdicombe JG. Regulation of human airway surface liquid. Respir Physiol 1995;99: 3-12

[69] Chambers LA, Rollins BM, Tarran R. Liquid movement across the surface epithelium of large airways. Respir Physiol Neurobiol 2007;159: 256-70

[70] Khan TZ, Wagener JS, Bost T, Martinez J, Accurso FJ, Riches DWH. Early pulmonary inflammation in infants with cystic fibrosis. Am J Respir Crit Care Med 1995;151: 1075-82

[71] Muhlebach MS, Stewart PW, Leigh MW, Noah TL. Quantitation of inflammatory responses to bacteria in young cystic fibrosis and control patients. Am J Respir Crit Care Med 1999;160: 186-91

[72] Balough K, McCubbin M, Weinberger M, Smits W, Ahrens R, Fick R. The relationship between infection and inflammation in the early stages of lung disease from cystic fibrosis. Pediatr Pulmonol 1995;20: 63-70

[73] Hayes E, Pohl K, McElvaney NG, Reeves EP. The cystic fibrosis neutrophil: a specialized yet potentially defective cell. Arch Immunol Ther Exp (Warsz) 2011;59: 97-112

[74] Sheppard MN. The pathology of cystic fibrosis. In: Hodson ME, Geddes DM, editors. Cystic fibrosis. London: Chapman & Hall; 1995. p. 131-49.

[75] Tomashefski JF, Jr., Konstan MW, Bruce MC, Abramowsky CR. The pathologic characteristics of interstitial pneumonia cystic fibrosis. A retrospective autopsy study. Am J Clin Pathol 1989;91: 522-30

[76] Chmiel JF, Davis PB. State of the art: why do the lungs of patients with cystic fibrosis become infected and why can't they clear the infection? Respir Res 2003;4: 8

[77] Konradova V, Vavrova V, Hlouskova Z, Copova M, Tomanek A, Houstek J. Ultrastructure of bronchial epithelium in children with chronic or recurrent respiratory diseases. Eur J Respir Dis 1982;63: 516-25

[78] Leigh MW, Kylander JE, Yankaskas JR, Boucher RC. Cell proliferation in bronchial epithelium and submucosal glands of cystic fibrosis patients. Am J Respir Cell Mol Biol 1995;12: 605-12

[79] Li JD, Feng W, Gallup M, Kim JH, Gum J, Kim Y, et al. Activation of NF-kappaB via a Src-dependent Ras-MAPK-pp90rsk pathway is required for Pseudomonas aeruginosa-induced mucin overproduction in epithelial cells. Proc Natl Acad Sci U S A 1998;95: 5718-23

[80] Hauber HP, Tsicopoulos A, Wallaert B, Griffin S, McElvaney NG, Daigneault P, et al. Expression of HCLCA1 in cystic fibrosis lungs is associated with mucus overproduction. Eur Respir J 2004;23: 846-50

[81] Voynow JA, Young LR, Wang Y, Horger T, Rose MC, Fischer BM. Neutrophil elastase increases MUC5AC mRNA and protein expression in respiratory epithelial cells. Am J Physiol 1999;276: L835-43

[82] Hajj R, Lesimple P, Nawrocki-Raby B, Birembaut P, Puchelle E, Coraux C. Human airway surface epithelial regeneration is delayed and abnormal in cystic fibrosis. J Pathol 2007;211: 340-50

[83] Matsui H, Grubb BR, Tarran R, Randell SH, Gatzy JT, Davis CW, et al. Evidence for periciliary liquid layer depletion, not abnormal ion composition, in the pathogenesis of cystic fibrosis airway disease. Cell 1998;95: 1005-15

[84] Zabner J, Smith JJ, Karp PH, Widdicombe JH, Welsh MJ. Loss of CFTR chloride channels alters salt absorption by cystic fibrosis airway epithelia in vitro. Mol Cell 1998;2: 397-403.

[85] Clary-Meinesz C, Mouroux J, Cosson J, Huitorel P, Blaive B. Influence of external pH on ciliary beat frequency in human bronchi and bronchioles. Eur Respir J 1998;11: 330-3

[86] Coakley RD, Boucher RC. Regulation and functional significance of airway surface liquid pH. JOP 2001;2: 294-300

[87] Worlitzsch D, Tarran R, Ulrich M, Schwab U, Cekici A, Meyer KC, et al. Effects of reduced mucus oxygen concentration in airway *Pseudomonas* infections of cystic fibrosis patients. J Clin Invest 2002;109: 317-25

[88] Jayaraman S, Joo NS, Reitz B, Wine JJ, Verkman AS. Submucosal gland secretions in airways from cystic fibrosis patients have normal [Na(+)] and pH but elevated viscosity. Proc Natl Acad Sci U S A 2001;98: 8119-23

[89] Tarran R, Trout L, Donaldson SH, Boucher RC. Soluble mediators, not cilia, determine airway surface liquid volume in normal and cystic fibrosis superficial airway epithelia. J Gen Physiol 2006;127: 591-604

[90] Watt WC, Lazarowski ER, Boucher RC. Cystic fibrosis transmembrane regulator-independent release of ATP. Its implications for the regulation of P2Y2 receptors in airway epithelia. J Biol Chem 1998;273: 14053-8

[91] Lazarowski ER, Tarran R, Grubb BR, van Heusden CA, Okada S, Boucher RC. Nucleotide release provides a mechanism for airway surface liquid homeostasis. J Biol Chem 2004;279: 36855-64

[92] Picher M, Burch LH, Boucher RC. Metabolism of P2 receptor agonists in human airways: implications for mucociliary clearance and cystic fibrosis. J Biol Chem 2004;279: 20234-41

[93] Cheung KH, Leung CT, Leung GP, Wong PY. Synergistic effects of cystic fibrosis transmembrane conductance regulator and aquaporin-9 in the rat epididymis. Biol Reprod 2003;68: 1505-10

[94] Pietrement C, Da Silva N, Silberstein C, James M, Marsolais M, Van Hoek A, et al. Role of NHERF1, cystic fibrosis transmembrane conductance regulator, and cAMP in the regulation of aquaporin 9. J Biol Chem 2008;283: 2986-96

[95] Donaldson SH, Bennett WD, Zeman KL, Knowles MR, Tarran R, Boucher RC. Mucus clearance and lung function in cystic fibrosis with hypertonic saline. N Engl J Med 2006;354: 241-50

[96] Levin MH, Sullivan S, Nielson D, Yang B, Finkbeiner WE, Verkman AS. Hypertonic saline therapy in cystic fibrosis: Evidence against the proposed mechanism involving aquaporins. J Biol Chem 2006;281: 25803-12

[97] Pedersen PS, Braunstein TH, Jorgensen A, Larsen PL, Holstein-Rathlou NH, Frederiksen O. Stimulation of aquaporin-5 and transepithelial water permeability in human airway epithelium by hyperosmotic stress. Pflugers Arch 2007;453: 777-85

[98] Skowron-zwarg M, Boland S, Caruso N, Coraux C, Marano F, Tournier F. Interleukin-13 interferes with CFTR and AQP5 expression and localization during human airway epithelial cell differentiation. Exp Cell Res 2007;313: 2695-702

[99] Vanthanouvong V, Kozlova I, Johannesson M, Naas E, Nordvall SL, Dragomir A, et al. Composition of nasal airway surface liquid in cystic fibrosis and other airway diseases determined by X-ray microanalysis. Microsc Res Tech 2006;69: 271-6

[100] Grubb BR, Boucher RC. Pathophysiology of gene-targeted mouse models for cystic fibrosis. Physiol Rev 1999;79: S193-S214

[101] Reddy MM, Light MJ, Quinton PM. Activation of the epithelial Na+ channel (ENaC) requires CFTR Cl- channel function. Nature 1999;402: 301-4.

[102] Strazzabosco M, Fabris L. Functional anatomy of normal bile ducts. Anat Rec (Hoboken) 2008;291: 653-60

[103] Sell S. Heterogeneity and plasticity of hepatocyte lineage cells. Hepatology 2001;33: 738-50

[104] Banales JM, Prieto J, Medina JF. Cholangiocyte anion exchange and biliary bicarbonate excretion. World J Gastroenterol 2006;12: 3496-511

[105] Martinez-Anso E, Castillo JE, Diez J, Medina JF, Prieto J. Immunohistochemical detection of chloride/bicarbonate anion exchangers in human liver. Hepatology 1994;19: 1400-6

[106] Banales JM, Arenas F, Rodriguez-Ortigosa CM, Saez E, Uriarte I, Doctor RB, et al. Bicarbonate-rich choleresis induced by secretin in normal rat is taurocholate-dependent and involves AE2 anion exchanger. Hepatology 2006;43: 266-75

[107] Fitz JG, Basavappa S, McGill J, Melhus O, Cohn JA. Regulation of membrane chloride currents in rat bile duct epithelial cells. J Clin Invest 1993;91: 319-28

[108] Cohn JA, Strong TV, Picciotto MR, Nairn AC, Collins FS, Fitz JG. Localization of the cystic fibrosis transmembrane conductance regulator in human bile duct epithelial cells. Gastroenterology 1993;105: 1857-64

[109] Kim D, Steward MC. The role of CFTR in bicarbonate secretion by pancreatic duct and airway epithelia. J Med Invest 2009;56 Suppl: 336-42

[110] Alvaro D, Cho WK, Mennone A, Boyer JL. Effect of secretion on intracellular pH regulation in isolated rat bile duct epithelial cells. J Clin Invest 1993;92: 1314-25

[111] Spirli C, Fabris L, Duner E, Fiorotto R, Ballardini G, Roskams T, et al. Cytokine-stimulated nitric oxide production inhibits adenylyl cyclase and cAMP-dependent secretion in cholangiocytes. Gastroenterology 2003;124: 737-53

[112] McGill JM, Basavappa S, Mangel AW, Shimokura GH, Middleton JP, Fitz JG. Adenosine triphosphate activates ion permeabilities in biliary epithelial cells. Gastroenterology 1994;107: 236-43

[113] Clarke LL, Harline MC, Gawenis LR, Walker NM, Turner JT, Weisman GA. Extracellular UTP stimulates electrogenic bicarbonate secretion across CFTR knockout gallbladder epithelium. Am J Physiol Gastrointest Liver Physiol 2000;279: G132-8

[114] Tietz PS, Marinelli RA, Chen XM, Huang B, Cohn J, Kole J, et al. Agonist-induced coordinated trafficking of functionally related transport proteins for water and ions in cholangiocytes. J Biol Chem 2003;278: 20413-9

[115] Colombo C, Battezzati PM, Crosignani A, Morabito A, Costantini D, Padoan R, et al. Liver disease in cystic fibrosis: A prospective study on incidence, risk factors, and outcome. Hepatology 2002;36: 1374-82

[116] Wilschanski M. Patterns of gastrointestinal disease associated with mutations of CFTR. Curr Gastroenterol Rep 2008;10: 316-23

[117] Lindblad A, Glaumann H, Strandvik B. Natural history of liver disease in cystic fibrosis. Hepatology 1999;30: 1151-8

[118] Moyer K, Balistreri W. Hepatobiliary disease in patients with cystic fibrosis. Curr Opin Gastroenterol 2009;25: 272-8

[119] Herrmann U, Dockter G, Lammert F. Cystic fibrosis-associated liver disease. Best Pract Res Clin Gastroenterol 2010;24: 585-92

[120] Colombo C, S. BP, Motta V, Zazzeron L. Liver disease in cystic fibrosis. In: Blum HE, Cox DW, Haussinger D, Jansen PL, Kullak-Ublick GA, editors. Genetics in liver diseases Proceedings of the Falk Symposium. Dordrecht: Springer; 2007. p. 102-18.

[121] Freudenberg F, Broderick AL, Yu BB, Leonard MR, Glickman JN, Carey MC. Pathophysiological basis of liver disease in cystic fibrosis employing a DeltaF508 mouse model. Am J Physiol Gastrointest Liver Physiol 2008;294: G1411-20

[122] Freudenberg F, Leonard MR, Liu SA, Glickman JN, Carey MC. Pathophysiological preconditions promoting mixed "black" pigment plus cholesterol gallstones in a DeltaF508 mouse model of cystic fibrosis. Am J Physiol Gastrointest Liver Physiol 2010;299: G205-14

[123] Minagawa N, Nagata J, Shibao K, Masyuk AI, Gomes DA, Rodrigues MA, et al. Cyclic AMP regulates bicarbonate secretion in cholangiocytes through release of ATP into bile. Gastroenterology 2007;133: 1592-602

[124] Fiorotto R, Spirli C, Fabris L, Cadamuro M, Okolicsanyi L, Strazzabosco M. Ursodeoxycholic acid stimulates cholangiocyte fluid secretion in mice via CFTR-dependent ATP secretion. Gastroenterology 2007;133: 1603-13

[125] Woo K, Dutta AK, Patel V, Kresge C, Feranchak AP. Fluid flow induces mechanosensitive ATP release, calcium signalling and Cl- transport in biliary epithelial cells through a PKCzeta-dependent pathway. J Physiol 2008;586: 2779-98

[126] Beuers U, Maroni L, Elferink RO. The biliary HCO(3)(-) umbrella: experimental evidence revisited. Curr Opin Gastroenterol 2012;28: 253-7

[127] Hohenester S, Wenniger LM, Paulusma CC, van Vliet SJ, Jefferson DM, Elferink RP, et al. A biliary HCO3- umbrella constitutes a protective mechanism against bile acid-induced injury in human cholangiocytes. Hepatology 2012;55: 173-83

[128] Parolini O, Alviano F, Bagnara GP, Bilic G, Buhring HJ, Evangelista M, et al. Concise review: isolation and characterization of cells from human term placenta: outcome of the first international Workshop on Placenta Derived Stem Cells. Stem Cells 2008;26: 300-11

[129] Evangelista M, Soncini M, Parolini O. Placenta-derived stem cells: new hope for cell therapy? Cytotechnology 2008;58: 33-42

[130] Portmann-Lanz CB, Schoeberlein A, Huber A, Sager R, Malek A, Holzgreve W, et al. Placental mesenchymal stem cells as potential autologous graft for pre- and perinatal neuroregeneration. Am J Obstet Gynecol 2006;194: 664-73

[131] Sakuragawa N, Kakinuma K, Kikuchi A, Okano H, Uchida S, Kamo I, et al. Human amnion mesenchyme cells express phenotypes of neuroglial progenitor cells. J Neurosci Res 2004;78: 208-14

[132] Portmann-Lanz CB, Schoeberlein A, Portmann R, Mohr S, Rollini P, Sager R, et al. Turning placenta into brain: placental mesenchymal stem cells differentiate into neurons and oligodendrocytes. Am J Obstet Gynecol 2010;202: 294 e1- e11

[133] Mohr S, Portmann-Lanz CB, Schoeberlein A, Sager R, Surbek DV. Generation of an osteogenic graft from human placenta and placenta-derived mesenchymal stem cells. Reprod Sci 2010;17: 1006-15

[134] Alviano F, Fossati V, Marchionni C, Arpinati M, Bonsi L, Franchina M, et al. Term Amniotic membrane is a high throughput source for multipotent Mesenchymal Stem

Cells with the ability to differentiate into endothelial cells in vitro. BMC Dev Biol 2007;7: 11

[135] Miki T, Marongiu F, Ellis EC, Dorko K, Mitamura K, Ranade A, et al. Production of hepatocyte-like cells from human amnion. Methods Mol Biol 2009;481: 155-68

[136] Paracchini V, Carbone A, Colombo F, Castellani S, Mazzucchelli S, Di Gioia S, et al. Amniotic mesenchymal stem cells: a new source for hepatocyte-like cells and induction of CFTR expression by coculture with cystic fibrosis airway epithelial cells. J Biomed Biotechnol 2012;2012: 575471

[137] Stadler G, Hennerbichler S, Lindenmair A, Peterbauer A, Hofer K, van Griensven M, et al. Phenotypic shift of human amniotic epithelial cells in culture is associated with reduced osteogenic differentiation in vitro. Cytotherapy 2008;10: 743-52

[138] Bilic G, Zeisberger SM, Mallik AS, Zimmermann R, Zisch AH. Comparative characterization of cultured human term amnion epithelial and mesenchymal stromal cells for application in cell therapy. Cell Transplant 2008;17: 955-68

[139] Wolbank S, Stadler G, Peterbauer A, Gillich A, Karbiener M, Streubel B, et al. Telomerase immortalized human amnion- and adipose-derived mesenchymal stem cells: maintenance of differentiation and immunomodulatory characteristics. Tissue Eng Part A 2009;15: 1843-54

[140] Vogel JP, Szalay K, Geiger F, Kramer M, Richter W, Kasten P. Platelet-rich plasma improves expansion of human mesenchymal stem cells and retains differentiation capacity and in vivo bone formation in calcium phosphate ceramics. Platelets 2006;17: 462-9

[141] Lange C, Cakiroglu F, Spiess AN, Cappallo-Obermann H, Dierlamm J, Zander AR. Accelerated and safe expansion of human mesenchymal stromal cells in animal serum-free medium for transplantation and regenerative medicine. J Cell Physiol 2007;213: 18-26

[142] Barlow S, Brooke G, Chatterjee K, Price G, Pelekanos R, Rossetti T, et al. Comparison of human placenta- and bone marrow-derived multipotent mesenchymal stem cells. Stem Cells Dev 2008;17: 1095-107

[143] Brooke G, Tong H, Levesque JP, Atkinson K. Molecular trafficking mechanisms of multipotent mesenchymal stem cells derived from human bone marrow and placenta. Stem Cells Dev 2008;17: 929-40

[144] Brooke G, Rossetti T, Pelekanos R, Ilic N, Murray P, Hancock S, et al. Manufacturing of human placenta-derived mesenchymal stem cells for clinical trials. Br J Haematol 2009;144: 571-9

[145] Chang CJ, Yen ML, Chen YC, Chien CC, Huang HI, Bai CH, et al. Placenta-derived multipotent cells exhibit immunosuppressive properties that are enhanced in the presence of interferon-gamma. Stem Cells 2006;24: 2466-77

[146] Miki T. Amnion-derived stem cells: in quest of clinical applications. Stem Cell Res Ther 2011;2: 25

[147] Parolini O, Alviano F, Bergwerf I, Boraschi D, De Bari C, De Waele P, et al. Toward cell therapy using placenta-derived cells: disease mechanisms, cell biology, preclinical studies, and regulatory aspects at the round table. Stem Cells Dev 2010;19: 143-54

[148] Manuelpillai U, Moodley Y, Borlongan CV, Parolini O. Amniotic membrane and amniotic cells: potential therapeutic tools to combat tissue inflammation and fibrosis? Placenta 2011;32 Suppl 4: S320-5

[149] Li C, Zhang W, Jiang X, Mao N. Human-placenta-derived mesenchymal stem cells inhibit proliferation and function of allogeneic immune cells. Cell Tissue Res 2007;330: 437-46

[150] Wolbank S, Peterbauer A, Fahrner M, Hennerbichler S, van Griensven M, Stadler G, et al. Dose-dependent immunomodulatory effect of human stem cells from amniotic membrane: a comparison with human mesenchymal stem cells from adipose tissue. Tissue Eng 2007;13: 1173-83

[151] Magatti M, De Munari S, Vertua E, Gibelli L, Wengler GS, Parolini O. Human amnion mesenchyme harbors cells with allogeneic T-cell suppression and stimulation capabilities. Stem Cells 2008;26: 182-92

[152] Bailo M, Soncini M, Vertua E, Signoroni PB, Sanzone S, Lombardi G, et al. Engraftment potential of human amnion and chorion cells derived from term placenta. Transplantation 2004;78: 1439-48

[153] Banas A, Teratani T, Yamamoto Y, Tokuhara M, Takeshita F, Osaki M, et al. IFATS collection: in vivo therapeutic potential of human adipose tissue mesenchymal stem cells after transplantation into mice with liver injury. Stem Cells 2008;26: 2705-12

[154] Jones BJ, McTaggart SJ. Immunosuppression by mesenchymal stromal cells: from culture to clinic. Exp Hematol 2008;36: 733-41

[155] Roelen DL, van der Mast BJ, in't Anker PS, Kleijburg C, Eikmans M, van Beelen E, et al. Differential immunomodulatory effects of fetal versus maternal multipotent stromal cells. Hum Immunol 2009;70: 16-23

[156] Magatti M, De Munari S, Vertua E, Nassauto C, Albertini A, Wengler GS, et al. Amniotic mesenchymal tissue cells inhibit dendritic cell differentiation of peripheral blood and amnion resident monocytes. Cell Transplant 2009;18: 899-914

[157] Nauta AJ, Kruisselbrink AB, Lurvink E, Willemze R, Fibbe WE. Mesenchymal stem cells inhibit generation and function of both CD34+-derived and monocyte-derived dendritic cells. J Immunol 2006;177: 2080-7

[158] Wang M, Yoshida A, Kawashima H, Ishizaki M, Takahashi H, Hori J. Immunogenicity and antigenicity of allogeneic amniotic epithelial transplants grafted to the cornea, conjunctiva, and anterior chamber. Invest Ophthalmol Vis Sci 2006;47: 1522-32

[159] Kubo M, Sonoda Y, Muramatsu R, Usui M. Immunogenicity of human amniotic membrane in experimental xenotransplantation. Invest Ophthalmol Vis Sci 2001;42: 1539-46

[160] Dua HS, Azuara-Blanco A. Amniotic membrane transplantation. Br J Ophthalmol 1999;83: 748-52

[161] Faulk WP, Matthews R, Stevens PJ, Bennett JP, Burgos H, Hsi BL. Human amnion as an adjunct in wound healing. Lancet 1980;1: 1156-8

[162] Bennett JP, Matthews R, Faulk WP. Treatment of chronic ulceration of the legs with human amnion. Lancet 1980;1: 1153-6

[163] Kesting MR, Wolff KD, Hohlweg-Majert B, Steinstraesser L. The role of allogenic amniotic membrane in burn treatment. J Burn Care Res 2008;29: 907-16

[164] Fernandes M, Sridhar MS, Sangwan VS, Rao GN. Amniotic membrane transplantation for ocular surface reconstruction. Cornea 2005;24: 643-53

[165] Kong XY, Cai Z, Pan L, Zhang L, Shu J, Dong YL, et al. Transplantation of human amniotic cells exerts neuroprotection in MPTP-induced Parkinson disease mice. Brain Res 2008;1205: 108-15

[166] Bankiewicz KS, Palmatier M, Plunkett RJ, Cummins A, Oldfield EH. Reversal of hemiparkinsonian syndrome in nonhuman primates by amnion implantation into caudate nucleus. J Neurosurg 1994;81: 869-76

[167] Kakishita K, Nakao N, Sakuragawa N, Itakura T. Implantation of human amniotic epithelial cells prevents the degeneration of nigral dopamine neurons in rats with 6-hydroxydopamine lesions. Brain Res 2003;980: 48-56

[168] Wu ZY, Hui GZ, Lu Y, Wu X, Guo LH. Transplantation of human amniotic epithelial cells improves hindlimb function in rats with spinal cord injury. Chin Med J (Engl) 2006;119: 2101-7

[169] Prather WR, Toren A, Meiron M, Ofir R, Tschope C, Horwitz EM. The role of placental-derived adherent stromal cell (PLX-PAD) in the treatment of critical limb ischemia. Cytotherapy 2009;11: 427-34

[170] Lanzoni G, Alviano F, Marchionni C, Bonsi L, Costa R, Foroni L, et al. Isolation of stem cell populations with trophic and immunoregulatory functions from human intestinal tissues: potential for cell therapy in inflammatory bowel disease. Cytotherapy 2009;11: 1020-31

[171] Ventura C, Cantoni S, Bianchi F, Lionetti V, Cavallini C, Scarlata I, et al. Hyaluronan mixed esters of butyric and retinoic Acid drive cardiac and endothelial fate in term

placenta human mesenchymal stem cells and enhance cardiac repair in infarcted rat hearts. J Biol Chem 2007;282: 14243-52

[172] Cargnoni A, Gibelli L, Tosini A, Signoroni PB, Nassuato C, Arienti D, et al. Transplantation of allogeneic and xenogeneic placenta-derived cells reduces bleomycin-induced lung fibrosis. Cell Transplant 2009;18: 405-22

[173] Kinder BW, Brown KK, Schwarz MI, Ix JH, Kervitsky A, King TE, Jr. Baseline BAL neutrophilia predicts early mortality in idiopathic pulmonary fibrosis. Chest 2008;133: 226-32

[174] Cargnoni A, Ressel L, Rossi D, Poli A, Arienti D, Lombardi G, et al. Conditioned medium from amniotic mesenchymal tissue cells reduces progression of bleomycin-induced lung fibrosis. Cytotherapy 2012;14: 153-61

[175] Timmers L, Lim SK, Arslan F, Armstrong JS, Hoefer IE, Doevendans PA, et al. Reduction of myocardial infarct size by human mesenchymal stem cell conditioned medium. Stem Cell Res 2007;1: 129-37

[176] van Poll D, Parekkadan B, Cho CH, Berthiaume F, Nahmias Y, Tilles AW, et al. Mesenchymal stem cell-derived molecules directly modulate hepatocellular death and regeneration in vitro and in vivo. Hepatology 2008;47: 1634-43

[177] Gharaee-Kermani M, Gyetko MR, Hu B, Phan SH. New insights into the pathogenesis and treatment of idiopathic pulmonary fibrosis: a potential role for stem cells in the lung parenchyma and implications for therapy. Pharm Res 2007;24: 819-41

[178] Wang G, Bunnell BA, Painter RG, Quiniones BC, Tom S, Lanson NA, Jr., et al. Adult stem cells from bone marrow stroma differentiate into airway epithelial cells: potential therapy for cystic fibrosis. Proc Natl Acad Sci U S A 2005;102: 186-91

[179] Farmen SL, Karp PH, Ng P, Palmer DJ, Koehler DR, Hu J, et al. Gene transfer of CFTR to airway epithelia: low levels of expression are sufficient to correct Cl- transport and overexpression can generate basolateral CFTR. Am J Physiol Lung Cell Mol Physiol 2005;289: L1123-30

[180] Mo XT, Guo SC, Xie HQ, Deng L, Zhi W, Xiang Z, et al. Variations in the ratios of co-cultured mesenchymal stem cells and chondrocytes regulate the expression of cartilaginous and osseous phenotype in alginate constructs. Bone 2009;45: 42-51

[181] Bian L, Zhai DY, Mauck RL, Burdick JA. Coculture of human mesenchymal stem cells and articular chondrocytes reduces hypertrophy and enhances functional properties of engineered cartilage. Tissue Eng Part A 2011;17: 1137-45

[182] Badri L, Walker NM, Ohtsuka T, Wang Z, Delmar M, Flint A, et al. Epithelial Interactions and Local Engraftment of Lung-resident Mesenchymal Stem Cells. Am J Respir Cell Mol Biol 2011:

[183] Takashima S, Ise H, Zhao P, Akaike T, Nikaido T. Human amniotic epithelial cells possess hepatocyte-like characteristics and functions. Cell Struct Funct 2004;29: 73-84

[184] Sakuragawa N, Enosawa S, Ishii T, Thangavel R, Tashiro T, Okuyama T, et al. Human amniotic epithelial cells are promising transgene carriers for allogeneic cell transplantation into liver. J Hum Genet 2000;45: 171-6

[185] Marongiu F, Gramignoli R, Dorko K, Miki T, Ranade AR, Paola Serra M, et al. Hepatic differentiation of amniotic epithelial cells. Hepatology 2011;53: 1719-29

[186] Puglisi MA, Tesori V, Lattanzi W, Piscaglia AC, Gasbarrini GB, D'Ugo DM, et al. Therapeutic implications of mesenchymal stem cells in liver injury. J Biomed Biotechnol 2011;2011: 860578

[187] Cao H, Yang J, Yu J, Pan Q, Li J, Zhou P, et al. Therapeutic potential of transplanted placental mesenchymal stem cells in treating Chinese miniature pigs with acute liver failure. BMC Med 2012;10: 56

[188] Takami T, Terai S, Sakaida I. Stem cell therapy in chronic liver disease. Curr Opin Gastroenterol 2012;28: 203-8

[189] Kuo TK, Hung SP, Chuang CH, Chen CT, Shih YR, Fang SC, et al. Stem cell therapy for liver disease: parameters governing the success of using bone marrow mesenchymal stem cells. Gastroenterology 2008;134: 2111-21, 21 e1-3

[190] di Bonzo LV, Ferrero I, Cravanzola C, Mareschi K, Rustichell D, Novo E, et al. Human mesenchymal stem cells as a two-edged sword in hepatic regenerative medicine: engraftment and hepatocyte differentiation versus profibrogenic potential. Gut 2008;57: 223-31

[191] Zhou P, Hohm S, Olusanya Y, Hess DA, Nolta J. Human progenitor cells with high aldehyde dehydrogenase activity efficiently engraft into damaged liver in a novel model. Hepatology 2009;49: 1992-2000

[192] Parekkadan B, van Poll D, Megeed Z, Kobayashi N, Tilles AW, Berthiaume F, et al. Immunomodulation of activated hepatic stellate cells by mesenchymal stem cells. Biochem Biophys Res Commun 2007;363: 247-52

[193] Zhao DC, Lei JX, Chen R, Yu WH, Zhang XM, Li SN, et al. Bone marrow-derived mesenchymal stem cells protect against experimental liver fibrosis in rats. World J Gastroenterol 2005;11: 3431-40

[194] Abdel Aziz MT, Atta HM, Mahfouz S, Fouad HH, Roshdy NK, Ahmed HH, et al. Therapeutic potential of bone marrow-derived mesenchymal stem cells on experimental liver fibrosis. Clin Biochem 2007;40: 893-9

[195] Li C, Kong Y, Wang H, Wang S, Yu H, Liu X, et al. Homing of bone marrow mesenchymal stem cells mediated by sphingosine 1-phosphate contributes to liver fibrosis. J Hepatol 2009;50: 1174-83

[196] Chang YJ, Liu JW, Lin PC, Sun LY, Peng CW, Luo GH, et al. Mesenchymal stem cells facilitate recovery from chemically induced liver damage and decrease liver fibrosis. Life Sci 2009;85: 517-25

[197] Sakaida I, Terai S, Yamamoto N, Aoyama K, Ishikawa T, Nishina H, et al. Transplantation of bone marrow cells reduces CCl4-induced liver fibrosis in mice. Hepatology 2004;40: 1304-11

[198] Higashiyama R, Inagaki Y, Hong YY, Kushida M, Nakao S, Niioka M, et al. Bone marrow-derived cells express matrix metalloproteinases and contribute to regression of liver fibrosis in mice. Hepatology 2007;45: 213-22

[199] Pulavendran S, Vignesh J, Rose C. Differential anti-inflammatory and anti-fibrotic activity of transplanted mesenchymal vs. hematopoietic stem cells in carbon tetrachloride-induced liver injury in mice. Int Immunopharmacol 2010;10: 513-9

[200] Xu R, Harrison PM, Chen M, Li L, Tsui TY, Fung PC, et al. Cytoglobin overexpression protects against damage-induced fibrosis. Mol Ther 2006;13: 1093-100

[201] Zhao W, Li JJ, Cao DY, Li X, Zhang LY, He Y, et al. Intravenous injection of mesenchymal stem cells is effective in treating liver fibrosis. World J Gastroenterol 2012;18: 1048-58

[202] Zheng WD, Zhang LJ, Shi MN, Chen ZX, Chen YX, Huang YH, et al. Expression of matrix metalloproteinase-2 and tissue inhibitor of metalloproteinase-1 in hepatic stellate cells during rat hepatic fibrosis and its intervention by IL-10. World J Gastroenterol 2005;11: 1753-8

[203] Zhang LJ, Yu JP, Li D, Huang YH, Chen ZX, Wang XZ. Effects of cytokines on carbon tetrachloride-induced hepatic fibrogenesis in rats. World J Gastroenterol 2004;10: 77-81

[204] Zhang D, Jiang M, Miao D. Transplanted human amniotic membrane-derived mesenchymal stem cells ameliorate carbon tetrachloride-induced liver cirrhosis in mouse. PLoS One 2011;6: e16789

[205] Sant'Anna LB, Cargnoni A, Ressel L, Vanosi G, Parolini O. Amniotic membrane application reduces liver fibrosis in a bile duct ligation rat model. Cell Transplant 2011;20: 441-53

[206] Griesenbach U, Alton EWFW. Cystic fibrosis gene therapy: successes, failures and hopes for the future. Exp Rev Resp Med 2009;3: 363-71

[207] Conese M, Ascenzioni F, Boyd AC, Coutelle C, De Fino I, De Smedt S, et al. Gene and cell therapy for cystic fibrosis: from bench to bedside. J Cyst Fibros 2011;10 Suppl 2: S114-28

[208] Sueblinvong V, Weiss DJ. Stem cells and cell therapy approaches in lung biology and diseases. Transl Res 2010;156: 188-205

[209] Bruscia EM, Price JE, Cheng E-C, Weiner S, Caputo C, Ferreira EC, et al. Assessment of cystic fibrosis transmembrane conductance regulator (CFTR) activity in CFTR-null mice after bone marrow transplantation. Proc Natl Acad Sci U S A 2006;103: 2965-70

[210] Kotton DN. Next-generation regeneration: the hope and hype of lung stem cell research. Am J Respir Crit Care Med 2012;185: 1255-60

[211] Wetsel RA, Wang D, Calame DG. Therapeutic potential of lung epithelial progenitor cells derived from embryonic and induced pluripotent stem cells. Annu Rev Med 2011;62: 95-105

[212] Laurson J, Selden C, Hodgson HJ. Hepatocyte progenitors in man and in rodents--multiple pathways, multiple candidates. Int J Exp Pathol 2005;86: 1-18

[213] Alison MR, Islam S, Lim S. Stem cells in liver regeneration, fibrosis and cancer: the good, the bad and the ugly. J Pathol 2009;217: 282-98

[214] Dai LJ, Li HY, Guan LX, Ritchie G, Zhou JX. The therapeutic potential of bone marrow-derived mesenchymal stem cells on hepatic cirrhosis. Stem Cell Res 2009;2: 16-25

[215] Lin H, Xu R, Zhang Z, Chen L, Shi M, Wang FS. Implications of the immunoregulatory functions of mesenchymal stem cells in the treatment of human liver diseases. Cell Mol Immunol 2011;8: 19-22

Isolation of Bone Marrow Stromal Cells: Cellular Composition is Technique-Dependent

Hideki Agata

Additional information is available at the end of the chapter

1. Introduction

Bone marrow contains a colony-forming, fibroblast-like cell population called bone marrow mesenchymal stem cells or bone marrow stromal cells (BMSCs) [1, 2]. Since BMSCs are capable of differentiating into multiple lineages (osteogenic, chondrogenic, adipogenic, neurogenic, and myogenic lineages), they have attracted significant interest as useful somatic stem cells for use in tissue engineering and regenerative medicine [3 - 7]. As BMSCs adhere to tissue culture-treated plastic, they are usually isolated by adherent cultivation of untreated whole bone marrow [8 - 10]. However, this technique may be inefficient for the isolation of BMSCs because untreated bone marrow contains a large proportion of erythrocytes and their presence may interfere with the initial adherence of BMSCs. The removal of unwanted high density blood cells by density gradient centrifugation increases the number of colony-forming units (CFUs) in primary BMSC culture [11]. Removal of erythrocytes by hemolysis treatment is also effective at increasing the number of CFUs [12]. However, recent studies have shown that BMSCs isolated by these techniques are different from those isolated by adherent culture techniques [13]. Since BMSCs consist of a heterogeneous mixture of cells with varying potentials at different stages of differentiation, the characteristics of the cultured cells depend on the initial composition of the cell population [14, 15]. Therefore, the final cellular composition of BMSCs will vary significantly with the isolation technique used. Few studies have focused on the importance of the initial cellular composition of isolated BMSCs. In this chapter, possible differences in the cellular composition of BMSCs isolated from untreated, hemolysed, or density gradient fractionated bone marrow will be discussed. Furthermore, the optimal technique for the isolation of BMSCs for use in tissue engineering and regenerative medicine will be discussed from a clinical point of view.

2. Bone marrow stromal cells

BMSCs are a plastic-adherent, non-hematopoietic cell population residing in the bone marrow [16]. As BMSCs are morphologically similar to skin fibroblasts and can be expanded in a culture medium for fibroblasts, they were initially described as stromal fibroblasts [17], though their differentiation potentials are far different from those of skin fibroblasts [18]. While skin fibroblasts are incapable of differentiating into other cell types, BMSCs are capable of differentiating into cells of multiple mesenchymal tissues such as bone, cartilage, fat, tendon, muscle, and marrow stroma [19]. To emphasize this property, BMSCs are also called mesenchymal stem cells or multipotent mesenchymal stromal cells [20], though they can also differentiate into non-mesenchymal (non-mesodermal) cell types such as neurons [21] and insulin-producing cells [22]. Although BMSCs do not possess totipotencies like embryonic stem cells (ESCs) or induced pluripotent stem cells (iPSCs), they are clinically more useful than these totipotent stem cells because they can be easily isolated from a small volume of bone marrow aspirate and do not require gene transfections to demonstrate their differentiation abilities [23]. Thus, BMSCs have attracted significant interest as potent stem cells for use in tissue engineering and regenerative medicine of various tissues. In fact, clinical studies have shown that BMSCs are useful for the treatment of bone, cartilage, heart, and the central nervous system [24-27]. In addition, BMSCs recently attracted attention as immuno-modulatory cells useful for the treatment of immue diseases such as graft versus host disease (GVHD) [28, 29]. Therefore, clinical use of BMSCs should increase over the next few years.

3. Animal-derived BMSC as a model of human BMSC

BMSCs are present in the bone marrow of humans as well as other animals such as mice, rats, rabbits, dogs, pigs, sheeps, horses, and cows [4, 8, 30 - 35]. As BMSCs seem to be postnatal stem cells that are common among mammalian species, these animals have been used to investigate the origin and *in vivo* functions of BMSCs [36, 37]. In addition, these animal-derived BMSCs are considered useful as a models of human BMSCs because it is not always easy to recruit a sufficient number of human BMSC donors for experimental use. Furthermore, more reliable results can be obtained by using animal-derived BMSCs because experimental animals have uniform genetic backgrounds and are housed under controlled conditions, eliminating behavioral and environmental variations that could influence BMSC properties. In fact, several studies have reported that the characteristics of human BMSCs varied significantly among donors [15, 38, 39], while such variations are not observed in animal-derived BMSCs. Therefore, animal-derived BMSCs are considered to be useful alternatives to human BMSCs for laboratory experimentation. However, it remains unknown which animal's BMSCs offer the best model system to represent human BMSCs. In general, donor animals of BMSCs are chosen based on their costs and availabilities. However, it has been shown that there are a number of characteristic differences in the BMSCs among species [40]. Therefore, it is important to consider species difference in addition to the costs and availabilities when selecting model systems for human BMSCs.

Considering their costs and availabilities, mice are more attractive candidates than other laboratory animals. However, rat BMSCs are used as a model of human BMSCs in our laboratory because mouse BMSC characteristics differ from those of human BMSCs. For example, mouse BMSCs need the support of feeder cells for their stable growth, while human BMSCs are able to grow in a feeder cell-independent manner [40]. Responses to differentiation stimuli are also different. While human BMSCs are readily induced to differentiate into the osteogenic lineage by dexamethasone, mouse BMSCs are less responsive to dexthamethasone treatment [41]. Although the reasons why mouse BMSCs differ from human BMSCs remain unknown, it has been suggested that mouse BMSCs are very rare in the bone marrow and need support by other cells for their growth and differentiation [40]. On the contrary, rat BMSCs can be easily isolated from bone marrow and they are able to grow without feeder cells, as do human BMSCs [13]. In addition, rat BMSCs are able to differentiate into multiple lineages under induction protocols used for human BMSCs [42]. Therefore, we believe that rat BMSCs offer a more appropriate model of human BMSCs, though fewer reagents and antibodies are available for rat cells than for mouse cells.

4. Isolation of BMSCs

Since BMSCs form adherent colonies in plastic culture vessels, BMSCs are generally obtained from adherent cultures of untreated whole bone marrow [2 - 4]. However, it has been suggested that this technique is inefficient for the isolation of BMSCs because untreated bone marrow contains a large proportion of erythrocytes and their presence may interfere with the initial colony formation of BMSCs [11 - 13]. As human BMSCs are a rare population in the bone marrow (0.01 - 0.1% of whole marrow), it is possible that the efficacy of initial colony formation directly affects the total yield of BMSCs. Inefficient colony formation may also lead to the reduced potentials of BMSCs because previous studies have shown that BMSCs lose their differentiation abilities depending on the duration of *ex vivo* culture [39]. Accordingly, it is important to investigate whether BMSCs can be more efficiently isolated by the removal of unwanted cells. Both density gradient centrifugation and hemolysis (red blood cell lysis) treatment remove erythrocytes for the efficient isolation of the mononuclear cell fraction of bone marrow. Although both these techniques were originally developed for the isolation of white blood cells such as lymphocytes, they can also be used for the isolation of BMSCs because they are contained within the mononuclear cell fraction. In fact, several studies have used either or both of these techniques for the isolation of BMSCs; they reported that BMSCs were more efficiently isolated by these techniques (Table 1) [12, 32, 34, 43].

However, it remains unknown whether BMSCs isolated by these techniques are identical to those isolated from untreated whole bone marrow because BMSCs are composed of hetero-geneous cells with varying growth and differentiation potentials [15]. Thus, the cellular composition of BMSC populations could be dependent upon the isolation technique. Although it remains unknown how many different types of cells constitute the BMSC fraction, at least committed osteogenic cells as well as uncommitted stem cells are present when BMSCs are

Target cells	Compared isolation techniques	The most efficient isolation technique	Reference
Human BMSCs	• Hemolysis (red blood cell lysis) • Density gradient centrifugation • Adherent culture of whole bone marrow	Hemolysis	[12] Horn et al., 2008.
Pig BMSCs	• Hemolysis • Dextran sedimentation • Density gradient centrifugation	Hemolysis	[32] Peterbauer-Scherb et al., 2010
Rat BMSCs	• Density gradient centrifugation • Adherent culture of whole bone marrow	Density gradient centrifugation	[43] Polisetti et al., 2010
Equine BMSCs	• Density gradient centrifugation • Adherent culture of whole bone marrow	Density gradient centrifugation	[34] Bourzac et al., 2010

Table 1. Removal of erythrocytes by hemolysis or density gradient centrifugation may enable the efficient isolation of BMSCs.

isolated from untreated whole bone marrow [44]. Changes in the relative sizes of these two cell populations greatly influence the characteristics of BMSCs. In other words, a greater number of committed osteogenic cells makes the BMSC fraction more osteogenic, while a greater number of uncommitted stem cells makes them more stem-cell like. Thus, we investigated differences in the cellular composition of BMSCs isolated from untreated, density-gradient-centrifuged, and hemolysed bone marrow, with a special reference to committed osteogenic cells and uncommitted stem cells. For these experiments, rat bone marrow was used instead of human bone marrow to avoid the influence of variations among donors.

5. The number of committed osteogenic cells contained in BMSCs varies with the isolation technique

Committed osteogenic cells can be defined as a cell population that is capable of forming bone without osteogenic induction. Because of the presence of this cell population, *in vivo* transplantation of untreated whole bone marrow to ectopic sites usually results in the formation of new bone [45]. If this cell population is decreased or lost by the hemolysis or density gradient centrifugation steps, new bone formation may not be observed in the transplants. On the contrary, if this cell population is enriched by these techniques, more significant bone formation should be observed. Therefore, we investigated the *in vivo* bone-forming ability of three populations: marrow that was untreated, marrow that was hemolysed with ammonium chloride, and marrow that was fractionated by density-gradient-centrifugation over Ficoll® (Ficoll-treated). As shown in Figure 1A, the percentage of bone-forming transplants (transplants containing ectopic bone/ total transplants) was the lowest in the Ficoll-treated group. The amount of new bone formation, which was scored on a semi-quantitative scale from zero to three (Table 2), was also lowest in the Ficoll-treated group (Figure 1B). The hemolysed group also showed less bone-forming ability than did the untreated group, though its ability was still greater than that of the Ficoll-treated group (Figure 1 A and 1B).

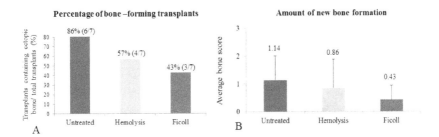

Figure 1. *In vivo* bone-forming ability of untreated, hemolysed, or Ficoll-treated bone marrow. (A) The percentage of bone-forming transplants (transplants containing ectopic bone/ total transplants), which was calculated from the results of seven independent experiments, was greatest in the untreated group, followed by the hemolyzed group, and lowest in the Ficoll-treated group. (B) The amount of new bone formation (total bone score/ total transplants) was greatest in the hemolyzed group, followed by the untreated group, and lowest in the Ficoll-treated group (n = 7). (Modified from Agata et al., 2012 [13] with permission)

	Bone score (Percentage of new bone area in the transplant)
0	No bone evident
1	Bone area < 5%
2	5% < Bone area < 10%
3	Bone area > 10%

Table 2. Bone score of each sample was determined from the percentage of the area containing bone (new bone area/ total area) (Modified from Agata et al., 2012 [13] with permission)

As these results showed that Ficoll-treated bone marrow contains fewer committed osteogenic cells than either untreated or hemolysed bone marrow, we next investigated whether BMSCs isolated from Ficoll-treated bone marrow actually contains lower numbers of committed osteogenic cells. Untreated, hemolysed, or Ficoll-treated rat bone marrow was plated on cell culture dishes, and adherent colony-forming cells were expanded as BMSCs. Although these BMSCs did not show significant differences in their morphology or their expression of cell-surface CD54 and CD90 (Figure 2), they showed a significant difference in the expression of cell-surface alkaline phosphatase (ALP) (Figure 3A). The difference in ALP expression was also confirmed by quantitative ALP assays (Figure 3B).

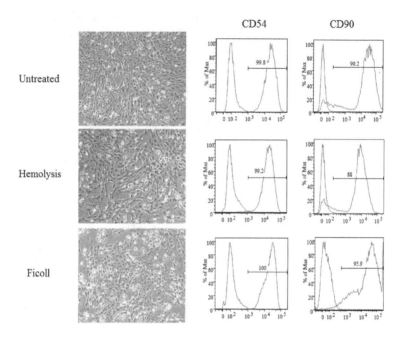

Figure 2. Morphology and expression of cell surface CD54 and CD90 of BMSCs that were isolated from untreated, hemolysed, or Ficoll-treated bone marrows. (Modified from Agata et al., 2012 [13] with permission)

Since these BMSCs were simply cultured in non-induction medium, the expression of cell surface ALP directly indicates the number of committed osteogenic cells contained in each BMSC. Therefore, it can be concluded that BMSCs isolated from Ficoll-treated bone marrow contain lower numbers of committed osteogenic cells than those isolated from untreated or hemolysed bone marrow.

6. The number of uncommitted stem cells contained in BMSCs also varies with the isolation technique

Although it remains unknown whether BMSCs contain committed progenitors of other lineages, their multi-lineage differentiation potentials are mainly attributed to the presence of uncommitted stem cells among heterogeneous BMSC populations. Therefore, it is important to investigate whether the number of uncommitted stem cells contained in BMSCs varies with the isolation techniques. Note, however, that it is difficult to calculate their numbers accurately because no specific markers for uncommitted stem cells are currently available. However, the abundance of these cells in BMSCs populations can be determined by analyzing the responsiveness to differentiation-inducing media (induction media), since uncommitted stem cells are highly responsive to differentiation stimuli. Thus, BMSCs that are rich in these cells show

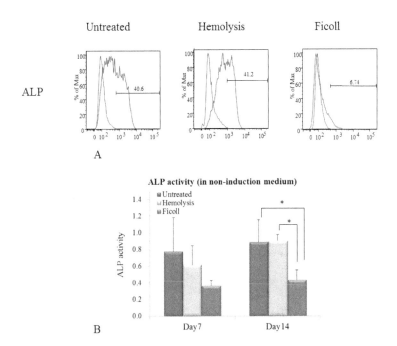

Figure 3. Differences among committed osteogenic cell populations from BMSCs isolated without treatment, or after hemolysis, or Ficoll separation. (A) The expression of cell surface alkaline phosphatase (ALP) of non-induced BMSCs was greatest in the untreated group, followed by the hemolyzed group, and lowest in the Ficoll-treated group. (B) Quantitative ALP assays confirmed the lowest ALP activity in the Ficoll-treated group. Data are presented as the means ± standard deviation (n = 3). *: P < 0.05. (Modified from Agata et al., 2012 [13] with permission).

great responsiveness when culture medium is changed from non-induction medium to induction medium. Accordingly, we investigated BMSCs isolated from untreated, hemolysed, or Ficoll-treated bone marrow for their responses to osteogenic induction medium. As shown in Figure 4A, the Ficoll-treated group showed the lowest ALP activity on day seven. However, this group significantly upregulated ALP activity and showed the greatest activity after 14 days of culture in osteogenic medium, though the difference did not reach a statistically significant level.

Since the Ficoll-treated group constantly showed the lowest ALP activity when cultured in non-induction medium (Figure 3B), the ratio of ALP upregulation (ALP activity in osteogenic induction medium/ ALP activity in non-induction medium) was also the greatest in this group. Gene expression analyses of osteopontin and core-binding factor subunit alpha-1 (*Cbfa1*), both of which are indicators of osteogenic differentiation, also showed the greatest responsiveness in the Ficoll-treated group (Figure 3B - 3E). These results indicate that BMSCs isolated from Ficoll-treated bone marrow contain greater numbers or higher concentrations of uncommitted stem cells than those isolated from untreated or hemolysed bone marrow.

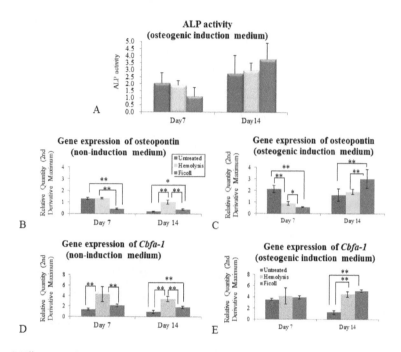

Figure 4. Differences in the responses to osteogenic induction medium among BMSCs isolated from untreated, hemo-lysed, or Ficoll-treated bone marrow. (A) ALP activities in osteogenic induction medium. (B) Gene expression of osteo-pontin in non-induction medium. (C) Gene expression of osteopontin in osteogenic induction medium. (D) Gene expression of *Cbfa-1* in non-induction medium. (E) Gene expression of *Cbfa-1* in osteogenic induction medium. Data are presented as the means ± standard deviation (n = 3). *: $P < 0.05$, **: $P < 0.01$. (Modified from Agata et al., 2012 [13] with permission)

7. Potential merits of hemolysis treatment or density gradient centrifugation of bone marrow to isolate BMSCs

Although hemolysis treatment of bone marrow with ammonium chloride primarily removes only erythrocytes from bone marrow, *in vivo* transplantation experiments indicated that some of the committed osteogenic cells contained in bone marrow are lost or damaged during the hemolysis treatment (Figure 1A and 1B). Thus, we hypothesized that BMSCs grown from hemolysed bone marrow might contain lower numbers of committed osteogenic cells and their cellular composition would differ from that of normal BMSCs (BMSCs grown from untreated bone marrow). However, contrary to the hypothesis, flow cytometric analyses revealed that these BMSCs contained equivalent numbers of committed osteogenic cells (Figure 3A). Since these BMSCs showed similar responses to osteogenic induction medium (Figure 4A), they seem to contain similar numbers of uncommitted stem cells as well. Therefore, it is likely that the cellular composition of BMSCs grown from hemolysed bone marrow is relatively close to that of normal BMSCs. As the cell yield in primary culture (harvested cell number after primary culture/ days of primary culture/ initially seeded cell number) was greater in the hemolysis group (0.52 in the hemolysed group and 0.44 in the untreated group), it can be concluded that hemolysis treatment of bone marrow is an efficient approach to the isolation of BMSCs.

After centrifugation over Ficoll®, bone marrow is separated into several fractions such as plasma, mononuclear cells, granulocytes, and erythrocytes. Since BMSCs belong to the mononuclear cell fraction in the bone marrow, it is likely that BMSCs are efficiently enriched in this fraction even though this isolate contains significantly lower cell numbers than untreated or hemolysed bone marrow (Figure 5).

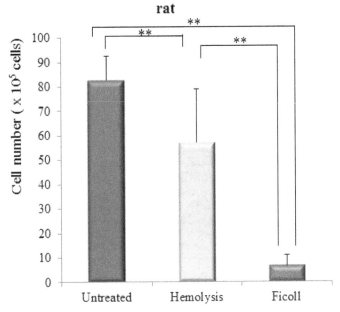

Figure 5. Rat bone marrow was divided into three portions and the suspensions were either hemolyzed, or subjected to Ficoll fractionation, or left without treatment (untreated). Significant differences were observed in the average numbers of cells isolated among the groups. Data are presented as the mean ± standard deviation (n=6). **: p < 0.01 (Modified from Agata et al., 2012 [13] with permission).

However, in contrast to expectations, the cell yield in primary culture was the lowest in this group (0.13 in the Ficoll-treated group). In addition, the cellular composition of this group's BMSCs seemed to be different from that of normal BMSCs, because these BMSCs showed significant differences in the percentage of cell-surface ALP-positive cells and the responses to osteogenic induction medium (Figure 3A and 4A), though they showed similarities in the morphologies and the expression of cell-surface CD54 and CD90 (Figure 2). Therefore, it can be concluded that density gradient centrifugation of bone marrow is not an efficient approach to the isolation of BMSCs that possess normal characteristics. However, this technique may be useful for the isolation of more potent (more primitive) BMSCs because BMSCs grown from Ficoll-treated bone marrow seem to contain greater numbers or higher concentrations of uncommitted stem cells.

8. Conclusion

As the cellular composition of BMSCs varies significantly with the isolation technique, it is important to select an appropriate isolation technique for the purpose that is intended. For example, if BMSCs are used for bone tissue engineering, it might be better to isolate BMSCs by hemolysis, because BMSCs that contain greater numbers of committed osteogenic cells are efficiently obtained by this technique. On the contrary, if BMSCs are used for the stem cell therapies of non-bone diseases such as stroke, it might be better to isolate BMSCs by density gradient centrifugation, because BMSCs obtained by this technique contain greater numbers of uncommitted stem cells. Flow cytometric or magnetic cell sorting with antibodies might also be useful for the isolation of BMSCs for use in stem cell therapies because BMSCs isolated by this technique possess greater multi-lineage potency. However, most of the current clinical studies still use the conventional adherence technique for the isolation of BMSCs because the fact that the characteristics of BMSCs varies with the isolation techniques remains largely unknown. Since the results of clinical studies are greatly affected by the potentials of the BMSCs used, selection of an appropriate isolation technique may lead to a better outcome. Nonetheless, further investigations are required to use these new techniques in clinical studies because available information concerning the safety, feasibility, and efficacy of these techniques is still limited. Furthermore, the cost effectiveness of these techniques should be investigated, since the conventional technique does not require any special reagents. Continuing investigations are important for the establishment of truly reliable new therapies using BMSCs.

Acknowledgements

This work was supported in part by a grant-in-aid (KAKENHI) for Young Scientist A from the Japan Society for the Promotion of Science (Japan).

Author details

Hideki Agata[*]

Address all correspondence to: agata@ims.u-tokyo.ac.jp

Tissue Engineering Research Group, Division of Molecular Therapy, The Institute of Medical Science, The University of Tokyo, Tokyo, Japan

References

[1] Caplan, A. I. Osteogenesis imperfecta, rehabilitation medicine, fundamental research and mesenchymal stem cells. Connect Tissue Res (1995). S, 9-14.

[2] Friedenstein, A. J, Chailakhjan, R. K, & Lalykina, K. S. The development of fibroblast colonies in monolayer cultures of guinea-pig bone marrow and spleen cells. Cell Tissue Kinet (1970). , 3(4), 393-403.

[3] Ashton, B. A, Allen, T. D, Howlett, C. R, Eaglesom, C. C, Hattori, A, & Owen, M. Formation of bone and cartilage by marrow stromal cells in diffusion chambers *in vivo*. Clin Orthop Relat Res (1980).

[4] Leboy, P. S, Beresford, J. N, Devlin, C, & Owen, M. E. Dexamethasone induction of osteoblast mRNAs in rat marrow stromal cell cultures. J Cell Physiol (1991). , 146(3), 370-8.

[5] Bianco, P, Riminucci, M, Kuznetsov, S, & Robey, P. G. Multipotential cells in the bone marrow stroma: regulation in the context of organ physiology. Crit Rev Eukaryot Gene Expr (1999). , 9(2), 159-73.

[6] Pittenger, M. F, Mackay, A. M, Beck, S. C, Jaiswal, R. K, Douglas, R, Mosca, J. D, Moorman, M. A, Simonetti, D. W, Craig, S, & Marshak, D. R. Multilineage potential of adult human mesenchymal stem cells. Science. (1999). , 284(5411), 143-7.

[7] Makino, S, Fukuda, K, Miyoshi, S, Konishi, F, Kodama, H, Pan, J, Sano, M, Takahashi, T, Hori, S, Abe, H, Hata, J, Umezawa, A, & Ogawa, S. Cardiomyocytes can be generated from marrow stromal cells *in vitro*. J Clin Invest (1999). , 103(5), 697-705.

[8] Pereira, R. F, Hara, O, Laptev, M. D, Halford, A. V, Pollard, K. W, Class, M. D, Simon, R, Livezey, D, & Prockop, K. DJ. Marrow stromal cells as a source of progenitor cells for nonhematopoietic tissues in transgenic mice with a phenotype of osteogenesis imperfecta. Proc Natl Acad Sci U S A (1998). , 95(3), 1142-7.

[9] Honmou, O, Houkin, K, Matsunaga, T, Niitsu, Y, Ishiai, S, Onodera, R, Waxman, S. G, & Kocsis, J. D. Intravenous administration of auto serum-expanded autologous mesenchymal stem cells in stroke. Brain (2011). Pt 6):1790-807.

[10] Ogiso, B, Hughes, F. J, Melcher, A. H, & Mcculloch, C. A. Fibroblasts inhibit mineralised bone nodule formation by rat bone marrow stromal cells in vitro. J Cell Physiol (1991). , 146(3), 442-50.

[11] Bourzac, C, Smith, L. C, Vincent, P, Beauchamp, G, Lavoie, J. P, & Laverty, S. Isolation of equine bone marrow-derived mesenchymal stem cells: a comparison between three protocols. Equine Vet J. (2010). , 42(6), 519-27.

[12] Horn, P, Bork, S, Diehlmann, A, Walenda, T, Eckstein, V, Ho, A. D, & Wagner, W. Isolation of human mesenchymal stromal cells is more efficient by red blood cell lysis. Cytotherapy (2008). , 10(7), 676-85.

[13] Agata, H, Yamazaki, M, Uehara, M, Hori, A, Sumita, Y, Tojo, A, & Kagami, H. Characteristic differences among osteogenic cell populations of rat bone marrow stromal cells isolated from untreated, hemolyzed or Ficoll-treated marrow. Cytotherapy (2012). , 14(7), 791-801.

[14] Liu, Z. J, Zhuge, Y, & Velazquez, O. C. Trafficking and differentiation of mesenchymal stem cells. J Cell Biochem (2009). , 106(6), 984-91.

[15] Phinney, D. G, Kopen, G, Righter, W, Webster, S, Tremain, N, & Prockop, D. J. Donor variation in the growth properties and osteogenic potential of human marrow stromal cells. J Cell Biochem (1999). , 75(3), 424-36.

[16] Kagami, H, Agata, H, & Tojo, A. Bone marrow stromal cells (bone marrow-derived multipotent mesenchymal stromal cells) for bone tissue engineering: basic science to clinical translation. Int J Biochem Cell Biol (2011). , 43(3), 286-9.

[17] Friedenstein, A. J. Marrow stromal fibroblasts. Calcif Tissue Int (1995). Suppl 1:S17.

[18] Igarashi, A, Segoshi, K, Sakai, Y, Pan, H, Kanawa, M, Higashi, Y, Sugiyama, M, Nakamura, K, Kurihara, H, Yamaguchi, S, Tsuji, K, Kawamoto, T, & Kato, Y. Selection of common markers for bone marrow stromal cells from various bones using real-time RT-PCR: effects of passage number and donor age. Tissue Eng. (2007). , 13(10), 2405-17.

[19] Bianco, P, & Robey, P. G. Marrow stromal stem cells. J Clin Invest (2000). , 105(12), 1663-8.

[20] Bianco, P, Robey, P. G, & Simmons, P. J. Mesenchymal stem cells: revisiting history, concepts, and assays. Cell Stem Cell (2008). , 2(4), 313-9.

[21] Sanchez-ramos, J, Song, S, Cardozo-pelaez, F, Hazzi, C, Stedeford, T, Willing, A, Freeman, T. B, Saporta, S, Janssen, W, Patel, N, Cooper, D. R, & Sanberg, P. R. Adult bone marrow stromal cells differentiate into neural cells in vitro. Exp Neurol (2000). , 164(2), 247-56.

[22] Lee, R. H, Seo, M. J, Reger, R. L, Spees, J. L, Pulin, A. A, Olson, S. D, & Prockop, D. J. Multipotent stromal cells from human marrow home to and promote repair of pancreatic islets and renal glomeruli in diabetic NOD/scid mice. Proc Natl Acad Sci U S A (2006). , 103(46), 17438-43.

[23] Pozzobon, M, Ghionzoli, M, De Coppi, P, & Ips, E. S. MSC, and AFS cells. Stem cells exploitation for Pediatric Surgery: current research and perspective. Pediatr Surg Int (2010). , 26(1), 3-10.

[24] Marcacci, M, Kon, E, Moukhachev, V, Lavroukov, A, Kutepov, S, Quarto, R, Mastrogiacomo, M, & Cancedda, R. Stem cells associated with macroporous bioceramics for

long bone repair: 6- to 7-year outcome of a pilot clinical study. Tissue Eng. (2007). , 13(5), 947-55.

[25] Wakitani, S, Okabe, T, Horibe, S, Mitsuoka, T, Saito, M, Koyama, T, Nawata, M, Tensho, K, Kato, H, Uematsu, K, Kuroda, R, Kurosaka, M, Yoshiya, S, Hattori, K, & Ohgushi, H. Safety of autologous bone marrow-derived mesenchymal stem cell transplantation for cartilage repair in 41 patients with 45 joints followed for up to 11 years and 5 months. J Tissue Eng Regen Med. (2011). , 5(2), 146-50.

[26] Yang, Z, Zhang, F, Ma, W, Chen, B, Zhou, F, Xu, Z, Zhang, Y, Zhang, D, Zhu, T, Wang, L, Wang, H, Ding, Z, & Zhang, Y. A novel approach to transplanting bone marrow stem cells to repair human myocardial infarction: delivery via a noninfarct-relative artery. Cardiovasc Ther (2010). Dec;, 28(6), 380-5.

[27] Lee, J. S, Hong, J. M, Moon, G. J, Lee, P. H, & Ahn, Y. H. Bang OY; Starting collaborators. A long-term follow-up study of intravenous autologous mesenchymal stem cell transplantation in patients with ischemic stroke. Stem Cells. (2010). , 28(6), 1099-106.

[28] Le Blanc K, Frassoni F, Ball L, Locatelli F, Roelofs H, Lewis I, Lanino E, Sundberg B, Bernardo ME, Remberger M, Dini G, Egeler RM, Bacigalupo A, Fibbe W, Ringdén O.Mesenchymal stem cells for treatment of steroid-resistant, severe, acute graft-versus-host disease: a phase II study. Lancet. (2008). , 371(9624), 1579-86.

[29] Ringdén, O, Uzunel, M, Rasmusson, I, Remberger, M, Sundberg, B, Lönnies, H, Marschall, H. U, Dlugosz, A, Szakos, A, Hassan, Z, Omazic, B, Aschan, J, & Barkholt, L. Le Blanc K. Mesenchymal stem cells for treatment of therapy-resistant graft-versus-host disease. Transplantation (2006). , 81(10), 1390-7.

[30] Howlett, C. R, Cavé, J, Williamson, M, Farmer, J, Ali, S. Y, Bab, I, & Owen, M. E. Mineralization in in vitro cultures of rabbit marrow stromal cells. Clin Orthop Relat Res (1986).

[31] Mankani, M. H, Kuznetsov, S. A, Shannon, B, Nalla, R. K, Ritchie, R. O, Qin, Y, & Robey, P. G. Canine cranial reconstruction using autologous bone marrow stromal cells. Am J Pathol (2006). , 168(2), 542-50.

[32] Peterbauer-scherb, A, Van Griensven, M, Meinl, A, Gabriel, C, Redl, H, & Wolbank, S. Isolation of pig bone marrow mesenchymal stem cells suitable for one-step procedures in chondrogenic regeneration. J Tissue Eng Regen Med (2010). , 4(6), 485-90.

[33] Giannoni, P, Mastrogiacomo, M, Alini, M, Pearce, S. G, Corsi, A, Santolini, F, Muraglia, A, Bianco, P, & Cancedda, R. Regeneration of large bone defects in sheep using bone marrow stromal cells. J Tissue Eng Regen Med (2008). , 2(5), 253-62.

[34] Bourzac, C, Smith, L. C, Vincent, P, Beauchamp, G, Lavoie, J. P, & Laverty, S. Isolation of equine bone marrow-derived mesenchymal stem cells: a comparison between three protocols. Equine Vet J (2010). , 42(6), 519-27.

[35] Kopesky, P. W, Vanderploeg, E. J, Sandy, J. S, Kurz, B, & Grodzinsky, A. J. Self-as-
      sembling peptide hydrogels modulate in vitro chondrogenesis of bovine bone mar-
      row stromal cells. Tissue Eng Part A (2010). , 16(2), 465-77.

[36] Takashima, Y, Era, T, Nakao, K, Kondo, S, Kasuga, M, Smith, A. G, & Nishikawa, S.
      Neuroepithelial cells supply an initial transient wave of MSC differentiation. Cell
      (2007). , 129(7), 1377-88.

[37] Mosca, J. D, Hendricks, J. K, Buyaner, D, Davis-sproul, J, Chuang, L. C, Majumdar,
      M. K, Chopra, R, Barry, F, Murphy, M, Thiede, M. A, Junker, U, Rigg, R. J, Forestell,
      S. P, Böhnlein, E, Storb, R, & Sandmaier, B. M. Mesenchymal stem cells as vehicles
      for gene delivery. Clin Orthop Relat Res (2000). Suppl):S, 71-90.

[38] Siddappa, R, Licht, R, Van Blitterswijk, C, & De Boer, J. Donor variation and loss of
      multipotency during in vitro expansion of human mesenchymal stem cells for bone
      tissue engineering. J Orthop Res (2007). , 25(8), 1029-41.

[39] Agata, H, Asahina, I, Watanabe, N, Ishii, Y, Kubo, N, Ohshima, S, Yamazaki, M, Tojo,
      A, & Kagami, H. Characteristic change and loss of in vivo osteogenic abilities of hu-
      man bone marrow stromal cells during passage. Tissue Eng Part A (2010). , 16(2),
      663-73.

[40] Kuznetsov, S, & Robey, P. G. Species differences in growth requirements for bone
      marrow stromal fibroblast colony formation In vitro. Calcif Tissue Int (1996). , 59(4),
      265-70.

[41] Mizuno, D, Agata, H, Furue, H, Kimura, A, Narita, Y, Watanabe, N, Ishii, Y, Ueda,
      M, Tojo, A, & Kagami, H. Limited but heterogeneous osteogenic response of human
      bone marrow mesenchymal stem cells to bone morphogenetic protein-2 and serum.
      Growth Factors (2010). , 28(1), 34-43.

[42] Tan, Q, Lui, P. P, Rui, Y. F, & Wong, Y. M. Comparison of potentials of stem cells
      isolated from tendon and bone marrow for musculoskeletal tissue engineering. Tis-
      sue Eng Part A. (2012).

[43] Polisetti, N, Chaitanya, V. G, Babu, P. P, & Vemuganti, G. K. Isolation, characteriza-
      tion and differentiation potential of rat bone marrow stromal cells. Neurol India
      (2010). , 58(2), 201-8.

[44] Aubin, J. E. Osteoprogenitor cell frequency in rat bone marrow stromal populations:
      role for heterotypic cell-cell interactions in osteoblast differentiation. J Cell Biochem
      (1999). , 72(3), 396-410.

[45] Ohgushi, H, Goldberg, V. M, & Caplan, A. I. Heterotopic osteogenesis in porous ce-
      ramics induced by marrow cells. J Orthop Res (1989). , 7(4), 568-78.

Chapter 4

Dental-Related Stem Cells and Their Potential in Regenerative Medicine

Razieh Karamzadeh and
Mohamadreza Baghaban Eslaminejad

Additional information is available at the end of the chapter

1. Introduction

Stem cells have been opening a promising future in clinical therapies because of their two remarkable features known as self-renewal and multi-lineage differentiation. These cells can be classified in terms of their origin (embryonic, prenatal and postnatal stem cells) as well as the differentiation commitments (pleuripotent, multipotent and unipotent). Postnatal stem cells, also known as the adult stem cells (ASCs), normally exist in almost every adult tissues, including bone marrow, skin, neural tissues, and dental epithelium, acting as supportive cells by their regeneration capacity. Among different stem cell types, ASCs seem to be more applicable in stem cell-mediated therapies and regenerative medicine because these cells lack ethical concerns, and possesses less tumorgenic potency than their embryonic counterparts.

Recently, human dental stem cells (DSCs), a subtype of ASCs, have drawn worldwide attention for future therapies due to their both technical and practical superiorities. In addition to having some mesenchymal stem cell (MSC) characteristics, including plastic adherent ability with formation of colonies in vitro, and also immunoprivileged properties, DSCs are easily-accessible cells with higher proliferation capacity than ordinary marrow-derived MSCs. Currently, there are six types of stem/progenitor cells determined in dental-related tissues. 1) dental pulp stem cell (DPSCs), 2) stem cells from human exfoliated deciduous teeth (SHED), 3) periodontal ligament stem cells (PDLSC), 4) stem cells from apical papilla (SCAP) of developing tooth, 5) dental follicle stem/progenitor cells (DFPCs) and 6) gingiva stem cells (GSCs). DPSCs, SHEDs and SCAPs are referred to as dental pulp-related stem cells, and PDLSCs & DFPCs as periodontium-related stem cells [1, 5].

This chapter focuses on different aspects of dental-derived adult stem cells, such as their classification, biological characterization, initiating culture, cultivation systems, cryopreservation and potential applications in tissue engineering and regenerative medicine. The data are organized as three main parts, including: 1) Dental-related stem cell biology: from the classification to the characterization and differentiation potential 2) Dental-related stem cell initiation culture, culture systems and cryopreservation 3) Dental-related stem cell- based tissue regeneration.

2. Dental-related stem cell biology: From the classification to the characterization & differentiation potential

According to the literature, there are several types of stem/progenitor cells existed in dental tissue. In this section, each of these cells will be described in terms of their main characteristics.

2.1. Dental Pulp Stem Cells (DPSCs)

The presence of stem cells in dental pulp tissue primarily have been reported in 1985 by Yamamura [3, 4, 6] (Figure 1). Later on, Caplan et al. have demonstrated that these cells presented osteogenic and chondrogenic potential in vitro, and could also differentiate into dentin, in vivo. In 2000, Gronthos et al. have isolated dental pulp stem cells from adult human dental pulp, which had the ability to regenerate a dentin-pulp-like complex [7]. Interestingly, some recent works have found the presence of stem cells in inflamed pulp with capacity to form mineralized matrix both in vitro and in vivo. These findings make dental pulp as an interesting tissue source of putative stem cells, even in diseased form.[8]

DPSCs are similar to MSCs in some ways: they are of fibroblastic morphology with selective adherence to solid surfaces, having good proliferative potential and capacity to differentiate in vitro, and the ability to repair tissues in vivo. It's interesting to note that DPSCs could differentiate into not only osteoblasts, chondrocytes & adipocytes, but also myocytes, neurons and hepatocytes lineages in vitro [4]. DPSCs are characterized by their negative expression of hematopoietic antigens (e.g., CD45, CD34, CD14), and positive expression of stromal-associated markers (e.g., CD90, CD29, CD73, CD105, CD44) (Table 1). They also express multipotent marker (STRO-1) and extracellular matrix proteins, such as collagen, vimentin, laminin, and fibronectin. [9-11]. Interestingly, some of the pluripotent stem cell markers, such as Oct4, Nanog, Sox2, Klf4, SSEA4 & c-Myc have been reported to express on DPSCs [12-14]. More recently, it was demonstrated that core transcription factor of the reprogramming Oct4, Nanog, Klf4 and c-Myc become significantly down-regulated following the DPSC differentiation [4].

Apart from stemness markers, DPSCs are also shown to express bone markers, such as bone sialoprotein, osteocalcin, alkaline phosphates (ALP), and type I collagen. This indicates their differentiation commitment into bone tissue [15]. On the other hand, the expression of dentin sialophosphoprotein (an odontoblast specific protein precursor) is not present in the cultures of hDPSCs implied that these cells represent an undifferentiated pre-odontogenic phenotype [7, 16].

From immunological perspective, it has been reported that DPSCs displayed more immnosuppressive activities than the BM-MSCs. This was obvious in inhibiting T cells response in vitro [17].

Based on some investigations, there is a sub-type of DPSCs referred to as "immature dental pulp stems cells" (IDPSCs), which have promising potential in future stem cell researches. IDPSCs were firstly, isolated from pulp tissue of the human exfoliated deciduous as well as permanent teeth [18]. These cells express both embryonic and MSC markers (see part 2.2). It has been indicated that transferring of human IDPSCs (hDPSCs) into mouse blastocysts resulted in formation of human/mouse chimera which was able to retain proliferation and differentiation capacity [19]. Furthermore, hIDPSCs possess the capacity to rapidly reprogrammed into induced pleuripotent stem cells (iPSc) which are able to produce primary hIDPSC-iPSC colonies even under feeder-free conditions [20].

2.2. Dental Stem cells from Human Exfoliated Deciduous teeth (SHED)

In 2003, Miura et al. have reported to isolate a stem cell population from the living pulp remnants of exfoliated deciduous teeth. These authors have termed the cells as stem cells from human exfoliated deciduous teeth (SHED) [21] (Figure 1). These cells which are believed to be of the neural crest origin are heterogeneous fibroblast-like population possessing an extensive proliferating capacity than either DPSCs or BM-MSCs [22]. In terms of surface epitopes, it has been found that they express markers of MSCs (STRO-1, CD146, SSEA4, CD90, CD73, CD 105, CD106 and CD 166) and lack of hematopoietic/endothelial markers (CD34, CD31) (Table 1). Under an appropriate culture conditions, SHED are able to differentiate into the variety of cell types, including neural cells, angiogenic endothelial cells, adipocytes, osteoblasts, and odontoblasts [23-25]. In vivo transplantation of SHED have been reported to result in formation of bone and dentin like-tissue. [18, 21, 26-29]. There are some studies suggested that SHED is different from IDPSCs in terms of expression of stem cell markers (see part 1.1)[18, 30]. Moreover, some research works have been reported that SHED would possess immunomodulatory function as seen in BM-MSCs [28].

2.3. Periodontal Ligament Stem Cells (PDLSC)

Periodontal ligament stem cells (PDLSCs) have first been introduced by Seo et al. [31] (Figure 1). Like MSCs, PDLSCs have been reported to form adherent clonogenic population of fibroblast-like cells in the culture. They express both early MSC markers such as, STRO-1 and CD146, and other MSC and pluripotent makers, such as CD44, CD90, CD105, CD73, CD26, CD10, CD29 and CD166; meanwhile, they have no expression for CD40, CD80, and CD86[31-33] (Table 1). Some investigations have revealed that PDLSCs may be positive for embryonic stem cell markers, as well, including SSEA1, SSEA3, SSEA4, TRA-1-60, TRA-1-81, Oct4, Nanog, Sox2 and Rex1, and ALP [34]. Based on some research works, SSEA4-positive PDLSCs displayed the potential to generate adipocytes, osteoblasts, chondrocytes (from mesodermal layer), neurons (from ectodermal layer), and hepatocytes (from endodermal lineage) in vitro [31, 34, 35]. Furthermore, it has been shown that transplantation of PDLSCs into immunocompromised rodents resulted in the generation of cementum/PDL-like structure and contributes to periodontal tissue repair [31].

PDLSCs show immunomodulatory activity by up-regulation of soluble immunosuppressive factors (TGF-β1, hepatocyte growth factor (HGF) and indoleamine 2, 3-dioxygenase (IDO) in the presence of activated peripheral blood mononuclear cells (PBMNCs). Similar to the DPSCs, PDLSCs are positive for HLA-ABC (MHC class I antigen) while negative for HLA-DR (MHC class II antigen) [32].

2.4. Dental Follicle Progenitor Cells (DFPCs)

In 2005 & 2007, Morsczeck et al. and Kémoun et al., respectively have identified unique undifferentiated lineage committed cells possessing mesenchymal progenitor features in the human dental follicle (Figure 1). The cells were referred to as "dental follicle precursor cells" (DFPCs) [36, 37]. Characteristically, DFPCs, similar to the bone marrow stem cells, are adherent and colony-forming cells. These cells have been reported to express Notch-1, CD13, CD44, CD73, CD105, and STRO-1 [1, 36] (Table 1). Human DFPCs has been believed to consist of precursor cells for cementoblasts, periodontal ligament cells, and osteoblasts. Under appropriate in vitro conditions, they are capable of differentiating into osteoblasts, cementoblasts, chondrocytes and adipocytes. Interestingly, although both DFPCs and SHED are of the neural crest origin, their neural differentiation potentials are different under the same culture conditions. It has been reported that SHED possess good differentiation potential than DFPCs in terms of the expression of Pax6 which is a marker of retinal stem cells [27].

2.5. Stem Cells from the Apical Papilla (SCAP)

Stem cells from dental apical papilla (SCAP) were first identified and characterized by Sonoyama et al. in human permanent immature teeth [38] (Figure 1). These authors described the cells as adherent clonogenic cells with mesenchymal stem cell features, which are expressed STRO-1, CD24, CD29, CD73, CD90, CD105, CD106, CD146, CD166, and ALP, and not expressing CD34; CD45; CD18; and CD150. Among these markers, CD24 would be of a specific marker for SCAP since it's not found in the other dental stem cells (Figure 2). Excitingly, some authors have reported that SCAP display higher telomerase expression than both DPSCs and BM-MSCs [38]. Furthermore, SCAP has been shown to positively stain with several neural markers implying their possible origin from the neural crest [39]. In terms of differentiation, SCAP are capable of generating osteoblasts, odontoblasts and adipocytes in vitro. An in vivo study has demonstrated that these cells form hard tissue when being loaded onto hydroxyapatite (HA) and implanted subcutaneously in immunocompromised rats [38-40]. Moreover, SCAP have been reported to possess a significantly higher mineralization potential as well as proliferation rate than DPSCs. This finding might be of some importance for their use in dental and/or bone tissue engineering and regeneration [41].

About the possibility of immunogenicity of SCAPs, an independent study have reported that swine SCAPs are non-immunogenic and suppressed T cells proliferation in vitro [42].

2.6. Stem Cells derived from Gingiva (GSCs)

The isolation of a stem cell population from gingiva was firstly reported by Zhang et al. in 2009 [43] (Figure 1). These authors derived the cells from the spinous layer of human gingiva and referred to them as gingival stem cells (GSCs). In terms of markers, it has been shown that GSCs are negative for CD45/CD34, but positive for CD29, CD44, CD73, CD90, CD105, CD146, STRO-1 and SSEA4 (Table 1). In addition, extracellular matrix proteins, such as collagen, vimentin, Collagen type-1, and fibronectin have been reported to express in these cells [43, 44]. Like MSCs, GSCs possess a differentiation potential into osteoblasts, adipocytes and chondrocytes in vitro [45]. Moreover, these cells have been found to be able to differentiate along endothelial as well as neural cell lineages. Furthermore, in vivo bone regeneration potential of GSCs was demonstrated by transplantation of GSCs/HA into immunocompromised mice [45]. More importantly, in a comparative study, it was demonstrated that GSCs showed stable phenotypes, maintain normal karyotype and telomerase activity in long-term cultures in comparison with BM-MSC [45].

As with other dental related stem cells, GSCs has been found to display immunomodulatory functions; they inhibit lymphocytes proliferation and express a wide range of immunosuppressive factors, including Interleukin-10 (IL-10), IDO, inducible NO synthase (iNOS), and cyclooxygenase 2 (COX-2) in response to the inflammatory cytokine, IFN- γ [43].

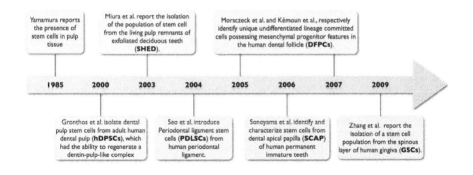

Figure 1. Timeline about the highlights in the history of the isolation of dental-related stem cells (see text).

	DPSCs	SHED	PDLSCs	DFPCs	SCAPs	GSCs
CD (+)	STRO-1	STRO-1	STRO-1	STRO-1	STRO-1	STRO-1
	CD10		CD10	CD10		
	CD13	CD13	CD13	CD13	CD13	CD13
					CD24	
			CD26			
	CD29	CD29	CD29	CD29	CD29	CD29
	CD44	CD44	CD44	CD44	CD44	CD44
	CD59		CD59	CD59		
	CD73	CD73	CD73	CD73	CD73	CD73
	CD90	CD90	CD90	CD90	CD90	CD90
	CD105	CD105	CD105	CD105	CD105	CD105
	CD106	CD106	CD106		CD106	CD106
	CD117					
	CD146	CD146			CD146	CD146
		CD166	CD166		CD166	CD166
CD (-)	CD14	CD14	CD14			
					CD18	
	CD19					
	CD24					
	CD34	CD34	CD34	CD34	CD34	CD34
			CD40			
	CD45	CD45	CD45	CD45	CD45	CD45
			CD80			
			CD86			
					CD150	
	HLA-DR		HLA-DR	HLA-DR		HLA-DR

Table 1. Cell Surface Marker Profiles of dental-related stem cells. DPSC; Dental pulp stem cell, SHED; Stem cells from human exfoliated deciduous teeth, PDLSC; Periodontal ligament stem cells, DFPC, Dental follicle precursor cells, SCAP; Stem cells from dental apical papilla, GSC; Gingival stem cells. [1-4]

3. Dental-related stem cell initiation culture, culture systems and cryopreservation

In dental related stem cell researches, the first step is to isolate cells from tissue sources. The next step is to expand the cells into sufficient number. In some occasion, it may be necessary to preserve the cells for future use since tissue sources would not be available on demand. In this section, we will describe the location of the certain teeth tissue from which the stem cell population can be derived and followed by description of common methods by which the isolation culture can be initiated. At the end, culture systems for the cell propagation as well as the main points regarding issue of cell cryopreservation will be explained.

3.1. Anatomical location of teeth tissue from which DSCs can be derived

Most of the human DSCs are come from teeth, which are subjected to the orthodontic treatments. Based on the studies, molars and premolars are mostly used for this purpose. Third molars (wisdom teeth) are the most common teeth for extraction in dental clinical practice. In addition, developing wisdom teeth during the adult life are the excellent candidates as the accessible source of developing tissue similar to those in embryonic development. There are a few studies considering the supernumerary teeth derived from other teeth, such as canine, for the isolation of DPSCs [12] In some cases, such as the isolation of DPSCs from inflamed dental pulps, endodontic treatments are used rather than orthodontics surgeries [46]. In any case, considering the precise location of the dental tissues in tooth anatomy is important to achieve certain types of DSCs with minimum cell contaminations. Hence, here is the brief description of the localization for the specific DSCs isolation.

3.1.1. Tissues contained dental pulp-related stem cells (DPSCs, SHED & SCAP)

Isolation of DPSCs following the pulp extraction could be achieved by either through the root or crown of the dental organ. In the case of SHEDs or DPSCs, which are derived from incompleted root teeth, the exposed pulp is accessible from the root without applying any specific procedure [21]. In other situation (extracted permanent or deciduous teeth), dental pulp extraction is accomplished through the dental crown by cutting the cementum-enamel junction (CEJ) using dental instruments, such as pliers (bone forceps), extirpation needle, Gracey curette, dental fissure burs, etc. [6] Moreover, in the case of inflamed teeth, pulp tissues are removed during the endodontic therapies [46] (Figure 2)

The isolation of SCAP is achieved by gentle separation of root apical papilla from the surface of the root with immature apex (i.e. located in the exterior of the root foramen area before the complete eruption of tooth in the oral cavity) during the extraction of third molars [47]. Root maturation results in the elimination of apical papilla; hence, the maturation period of teeth are important for isolation of SCAP. (Figure 2)

3.1.2. Tissues contained periodontium-related stem cells (PDLSCs & DFPCs) & GSCs isolation

PDLSC can be obtained from the middle third of the root surfaces of extracted PDL tissue, which is a soft connective tissue surrounded between the cementum and the inner wall of the alveolar bone socket. It's accomplished by scrapping surface of the middle third of the root [31].

DFPCs can be isolated by dissecting dental follicle from the upside of the dental crown from impacted teeth. Human dental follicle is an ectomesenchymal tissue that is derived from cranial neural crest. This tissue surrounds developing tooth germ and involves in the coordination of tooth eruption and periodontium formation. This tooth germ's tissue can easily be isolated after wisdom tooth extraction by routine orthodontical related surgeries. Impacted teeth, usually third molars, normally fail to erupt through the gum because of their encasement in the jawbone; therefore, routine surgical procedures are required for the extraction. [36, 37]. (Figure 2)

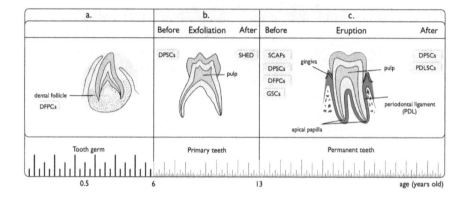

Figure 2. Overall view of dental-related stem cells based on different anatomical locations and stages during the human lifetime in. a. tooth germ, b. primary teeth, c. permanent teeth.

GSCs could be isolated from clinically healthy gingiva, which are obtained as remnant or discarded tissues following routine dental procedures [43]. (Figure 2)

3.2. DSCs culture initiation

In general, dental-related stem cells could isolate by either (1) enzymatic digestion (ED) of tissues or (2) outgrowth (OG) from tissue explant. In the case of enzymatic digestion, after the extraction, tissues are placed into the digestion enzymes, (generally, collagenase type-I & dispase) for about 30-60 minutes at 37 °C to achieve single-cell suspensions. In order to purify DSCs, single-cell suspensions could be subjected into (1) size-sieved isolation (using 3 μm strainer followed by 20 μm strainer), (2) stem cell colony cultivation (single colony culture of stem cells) or (3) magnetic/ fluorescence activated cell sorting (sorting based on surface markers) [48].

In the outgrowth method (OG), tissues are minced into 1-2 mm pieces and placed into the culture dishes to outgrowth [18]. More recently, Lizier and his co-workers established a scaled-up hIDPSCs culture system based on in vitro re-plating of pulp tissue explants followed by 3-4 days expansion [49].

There are some evidences, which suggested different behavior of DSCs according to the ED or OG isolation methods [41, 50, 51]. According to Huang et al. DPSC isolated by ED method (DPSC-ED) from permanent teeth showed higher proliferation rate than those isolated by the OG method (DPSC-OG) [50]. Moreover, STRO-1 & CD34 markers expressed more in DPSC-ED in comparison with DPSC-OG. DPSC-ED derived from deciduous and permanent teeth has been reported to display higher mineralization rate in the defined osteo/odonto medium [51, 52].

3.3. DSCs culture systems

Following the isolation of dental-related stem cells, the next step is to culture-expand the cells into the multiple copies since in the most strategies related to the cell-based-treatment of tissue defects, the copious amount of regenerating cells is needed. Many researchers have been focused on optimizing effective conditions under which DSCs can efficiently be propagated. On the other hand, differentiation potential of the multiplied cells must be determined because discovering the potential commitments of the cells may lead to better selection of them for future organ-targeted treatments [27, 48, 53]. Due to these considerations, this section opens up a brief overview for different DSC culture systems designed for the cell expansion and differentiation.

3.3.1. Serum free vs. serum rich culture systems

Normally, the isolation and expansion of DSC have depend on a high concentration of serum culture media (10%), which provide better cell adhesion during the initial isolation of the cells. Unfortunately, in long-term cultivation, the high level of serum might lead to spontaneous differentiation or malignant transformation of cells. In addition, use of serum in culture may result in contamination of cell culture with bovine pathogen for instance bovine spongiform encephalopathy (BSE). For these reasons, serum free culture systems are highly recommended [54-57]. In this regards, many attempt has been made to optimize DSC cultivation in serum-free or low serum medium. For example, Karbanova et al. have reported that DPSCs cultivated in low-serum medium exhibit less proliferation rate and different expression of stem cell markers compared to those cultivated in serum rich medium [14]. In contrast, Hirata et al have cultivated the cells in serum free media and have found the same survival rate of the cells as those cultivated in the serum containing medium [58].

In the case of DFPCs, studies indicated that applying serum replacement media didn't affect the expression of connective tissue markers, such as collagen type I and type III, and also neural stem progenitor marker, nestin [59]; however, there is no information about the possible changes in other markers in this regards.

It's interesting to note that SHEDs & PDLSCs cultivated in defined serum free media have been reported to display higher proliferation rate than those cultivated in the medium containing serum. Moreover such cells have found to express comparatively higher "stemness" markers [60]. Applying serum free media is one of the critical requirements for the future clinical treatments; therefore, additional works are needed for optimizing conditions to achieve final conclusion.

3.3.2. Neurosphere-forming vs. adherent culture systems

Sphere-forming culture systems are generally applied for neurogenic differentiation of stem cells. This culture system has also been used for DSC cultivation. The idea of applying such a system came from the consideration of neural crest origin of DSCs. It has been well established that neural stem/progenitor cells which are isolated from variety of sources are grown as neurospheres in defined serum-free culture medium supplemented with EGF and / or bFGF [61-63].

DSC Suspension culture was first suggested by Morita et al. (2007). These authors have cultivated PDLSCs in the sphere culture and found that PDLSC have the ability to form neurospheres in serum-free culture containing epidermal growth factor (EGF), basic fibroblast growth factor (bFGF) and leukemia inhibitory factor (LIF) with the ability to differentiate into both neural and mesodermal progeny [64].

In 2008, Sasaki et al. have cultivated DPSCs from the rat incisor in the sphere-culture and found that under these conditions, the cells expressed neural and glial markers. They have also noticed that CD81 positive DPSCs that were localized in odontoblast layer of apical portion of the dental pulp may have more potential to form neurospheres [65] Later on, it was demonstrated that sphere form of SCAP had multi-differentiation potential into mineralized cells, adipocytes and also myocytes under the defined media in vitro. Furthermore, In vivo studies have indicated that sphere SCAP showed more potential to generate mineralized tissues in comparison with the non-sphere SCAP [47].

3.3.3. Co-culture systems

Site-specific tissue interactions are essential for orchestration of proliferation, differentiation and also homeostasis of cells during the tooth germ development. In particular, epithelial-mesenchymal interactions are the most important developmental events, which are involved in reciprocal crosstalk between the ectodermal and mesenchymal tissues. These sequential interactions are critical for tooth morphogenesis and cell differentiation [66]. To imitate these in vivo interactions, co-culture systems have been developed.

Using co-culture systems, some attempts have been made to promote DSCs differentiation in vitro. In this regards different cell types have been examined as co-culture cells. For example, it has been demonstrated that co-culture of DFPCs/SCAP could lead to formation of bone-like structure in vivo and in vitro. This occurs since interaction between the cells stimulate cementogenic/osteogenic differentiation of DFPCs leading to up-regulation of bone intermediate proteins, such as bone morphogenetic protein 2 (BMP2), osteoprotegerin (OPG), bone sialoprotein (BSP) and osteocalcin (OCN), as well as down-regulation of receptor activator of nuclear factor κB ligand (RANKL) [67]. In other experiment, Arakaki et al. have co-cultured DPSCs with dental epithelial cells and found that in such a system, dental epithelial cells secret BMP2 and BMP4, thereby promote odontoblastic differentiation of DPSCs [68]. Interestingly, it has also been reported that co-culture of DPSCs with epithelial cells lead to epithelium invagination, as well [69]. Moreover, Wang et al. have established a co-culture of hDPSCs with osteoblasts and demonstrated that a higher mineralization and up-regulation of osteogenic-related genes in hDPSCs compared with those cultured in the absence of osteoblasts [70]. Furthermore, co-culture of DPSCs with non-dental MSCs, such as amniotic fluid-derived MSCs (AF-MSCs), has been reported to leads to the bone differentiation of AF-MSCs indicating the pre-commitment of DPSCs to induce osteogenic differentiation [71].

3.4. DSCs cryopreservation

According to the diversity of dental-related stem cells and their remarkable features for cell-mediated therapies and tissue engineering, developing a reliable method for cell banking have become a priority for future use. In this regard, cryopreservation could be established at the levels of teeth (organs), dental tissues or cells. In the case of teeth or dental tissues cryopreservation, minimal processing may needed for banking. There are some evidences which are demonstrated the successful cryopreservation of healthy and diseased teeth as well as dental tissues [72-78]. On the other hand, cryopreservation of DSCs still has been considered as an active area of the researches. There are several parameters which need to be considered prior to an establishment of a successful and more efficient protocol. The parameters which need to be determined include (1) DSCs-cultured passage(s), which leads to high-efficiency recovery post thaw, (2) concentration of cryoprotective agent, (3) cell concentration for high-efficient cryopreservation, (4) storage temperature, (5) the process of cryopreservation, and (6) evaluation of growth, surface markers and differentiation properties of DSCs after post thaw. So far, there have been many researches considering the comparative cryopreservation methods for optimizing the best protocols. More recently, it has been suggested that magnetic cryopreservation of DSCs was much better than conventional slow-freezing procedure in terms of cytotoxicity [76, 79, 80].

4. Dental-related stem cell based tissue regeneration

Although DSCs are newborn in the field of stem cell therapy and tissue engineering, they have opened the promising windows not only in tooth repair and regeneration studies but also in other organs. To date, most of DSCs mediated cell therapies and tissue-engineering studies have been focused on the animal models. However, more recently, a few clinical trial studies have also been accomplished. Meanwhile, the immunogenicity of these cells should be more considered for their allogeneic transplantation.

4.1. DSCs-based tooth engineering and regeneration of dental related tissue

In general, in the field of dentistry, the final goal of tissue engineering is to develop tooth-replacement therapies using the whole-bioengineered-tooth technology. To fulfill this, some authors have conducted the remarkable investigations. In this regard, there is some experiment in which either dissociated tooth germs or mesenchymal and epithelial cells derived from the tooth germs were prepared and loaded on to the prefabricated tooth-shaped scaffolds in order to fabricate a bioengineered tooth. Based on these investigations, tooth germ cells possessed a high potential to form dentin, enamel, pulp, and periodontal tissues in vivo [81-84]. However, using embryonic tooth germ and problems related to immunogenicity of animal transplantation, make this an unfeasible approach to clinical application of tooth regeneration [84].

Alternative cells would be DSCs. Using these cells, some preliminary studies have been accomplished to examine whether DSCs in combination with appropriate scaffold are able to promote regeneration of tooth tissues [85, 86]. For instance, transplantation of PDLSCs loaded onto HA/TCP have been shown to result in the production of cementum in mice while using gelfoam (collagen based gelatin sponge) as the carrier has been reported to fail creating cementum [31, 87]. Sonoyama and co-workers have reported the creation of a root/periodontal complex being capable of supporting a porcelain crown in swine by applying both SCAP and PDLSCs in HA/TCP as a carrier [38]. In a study on canine model, we have recently succeeded to achieve regeneration on an experimentally-created defect in peridontium using autologous DPSCs loaded onto Bio-Oss scaffolds [88]. Furthermore, Nakashima et al. have reported a successful induction of whole-pulp regeneration after pulpectomy in a dog model using autologous DPSCs loaded onto 3D scaffold of collagen-I & II and SDF-1 (stromal-cell-derived factor-1) as the morphogene [89, 90]. Moreover, a culture system termed as organ-engineering methods using PDLSCs have been developed to generate not only tooth root, but also the surrounding periodontal tissues, including PDL and alveolar bone in mouse model [84]. In addition to the above-mentioned animal studies, there is a published retrospective pilot study in human. According to this trial, autologous transplantation of PDL stem/progenitor cells might provide therapeutic improvement for the periodontal defects without any adverse effects during 32–72 months of follow-up [91].

4.2. DSCs-based tissue engineering and regeneration for other organs

Apart from the potential applications in dental tissue engineering and therapy, DSCs have been opened a dynamic field in repair and regeneration of non-dental tissues. In this context, there are many investigations indicating applicability of dental related stem cells in variety of disease models in the animal. For instance, SHED has been reported to exhibit a potential to improve parkinson's disease in rat by differentiating into dopaminergic neuron-like cells. Based on the different investigations, these cells have also the ability to promote wound healing in mice [92-94]. It has been demonstrated that SHED also contribute to repair of the critical-sized calvarial defects in mice model [95].

Transplantation of DPSCs has been shown to improve alzheimer's and parkinson's disease as well as acute myocardial infarction in a rat model [96-98]. Similarly, transplantation of hIDPSCs in canine model with golden retriever muscular dystrophy (GRMD) resulted in some improvement [99]. In addition, it has been reported that transplantation of tissue-engineered hIDPSC sheet was successfully reconstructed the corneal epithelium in rabbits with total limbal stem cell deficiency (LSCD) [100]. Applying PDLSCs with collagen based gelatin sponge carrier have been found to improve facial wrinkles by generating large amounts of collagen fibers in the mouse indicating the potential capacity of PDLSC in the field of plastic surgery. In the case of GSCs, *Intra-peritoneal (ip)* administration of the cells displayed improvement of inflammation-related tissue destruction in experimental colitis [43].

4.3. Immunogenicity of allogeneic transplantation of DSCs

According to the promising place of DSCs in clinical treatments in future, considering the immunogenicity of DSC transplantation is critical. Although autologous DSCs rather than allogenous ones are preferred for repair and regeneration purposes, several limitations such as inadequate cell numbers and donor site morbidity carry out problems. Thus, more studies will be needed to evaluate immunogenicity of allogenous DSCs for the future clinical applications. There are some evidences suggested that DSCs, as the mesenchymal stem cells, have immunomodulatory properties both in vitro and in vivo. These studies are almost considering in vitro immunogenicity of DSCs by evaluating the expression of pro/anti-inflammatory mediators, such as MHC classes, TGF-β, ODO, HGF, nitric oxide (NO), prostaglandin, immunosuppressive minor H antigen (HLA-G), and interferon (IFN)-γ as well as effect of DSCs in suppression of T cells proliferation [28, 101, 102].

In addition, in vivo studies also showed DSCs immunomodulatory functions. For instance, SHED transplantation up-regulated the ratio of Treg (regulatory T cells) and Th17 in MRL/ lpr mice model compared to the BM-MSCs; meanwhile, no change in the expression of IL-6 & IL-10 was detected. On the other hand, transplantation of human DPSCs into the rat model didn't initiate the immunologic responses in recipients [103]. Moreover, in another study, it was demonstrated that transplantation of hIDPSCs didn't show the immune reaction in the canine [99].

In spite of existing evidences, which suggested the immunomodulatory effect of DSCs, there are some data proposing that there is different expression of immune receptors, such as toll-like receptors (TLRs) on the cells. Presence of this receptor could affect the immumomodulatory phenotypes of DPSCs and DFPCs [101, 104, 105]; On the other hand, since some studies suggested that BM-MSCs may regain immunogenic property upon differentiation [106], the subject of immunogenicity of DSCs must be examined not only in an undifferentiated state but also in differentiated form.

5. Conclusion

Dental-related tissue contained several types of stem cells collectively referred to as dental stem cells (DSCs). In this stem cell family, there are 6 named member so far recognized and described. These include dental pulp stem cell (DPSCs), stem cells from human exfoliated deciduous teeth (SHED), periodontal ligament stem cells (PDLSCs), stem cells from apical papilla (SCAP) of developing tooth, dental follicle stem/progenitor cells (DFPCs) and gingival stem cells (GSCs). All these easily-accessible stem cells can be derived from dental tissue obtained from both young and adult patients. Furthermore the cells are described as having immunomodulatory function. These characteristics make DSCs a unique source for repair and regeneration of injured tissue. In this context, many studies have so far been conducted on the animal models and the reports together indicated the extensive potential of the cells in tissue repair and regeneration not only in teeth but also in other organs. After all these animal studies, some centers have started clinical trials to examine the cell potential in human diseases. To exploit the extensive regenerating potential of DSCs in clinic, many additional clinical trials must be planed and conducted till therapeutic protocols using these cells become established.

Author details

Razieh Karamzadeh and Mohamadreza Baghaban Eslaminejad*

*Address all correspondence to: eslami@royaninstitute.org; and bagesla@yahoo.com

Department of Stem Cell and Developmental Biology, Cell Science Research Center, Royan Institute for Stem Cell Biology and Technology, ACECR, Tehran, Iran

References

[1] Morsczeck C, Schmalz G, Reichert TE, Vollner F, Galler K, Driemel O. Somatic Stem Cells s for regenerative dentistry. Clin Oral Investig. 2008 Jun;12(2):113-8.

[2] Huang GT, Gronthos S, Shi S. Mesenchymal stem cells derived from dental tissues vs. those from other sources: their biology and role in regenerative medicine. J Dent Res. 2009 Sep;88(9):792-806.

[3] Zhang QZ, Nguyen AL, Yu WH, Le AD. Human oral mucosa and gingiva: a unique reservoir for mesenchymal stem cells. J Dent Res. 2012 Nov;91(11):1011-8.

[4] Ferro F, Spelat R, D'Aurizio F, Puppato E, Pandolfi M, Beltrami AP, et al. Dental Pulp Stem Cells Differentiation Reveals New Insights in Oct4A Dynamics. PLoS One. 2012;7(7):e41774.

[5] Rodriguez-Lozano FJ, Bueno C, Insausti CL, Meseguer L, Ramirez MC, Blanquer M, et al. Mesenchymal stem cells derived from dental tissues. Int Endod J. 2011 Sep; 44(9):800-6.

[6] Yamamura T. Differentiation of pulpal cells and inductive influences of various matrices with reference to pulpal wound healing. J Dent Res. 1985 Apr;64 Spec No: 530-40.

[7] Gronthos S, Mankani M, Brahim J, Robey PG, Shi S. Postnatal human dental pulp stem cells (DPSCs) in vitro and in vivo. Proc Natl Acad Sci U S A. 2000 Dec 5;97(25): 13625-30.

[8] Tandon S, Saha R, Rajendran R, Nayak R. Dental pulp stem cells from primary and permanent teeth: quality analysis. J Clin Pediatr Dent. 2010 Fall;35(1):53-8.

[9] Mitsiadis TA, Feki A, Papaccio G, Caton J. Dental pulp stem cells, niches, and notch signaling in tooth injury. Adv Dent Res. 2011 Jul;23(3):275-9.

[10] Shi S, Gronthos S. Perivascular niche of postnatal mesenchymal stem cells in human bone marrow and dental pulp. J Bone Miner Res. 2003 Apr;18(4):696-704.

[11] Eslaminejad MB, Vahabi S, Shariati M, Nazarian H. In vitro Growth and Characterization of Stem Cells from Human Dental Pulp of Deciduous Versus Permanent Teeth. J Dent (Tehran). 2010 Fall;7(4):185-95.

[12] Huang AH, Chen YK, Lin LM, Shieh TY, Chan AW. Isolation and characterization of dental pulp stem cells from a supernumerary tooth. J Oral Pathol Med. 2008 Oct; 37(9):571-4.

[13] Liu L, Wei X, Ling J, Wu L, Xiao Y. Expression pattern of Oct-4, Sox2, and c-Myc in the primary culture of human dental pulp derived cells. J Endod. 2011 Apr;37(4): 466-72.

[14] Karbanova J, Soukup T, Suchanek J, Pytlik R, Corbeil D, Mokry J. Characterization of dental pulp stem cells from impacted third molars cultured in low serum-containing medium. Cells Tissues Organs. 2011;193(6):344-65.

[15] Gronthos S, Brahim J, Li W, Fisher LW, Cherman N, Boyde A, et al. Stem cell properties of human dental pulp stem cells. J Dent Res. 2002 Aug;81(8):531-5.

[16] Shi S, Bartold PM, Miura M, Seo BM, Robey PG, Gronthos S. The efficacy of mesenchymal stem cells to regenerate and repair dental structures. Orthod Craniofac Res. 2005 Aug;8(3):191-9.

[17] Pierdomenico L, Bonsi L, Calvitti M, Rondelli D, Arpinati M, Chirumbolo G, et al. Multipotent mesenchymal stem cells with immunosuppressive activity can be easily isolated from dental pulp. Transplantation. 2005 Sep 27;80(6):836-42.

[18] Kerkis I, Kerkis A, Dozortsev D, Stukart-Parsons GC, Gomes Massironi SM, Pereira LV, et al. Isolation and characterization of a population of immature dental pulp stem cells expressing OCT-4 and other embryonic stem cell markers. Cells Tissues Organs. 2006;184(3-4):105-16.

[19] Siqueira da Fonseca SA, Abdelmassih S, de Mello Cintra Lavagnolli T, Serafim RC, Clemente Santos EJ, Mota Mendes C, et al. Human immature dental pulp stem cells' contribution to developing mouse embryos: production of human/mouse preterm chimaeras. Cell Prolif. 2009 Apr;42(2):132-40.

[20] Beltrao-Braga PI, Pignatari GC, Maiorka PC, Oliveira NA, Lizier NF, Wenceslau CV, et al. Feeder-free derivation of induced pluripotent stem cells from human immature dental pulp stem cells. Cell Transplant. 2011 Apr 1.

[21] Miura M, Gronthos S, Zhao M, Lu B, Fisher LW, Robey PG, et al. SHED: stem cells from human exfoliated deciduous teeth. Proc Natl Acad Sci U S A. 2003 May 13;100(10):5807-12.

[22] Nakamura S, Yamada Y, Katagiri W, Sugito T, Ito K, Ueda M. Stem cell proliferation pathways comparison between human exfoliated deciduous teeth and dental pulp stem cells by gene expression profile from promising dental pulp. J Endod. 2009 Nov;35(11):1536-42.

[23] Nourbakhsh N, Soleimani M, Taghipour Z, Karbalaie K, Mousavi SB, Talebi A, et al. Induced in vitro differentiation of neural-like cells from human exfoliated deciduous teeth-derived stem cells. Int J Dev Biol. 2011;55(2):189-95.

[24] Chadipiralla K, Yochim JM, Bahuleyan B, Huang CY, Garcia-Godoy F, Murray PE, et al. Osteogenic differentiation of stem cells derived from human periodontal ligaments and pulp of human exfoliated deciduous teeth. Cell Tissue Res. 2010 May; 340(2):323-33.

[25] Sakai VT, Zhang Z, Dong Z, Neiva KG, Machado MA, Shi S, et al. SHED differentiate into functional odontoblasts and endothelium. J Dent Res. 2010 Aug;89(8):791-6.

[26] Yamada Y, Nakamura S, Ito K, Sugito T, Yoshimi R, Nagasaka T, et al. A feasibility of useful cell-based therapy by bone regeneration with deciduous tooth stem cells, dental pulp stem cells, or bone-marrow-derived mesenchymal stem cells for clinical study using tissue engineering technology. Tissue Eng Part A. 2010 Jun;16(6): 1891-900.

[27] Morsczeck C, Vollner F, Saugspier M, Brandl C, Reichert TE, Driemel O, et al. Comparison of human dental follicle cells (DFCs) and stem cells from human exfoliated deciduous teeth (SHED) after neural differentiation in vitro. Clin Oral Investig. 2010 Aug;14(4):433-40.

[28] Yamaza T, Kentaro A, Chen C, Liu Y, Shi Y, Gronthos S, et al. Immunomodulatory properties of stem cells from human exfoliated deciduous teeth. Stem Cell Res Ther. 2010;1(1):5.

[29] Zheng Y, Liu Y, Zhang CM, Zhang HY, Li WH, Shi S, et al. Stem cells from deciduous tooth repair mandibular defect in swine. J Dent Res. 2009 Mar;88(3):249-54.

[30] Monteiro BG, Serafim RC, Melo GB, Silva MC, Lizier NF, Maranduba CM, et al. Human immature dental pulp stem cells share key characteristic features with limbal stem cells. Cell Prolif. 2009 Oct;42(5):587-94.

[31] Seo BM, Miura M, Gronthos S, Bartold PM, Batouli S, Brahim J, et al. Investigation of multipotent postnatal stem cells from human periodontal ligament. Lancet. 2004 Jul 10-16;364(9429):149-55.

[32] Wada N, Menicanin D, Shi S, Bartold PM, Gronthos S. Immunomodulatory properties of human periodontal ligament stem cells. J Cell Physiol. 2009 Jun;219(3):667-76.

[33] Trubiani O, Zalzal SF, Paganelli R, Marchisio M, Giancola R, Pizzicannella J, et al. Expression profile of the embryonic markers nanog, OCT-4, SSEA-1, SSEA-4, and frizzled-9 receptor in human periodontal ligament mesenchymal stem cells. J Cell Physiol. 2010 Oct;225(1):123-31.

[34] Kawanabe N, Murata S, Murakami K, Ishihara Y, Hayano S, Kurosaka H, et al. Isolation of multipotent stem cells in human periodontal ligament using stage-specific embryonic antigen-4. Differentiation. 2010 Feb;79(2):74-83.

[35] Gay IC, Chen S, MacDougall M. Isolation and characterization of multipotent human periodontal ligament stem cells. Orthod Craniofac Res. 2007 Aug;10(3):149-60.

[36] Morsczeck C, Gotz W, Schierholz J, Zeilhofer F, Kuhn U, Mohl C, et al. Isolation of precursor cells (PCs) from human dental follicle of wisdom teeth. Matrix Biol. 2005 Apr;24(2):155-65.

[37] Kemoun P, Laurencin-Dalicieux S, Rue J, Farges JC, Gennero I, Conte-Auriol F, et al. Human dental follicle cells acquire cementoblast features under stimulation by BMP-2/-7 and enamel matrix derivatives (EMD) in vitro. Cell Tissue Res. 2007 Aug; 329(2):283-94.

[38] Sonoyama W, Liu Y, Fang D, Yamaza T, Seo BM, Zhang C, et al. Mesenchymal stem cell-mediated functional tooth regeneration in swine. PLoS One. 2006;1:e79.

[39] Sonoyama W, Liu Y, Yamaza T, Tuan RS, Wang S, Shi S, et al. Characterization of the apical papilla and its residing stem cells from human immature permanent teeth: a pilot study. J Endod. 2008 Feb;34(2):166-71.

[40] Abe S, Yamaguchi S, Watanabe A, Hamada K, Amagasa T. Hard tissue regeneration capacity of apical pulp derived cells (APDCs) from human tooth with immature apex. Biochem Biophys Res Commun. 2008 Jun 20;371(1):90-3.

[41] Bakopoulou A, Leyhausen G, Volk J, Tsiftsoglou A, Garefis P, Koidis P, et al. Comparative analysis of in vitro osteo/odontogenic differentiation potential of human dental pulp stem cells (DPSCs) and stem cells from the apical papilla (SCAP). Arch Oral Biol. 2011 Jul;56(7):709-21.

[42] Ding G, Liu Y, An Y, Zhang C, Shi S, Wang W, et al. Suppression of T cell proliferation by root apical papilla stem cells in vitro. Cells Tissues Organs. 2010;191(5): 357-64.

[43] Zhang Q, Shi S, Liu Y, Uyanne J, Shi Y, Le AD. Mesenchymal stem cells derived from human gingiva are capable of immunomodulatory functions and ameliorate inflammation-related tissue destruction in experimental colitis. J Immunol. 2009 Dec 15;183(12):7787-98.

[44] Tang L, Li N, Xie H, Jin Y. Characterization of mesenchymal stem cells from human normal and hyperplastic gingiva. J Cell Physiol. 2011 Mar;226(3):832-42.

[45] Tomar GB, Srivastava RK, Gupta N, Barhanpurkar AP, Pote ST, Jhaveri HM, et al. Human gingiva-derived mesenchymal stem cells are superior to bone marrow-derived mesenchymal stem cells for cell therapy in regenerative medicine. Biochem Biophys Res Commun. 2010 Mar 12;393(3):377-83.

[46] Alongi DJ, Yamaza T, Song Y, Fouad AF, Romberg EE, Shi S, et al. Stem/progenitor cells from inflamed human dental pulp retain tissue regeneration potential. Regen Med. 2010 Jul;5(4):617-31.

[47] Abe S, Hamada K, Yamaguchi S, Amagasa T, Miura M. Characterization of the radio-
      response of human apical papilla-derived cells. Stem Cell Res Ther. 2011;2(1):2.

[48] Yan M, Yu Y, Zhang G, Tang C, Yu J. A journey from dental pulp stem cells to a bio-
      tooth. Stem Cell Rev. 2011 Mar;7(1):161-71.

[49] Lizier NF, Kerkis A, Gomes CM, Hebling J, Oliveira CF, Caplan AI, et al. Scaling-up
      of dental pulp stem cells isolated from multiple niches. PLoS One. 2012;7(6):e39885.

[50] Huang GT, Sonoyama W, Chen J, Park SH. In vitro characterization of human dental
      pulp cells: various isolation methods and culturing environments. Cell Tissue Res.
      2006 May;324(2):225-36.

[51] Bakopoulou A, Leyhausen G, Volk J, Tsiftsoglou A, Garefis P, Koidis P, et al. Assess-
      ment of the impact of two different isolation methods on the osteo/odontogenic dif-
      ferentiation potential of human dental stem cells derived from deciduous teeth.
      Calcif Tissue Int. 2011 Feb;88(2):130-41.

[52] Karamzadeh R, Eslaminejad MB, Aflatoonian R. Isolation, characterization and com-
      parative differentiation of human dental pulp stem cells derived from permanent
      teeth by using two different methods. J Vis Exp. 2012(69).

[53] Kim SH, Kim YS, Lee SY, Kim KH, Lee YM, Kim WK, et al. Gene expression profile
      in mesenchymal stem cells derived from dental tissues and bone marrow. J Periodon-
      tal Implant Sci. 2011 Aug;41(4):192-200.

[54] Tseng PY, Chen CJ, Sheu CC, Yu CW, Huang YS. Spontaneous differentiation of
      adult rat marrow stromal cells in a long-term culture. J Vet Med Sci. 2007 Feb;69(2):
      95-102.

[55] Torsvik A, Rosland GV, Svendsen A, Molven A, Immervoll H, McCormack E, et al.
      Spontaneous malignant transformation of human mesenchymal stem cells reflects
      cross-contamination: putting the research field on track - letter. Cancer Res. 2010 Aug
      1;70(15):6393-6.

[56] Gou S, Wang C, Liu T, Wu H, Xiong J, Zhou F, et al. Spontaneous differentiation of
      murine bone marrow-derived mesenchymal stem cells into adipocytes without ma-
      lignant transformation after long-term culture. Cells Tissues Organs. 2010;191(3):
      185-92.

[57] Ren Z, Wang J, Zhu W, Guan Y, Zou C, Chen Z, et al. Spontaneous transformation of
      adult mesenchymal stem cells from cynomolgus macaques in vitro. Exp Cell Res.
      2011 Dec 10;317(20):2950-7.

[58] Hirata TM, Ishkitiev N, Yaegaki K, Calenic B, Ishikawa H, Nakahara T, et al. Expres-
      sion of multiple stem cell markers in dental pulp cells cultured in serum-free media. J
      Endod. 2010 Jul;36(7):1139-44.

[59] Morsczeck C, Ernst W, Florian C, Reichert TE, Proff P, Bauer R, et al. Gene expression of nestin, collagen type I and type III in human dental follicle cells after cultivation in serum-free medium. Oral Maxillofac Surg. 2008 Jul;12(2):89-92.

[60] Tarle SA, Shi S, Kaigler D. Development of a serum-free system to expand dental-derived stem cells: PDLSCs and SHEDs. J Cell Physiol. 2011 Jan;226(1):66-73.

[61] Reynolds BA, Weiss S. Generation of neurons and astrocytes from isolated cells of the adult mammalian central nervous system. Science. 1992 Mar 27;255(5052): 1707-10.

[62] Kopen GC, Prockop DJ, Phinney DG. Marrow stromal cells migrate throughout forebrain and cerebellum, and they differentiate into astrocytes after injection into neonatal mouse brains. Proc Natl Acad Sci U S A. 1999 Sep 14;96(19):10711-6.

[63] Tropepe V, Coles BL, Chiasson BJ, Horsford DJ, Elia AJ, McInnes RR, et al. Retinal stem cells in the adult mammalian eye. Science. 2000 Mar 17;287(5460):2032-6.

[64] Techawattanawisal W, Nakahama K, Komaki M, Abe M, Takagi Y, Morita I. Isolation of multipotent stem cells from adult rat periodontal ligament by neurosphere-forming culture system. Biochem Biophys Res Commun. 2007 Jun 15;357(4):917-23.

[65] Sasaki R, Aoki S, Yamato M, Uchiyama H, Wada K, Okano T, et al. Neurosphere generation from dental pulp of adult rat incisor. Eur J Neurosci. 2008 Feb;27(3):538-48.

[66] Hargreaves KMaG, Harold E. Seltzer and Bender's Dental Pulp. 2002 ed: Quintessence Pub. Co., ; 2002. p. 500 pages.

[67] Bai Y, Matsuzaka K, Hashimoto S, Kokubu E, Wang X, Inoue T. Formation of bone-like tissue by dental follicle cells co-cultured with dental papilla cells. Cell Tissue Res. 2010 Nov;342(2):221-31.

[68] Arakaki M, Ishikawa M, Nakamura T, Iwamoto T, Yamada A, Fukumoto E, et al. Role of epithelial-stem cell interactions during dental cell differentiation. J Biol Chem. 2012 Mar 23;287(13):10590-601.

[69] Xiao L, Tsutsui T. Three-dimensional epithelial and mesenchymal cell co-cultures form early tooth epithelium invagination-like structures: expression patterns of relevant molecules. J Cell Biochem. 2012 Jun;113(6):1875-85.

[70] Wang Y, Yao J, Yuan M, Zhang Z, Hu W. Osteoblasts can induce dental pulp stem cells to undergo osteogenic differentiation. Cytotechnology. 2012 Jul 18.

[71] De Rosa A, Tirino V, Paino F, Tartaglione A, Mitsiadis T, Feki A, et al. Amniotic fluid-derived mesenchymal stem cells lead to bone differentiation when cocultured with dental pulp stem cells. Tissue Eng Part A. 2011 Mar;17(5-6):645-53.

[72] Chen YK, Huang AH, Chan AW, Shieh TY, Lin LM. Human dental pulp stem cells derived from different cryopreservation methods of human dental pulp tissues of diseased teeth. J Oral Pathol Med. 2011 Nov;40(10):793-800.

[73] Perry BC, Zhou D, Wu X, Yang FC, Byers MA, Chu TM, et al. Collection, cryopreservation, and characterization of human dental pulp-derived mesenchymal stem cells for banking and clinical use. Tissue Eng Part C Methods. 2008 Jun;14(2):149-56.

[74] Woods EJ, Perry BC, Hockema JJ, Larson L, Zhou D, Goebel WS. Optimized cryopreservation method for human dental pulp-derived stem cells and their tissues of origin for banking and clinical use. Cryobiology. 2009 Oct;59(2):150-7.

[75] Temmerman L, Beele H, Dermaut LR, Van Maele G, De Pauw GA. Influence of cryopreservation on the pulpal tissue of immature third molars in vitro. Cell Tissue Bank. 2010 Aug;11(3):281-9.

[76] Lee SY, Chiang PC, Tsai YH, Tsai SY, Jeng JH, Kawata T, et al. Effects of cryopreservation of intact teeth on the isolated dental pulp stem cells. J Endod. 2010 Aug;36(8):1336-40.

[77] Seo BM, Miura M, Sonoyama W, Coppe C, Stanyon R, Shi S. Recovery of stem cells from cryopreserved periodontal ligament. J Dent Res. 2005 Oct;84(10):907-12.

[78] Gioventu S, Andriolo G, Bonino F, Frasca S, Lazzari L, Montelatici E, et al. A novel method for banking dental pulp stem cells. Transfus Apher Sci. 2012 Jul 11.

[79] Kaku M, Kamada H, Kawata T, Koseki H, Abedini S, Kojima S, et al. Cryopreservation of periodontal ligament cells with magnetic field for tooth banking. Cryobiology. 2010 Aug;61(1):73-8.

[80] Lee SY, Huang GW, Shiung JN, Huang YH, Jeng JH, Kuo TF, et al. Magnetic cryopreservation for dental pulp stem cells. Cells Tissues Organs. 2012;196(1):23-33.

[81] Yen AH, Sharpe PT. Stem cells and tooth tissue engineering. Cell Tissue Res. 2008 Jan;331(1):359-72.

[82] Oshima M, Mizuno M, Imamura A, Ogawa M, Yasukawa M, Yamazaki H, et al. Functional tooth regeneration using a bioengineered tooth unit as a mature organ replacement regenerative therapy. PLoS One. 2011;6(7):e21531.

[83] Wang Y, Preston B, Guan G. Tooth bioengineering leads the next generation of dentistry. Int J Paediatr Dent. 2012 Jan 8.

[84] Nakahara T. Potential feasibility of dental stem cells for regenerative therapies: stem cell transplantation and whole-tooth engineering. Odontology. 2011 Jul;99(2):105-11.

[85] Mantesso A, Sharpe P. Dental stem cells for tooth regeneration and repair. Expert Opin Biol Ther. 2009 Sep;9(9):1143-54.

[86] Nakashima M, Akamine A. The application of tissue engineering to regeneration of pulp and dentin in endodontics. J Endod. 2005 Oct;31(10):711-8.

[87] Fang D, Seo BM, Liu Y, Sonoyama W, Yamaza T, Zhang C, et al. Transplantation of mesenchymal stem cells is an optimal approach for plastic surgery. Stem Cells. 2007 Apr;25(4):1021-8.

[88] Eslaminejad BM, Khorsand A, Arabsolghar M, Paknejad M, Ghaedi B, Rokn AR, et al. Autologous Dental Pulp Stem Cells in Regeneration of Defect Created in Canine Periodontal Tissue. J Oral Implantol. 2012 Aug 1.

[89] Nakashima M, Iohara K. Regeneration of dental pulp by stem cells. Adv Dent Res. 2011 Jul;23(3):313-9.

[90] Iohara K, Imabayashi K, Ishizaka R, Watanabe A, Nabekura J, Ito M, et al. Complete pulp regeneration after pulpectomy by transplantation of CD105+ stem cells with stromal cell-derived factor-1. Tissue Eng Part A. 2011 Aug;17(15-16):1911-20.

[91] Feng F, Akiyama K, Liu Y, Yamaza T, Wang TM, Chen JH, et al. Utility of PDL progenitors for in vivo tissue regeneration: a report of 3 cases. Oral Dis. 2010 Jan;16(1): 20-8.

[92] Wang J, Wang X, Sun Z, Yang H, Shi S, Wang S. Stem cells from human-exfoliated deciduous teeth can differentiate into dopaminergic neuron-like cells. Stem Cells Dev. 2010 Sep;19(9):1375-83.

[93] Nishino Y, Yamada Y, Ebisawa K, Nakamura S, Okabe K, Umemura E, et al. Stem cells from human exfoliated deciduous teeth (SHED) enhance wound healing and the possibility of novel cell therapy. Cytotherapy. 2011 May;13(5):598-605.

[94] Nishino Y, Ebisawa K, Yamada Y, Okabe K, Kamei Y, Ueda M. Human deciduous teeth dental pulp cells with basic fibroblast growth factor enhance wound healing of skin defect. J Craniofac Surg. 2011 Mar;22(2):438-42.

[95] Seo BM, Sonoyama W, Yamaza T, Coppe C, Kikuiri T, Akiyama K, et al. SHED repair critical-size calvarial defects in mice. Oral Dis. 2008 Jul;14(5):428-34.

[96] Apel C, Forlenza OV, de Paula VJ, Talib LL, Denecke B, Eduardo CP, et al. The neuroprotective effect of dental pulp cells in models of Alzheimer's and Parkinson's disease. J Neural Transm. 2009 Jan;116(1):71-8.

[97] Nesti C, Pardini C, Barachini S, D'Alessandro D, Siciliano G, Murri L, et al. Human dental pulp stem cells protect mouse dopaminergic neurons against MPP+ or rotenone. Brain Res. 2011 Jan 7;1367:94-102.

[98] Gandia C, Arminan A, Garcia-Verdugo JM, Lledo E, Ruiz A, Minana MD, et al. Human dental pulp stem cells improve left ventricular function, induce angiogenesis, and reduce infarct size in rats with acute myocardial infarction. Stem Cells. 2008 Mar; 26(3):638-45.

[99] Kerkis I, Ambrosio CE, Kerkis A, Martins DS, Zucconi E, Fonseca SA, et al. Early transplantation of human immature dental pulp stem cells from baby teeth to golden

retriever muscular dystrophy (GRMD) dogs: Local or systemic? J Transl Med. 2008;6:35.

[100] Gomes JA, Geraldes Monteiro B, Melo GB, Smith RL, Cavenaghi Pereira da Silva M, Lizier NF, et al. Corneal reconstruction with tissue-engineered cell sheets composed of human immature dental pulp stem cells. Invest Ophthalmol Vis Sci. 2010 Mar; 51(3):1408-14.

[101] Tomic S, Djokic J, Vasilijic S, Vucevic D, Todorovic V, Supic G, et al. Immunomodulatory properties of mesenchymal stem cells derived from dental pulp and dental follicle are susceptible to activation by toll-like receptor agonists. Stem Cells Dev. 2011 Apr;20(4):695-708.

[102] Bifari F, Pacelli L, Krampera M. Immunological properties of embryonic and adult stem cells. World J Stem Cells. 2010 Jun 26;2(3):50-60.

[103] de Mendonca Costa A, Bueno DF, Martins MT, Kerkis I, Kerkis A, Fanganiello RD, et al. Reconstruction of large cranial defects in nonimmunosuppressed experimental design with human dental pulp stem cells. J Craniofac Surg. 2008 Jan;19(1):204-10.

[104] Waterman RS, Tomchuck SL, Henkle SL, Betancourt AM. A new mesenchymal stem cell (MSC) paradigm: polarization into a pro-inflammatory MSC1 or an Immunosuppressive MSC2 phenotype. PLoS One. 2010;5(4):e10088.

[105] English K, Mahon BP. Allogeneic mesenchymal stem cells: agents of immune modulation. J Cell Biochem. 2011 Aug;112(8):1963-8.

[106] Liu H, Kemeny DM, Heng BC, Ouyang HW, Melendez AJ, Cao T. The immunogenicity and immunomodulatory function of osteogenic cells differentiated from mesenchymal stem cells. J Immunol. 2006 Mar 1;176(5):2864-71.

Chapter 5

Induce Differentiation of Embryonic Stem Cells by Co-Culture System

Fengming Yue, Sakiko Shirasawa, Hinako Ichikawa,
Susumu Yoshie, Akimi Mogi, Shoko Masuda,
Mika Nagai, Tadayuki Yokohama,
Tomotsune Daihachiro and Katsunori Sasaki

Additional information is available at the end of the chapter

1. Introduction

Stem cells, which are found in all multi-cellular organisms, can divide and differentiate into diverse special cell types and can self-renew to produce more stem cells. In mammals, two main broad types are included, such as embryonic stem (ES) cells and adult stem cells. The former are derived from the inner mass of blastocysts, and the latter have been found in various tissues from adult. In a developing embryo, stem cells can differentiate into all kinds of specialized cells, but also maintain the normal turnover of regenerative organs, such as blood, skin, or intestinal tissues. In adult organisms, stem cells and progenitor cells act as a repair system for the body.

ES cells, derived from the inner cell mass of pre-implantation embryos [1], can proliferate in culture and are able to give rise to all derivatives of the three primary germ layers: endoderm, mesoderm and ectoderm. In other words, they can develop into more than 200 cell types of the adult body when given stimulation for a specific cell type. The endoderm is composed of the entire gut tube and the lungs; the ectoderm gives rise to the nervous system and skin; and the mesoderm gives rise to muscle, bone, blood, and so on.

ES cells, being pluripotent cells, make them an excellent candidate as a source of functional differentiated cells for tissue replacement and regenerative medicine and after disease or injury. Using stem cell in regenerative therapy requires specific stimulation or signals for specific differentiation. If implanted directly, ES cells will randomly differentiate into many different types of cells and cause a teratoma eventually. ES cell researchers still face a few of the hurdles, including differentiating ES cells into specific cells while avoiding transplant immno-rejection [2].

Till to date, mouse embryonic stem (mES) cells and human embryonic stem (hES) cells have been used in researches. They require very different environments in order to maintain an undifferentiated state. Mouse ES cells are cultured on a layer of gelatin as an extracellular matrix and require the presence of feeder cells (STO or SNL) and leukemia inhibitory factor (LIF) [3]. Human ES cells are grown on a feeder layer of mouse embryonic fibroblasts (MEFs) and require the presence of basic fibroblast growth factor (bFGF or FGF-2) [4]. ES cells will rapidly differentiate without optimal culture conditions or genetic manipulation [5].

The multi-lineage differentiation potential of stem cells is not only an opportunity but also a challenge. An undesired cell type may lead to a pathophysiologic state or a non-functional tissue construct once that stem cells differentiate at the wrong time or place. In order to avoid such maladaptive responses, stem cells have evolved elaborate circuitry that triggers them to respond to differentiation cues only in an appropriate biological context. While most of researchers have been focusing on the role of soluble cues (e.g. growth factors and cytokines) in regulating stem cell differentiation, recent evidence demonstrated that the response to these stimuli are strongly modified by adhesive and mechanical cues, and that these microenvironment factors may be used explicitly to control stem cell differentiation in their own right[6]. With these advances in stem cell research, mimicking cellular microenvironment in vitro is becoming increasingly oriented toward to guide stem cell growth and differentiation.

In a living organism, cells are surrounded by peripheral other cells and embedded in an extracellular matrix (ECM) that defines the architecture, signaling, and biomechanics of the cellular microenvironment. As for stem cell, the word "niche" can be in reference to the in vivo and in vitro stem cell microenvironment. In architecture, the word niche refers to a recess, and in ecology it refers to a habitat where an organism can reside and reproduce. So, the grand position of the stem cell in popular concepts of science is appropriately humbled by the cells dwelling in a place where they might awaken with fleas. The concept of a niche as a specialized microenvironment housing stem cells was first proposed by Schofield, although experimental evidence was first provided by invertebrate models. In the gonads of Drosophila melanogaster and Caenorhabditis elegans, the germ stem cells reside at the distal end of a tapered structure, and have been shown to depend upon interactions with somatic cells so that stem-cell features could be maintained [7].

Stem cells are defined by their ability in complex multi-dimensional environment name as niche. Within the niche, several factors are important to regulate stem cell characteristics: (i) cell-cell interactions among stem cells; (ii) interactions between stem cells and neighboring differentiated cells; (iii) interactions between stem cells and extracellular matrix, adhesion molecules, soluble factors (growth factors, cytokines), oxygen tension, and other nature of the environment. Applying for regenerative medicine, specific differentiation of stem cells must be induced in vitro, and then specific graft with sufficient quantity and pure quality could be transplanted back into the patient. In order to archive this purpose, the researchers are trying to replicate the stem cell niche conditions in vitro. However, obviously, it is difficult to mimic the biological complexity of the native cell context in the laboratory under standard 2D culture conditions, since much of the complex interplay of mechanical and molecular factors present in vivo is absent in 2D culture status [8]. This is a major limitation to investigate cellular response in vitro. Therefore, we need generate a new culture system that would be "something between a culture dish and the cells", to represent cellular environment in a living organism and be more predictive of in vivo systems [9,10]. In particular, to stimulate stem cell potential and obtain biologically response in vitro, a new environment that are associated with their proliferation, differentiation, and assembly into tissues is desired. The researches should abide by the following premise: the function of the complicated factors is known to play a role during development or remodeling, and cellular responses to environment factors are predictable.

In our researches, we co-cultured ES cells with special cells to induce the specific differentiation. The co-culture system could supply stem cell for physical attachment (mechanical stretch), regulating signals, as well inducing factors such as cytokines (soluble or diffused). All these combined cues determined the differentiation of specific type of cells. The co-culture system recapitulated the combinations of parameters in the native environment to convert "collections of cells" into specific cell phenotypes. Hence, the design of co-culture system is necessarily inspired by stem cells research.

Co-culture system (ES cells and certain cell) supplied the physical, structural, and molecular factors to induce cellular differentiation. It opens several exciting possibilities: (i) establish functional implant which is suitable for transplantation and replace of degenerated tissues, (ii) investigate developmental processes and understand stem cell behavior in a native environment; (iii) avoid using biomaterials in order to escape from immuno-rejection. A variety of parameters were outlined in Fig.1. It included co-culture system and engineered 2D culture environment that influence stem cell behavior (e.g., self-renewal, migration, and differentiation).

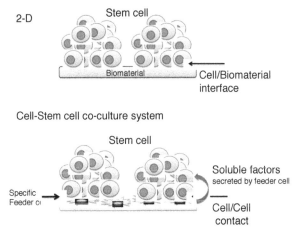

Figure 1. Manipulating the stem cell microenvironment in 2D and cell-stem cell co-culture system. Controllable parameters include matrix properties, cell/cell contact and soluble factors which were secreted by specific feeder cells.

The following section will review several important properties in the design co-culture system to control stem cell differentiation.

2. Interactions with stem cells

2.1. Direct attachment between stem cells and engineered materials

In tissue engineering, either natural or synthetic materials have been investigated for interaction with stem cells and to control their behavior [11]. The benefits to co-culture system include their ability to provide complicated signal to stem cells by physical attachment or chemical excretion. Compared to biological materials, natural or synthetic biomaterials, the former have poor mechanical properties and easily cause immune-response depending on the source of the materials; the later have wide diversity in properties that may be designed according to mechanics, chemistry, and degradation. The toxicity and a limited repertoire of cellular interactions are concerned.

As for the group of natural materials, collagen, matrigel, alginate, and hyaluronic acid (HA) have been used for stem cell researches. Collagen gels have been widely used in stem cell study, including mesenchymal stem cells (MSCs) [12,13] and ES cells [14]. Matrigel consists of a mixture of molecules derived from natural ECM and has been investigated for stem cell culture without feeder cells and inducing differentiation. An improved three-dimension (3D) and serum-free approach was established to differentiate hES cells into functional endothelial cells [16]. Alginate is a seaweed-derived polyanion that forms hydrogels through ionic cross-linking. ES cells have been induced in alginate hydrogels for a variety of applications, typically encapsulated stem cells for transplantation [15]. HA is a polysaccharide found in many tissues and has been modified to form hydrogels. HA hydrogels have been investigated for the culture and growth of undifferentiated human ES cells and MSCs [17, 18].

Synthetic materials were also widely used in stem cell cultures [19]. Materials that degrade through either hydrolytic or enzymatic mechanisms have been synthesized, and the advantage is the tenability and versatility of these physical properties. A hydroxyester has been extensively used in the field of tissue engineering, primarily due to their history of biocompatibility and use in medicine. One composition was seeded with human ES cells for the regeneration of numerous tissues, including vascular and neural structures [20].

2.2. Secreted Soluble factors

Cell and extracellular-matrix components in the stem-cell niche are relatively predictable, although the complexity and integration of these elements is far from known. Soluble mediators of cellular response would also be expected and a number of soluble factors such as growth factors and cytokines are important for stimulate and control the differentiation of stem cells. Adding relative molecules to the culture medium can induce the differentiation. For example, bone marrow stromal cells (BMSCs) have been directed into all kinds of cells [21]. Alternatively, it is advantageous to secrete the molecules directly from the specific cells. The molecules that can induce differentiation is various, such as basic fibroblast growth factor (FGF), members of the transforming growth factor family (TGF), small molecules such as retinoic acid. Molecule release is typically controlled through diffusion, degradation, or combination of factors. Multiple growth factors have been delivered from the same scaffold based on polymer degradation rates [22]. However, regards to co-culture system, the cells used as basement feeder open up the possibility to control molecule secretion for complex signaling cascades in stem cell differentiation, although the regulating mechanism is difficult to be cleared.

2.3. Mechanical and shape cues to control stem cell differentiation

Using soft lithography techniques, the influence of spatially patterned adhesion molecules on cell differentiation was investigated, such as cell spreading and shape on MSC differentiation, through control the cellular cytoskeleton. MSCs tended to the differentiation of osteoblasts, when they were patterned on larger islands of adhesion ligands, which allowed for cell spreading. On the other hand, MSCs on smaller islands stayed rounded and differentiated into adipocytes [23]. This study indicated that stem cell commitment could be regulated by adhesion molecules and is a consideration in design for inducing the differentiation of stem cells.

During the last decades, much progress has been made in the molecular understanding of early differentiation in stem cells. For example, neural inducer molecules, such as chordin, noggin, and retinoic acid (RA), were identified, and several intracellular mediators of neural differentiation have been characterized. Multiple-step method involving in embryoid body (EB) formation followed by different combination of growth factors was the most common method for inducing differentiation of ES cells [24, 25]. Although the methods can produce a good proportion of different type of specific cells, it has several apparent problems. (i) it is difficult to analyze and control each regulatory step of differentiation in this multiple-step because EBs contains many different kinds of cells, including endoderm, mesoderm, and ectoderm cells; (ii) growth factors have complicated function in vivo. For example, RA, a strong teratogen, is supposed to perturb neural patterning and neuronal identities in EBs as it does in vivo. RA treatment of early embryos causes suppression of forebrain development. It is therefore preferable to avoid RA treatment for therapeutic application unless RA induces the particular type of neurons of one's interest; (iii) in order to avoid infection and rejection, the serum of animal origin should be excluded; (iv) multiple-step method is cost-consuming.

3. Inducing specific differentiation of stem cells using with cell co-culture system

In our research, we introduce an efficient cell co-culture system for in vitro differentiation of specific cell type from ES cells in a serum-free condition that requires neither EBs nor complicated treatment with growth factors.

3.1. Induction of midbrain dopaminergic neurons from primate embryonic stem cells by co-culture with Sertoli cells

In the first study, we have established a new method for generating dopaminergic neurons from primate ES cells by co-culture with Sertoli cells. Neurodegenerative diseases present severe problems due to the limited repair capability of the nervous system [26]. Stem cells have a capacity for unlimited self-renewal, along with the ability to produce multiple different types of terminally differentiated descendants. They are candidate therapeutic tools in neurodegenerative disorders, such as Parkinson's disease, which is characterized by degeneration and death of midbrain neurons that produce dopamine. Transplantation of dopaminergic neurons taken from human fetuses into Parkinson's disease patients shows a remarkable, but inconsistent, ability to replace endogenous degenerated dopaminergic neurons and to ameliorate some of the disease symptoms [27, 28]. However, since treatment of a single Parkinson's disease patient requires dopamine neurons from 6 to 10 human fetuses, replacement therapy is not routinely available. Other sources of dopamine-producing cells, including those from the adrenal medulla or carotid bodies, have been examined for their ability to alleviate Parkinson's symptoms, but these sources are also limited in numbers and/or are not as effective as fetal dopamine neurons [29]. ES cells can proliferate indefinitely and are able to differentiate into cell types of all three germ layers in vivo and in vitro. These unique properties of ES cells make them an excellent candidate for the treatment of Parkinson's disease [30,31].

Our ES cell-Sertoli co-culture system is technically simple, cost-saving, and the induction is efficient and speedy. This protocol only used both of cells and treated without any inducing factors. After 3 weeks of induction, immuno-staining revealed that 90%±9% of the colonies contained tyrosine hydroxylase-positive (TH+) neurons, and 60% ±7% of the tubulin III-positive (Tuj III+) neurons were TH+ (Fig2. A-E). At the same time, the possible roles of Sertoli cell in the differentiation of ES cells into Dopaminergic Neurons were investigated. When cultured on the gelatin-coated dish in the same medium but without Sertoli cells, ES cells differentiated into neurons at a low frequency compared with the rate obtained with ES cells cultured on Sertoli cells (Fig2. F, lanes 1 and 2). This suggested that Sertoli cells had an active role in the promotion of neural differentiation of ES cells. We tested whether direct physical contact between ES cells and Sertoli cells was essential for the induction. ES cells cultured on gelatin-coated dishes and separated from co-cultured Sertoli cells by a 0.22-um filter membrane were still able to induce significant neural differentiation of ES cells (Fig2. F, lane3; Fig2.H). When Sertoli-conditioned medium was used to culture ES cells without Sertoli cells as a feeder layer, neural differentiation was still induced compared with ES cells cultured alone on gelatin-coated dishes (Fig2. F, lane4; Fig2.I)). Together these data suggest that Sertoli cells secrete one or more soluble neural-inducing factors.

Based on the known ability to promote neuronal differentiation [32], GDNF seemed to be a likely candidate for the Sertoli-induced differentiation of primate ES cells. We confirmed the presence of GDNF expression in Sertoli cells by immunohistochemistry (Fig. 2 J, Fig.2 K lane 1) and in the conditioned medium by Western blot analysis (Fig.2 K, lane 2). We therefore tested whether GDNF promoted dopaminergic neuron differentiation of primate ES cells. First, we added GDNF to ES/Sertoli cell co-cultures and compared results with ES cells on a gelatin

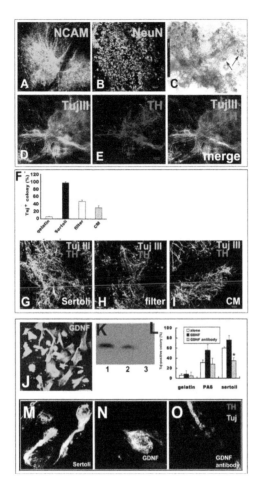

Figure 2. A-E. Sertoli-induced dopaminergic neural differentiation and of monkey embryonic stem cells. Characterization of monkey ES colony induced by Sertoli cells. Expression of NCAM (A), NeuN (B) confirmed the neural identity of cells in ES colony. After 3 weeks, approximately 97% of the ES cell colonies cultured with Sertoli cells were Tuj III+ **(D).** After 3 weeks of culture, immunostaining of Sertoli-induced neurons with anti-TH antibody **(E). (C):** Electron microscopy showed TH ImmunoGold particles (15nm) were associated with small vesicles presumably containing neurotransmitters located at the presynaptic terminal (arrow). **F-I.** The physical and chemical role of Sertoli cells in the induction of dopaminergic neurons. **(F):** Sertoli cells induced the expression of neuronal marker Tuj III in co-cultured monkey embryonic stem (ES) cells even when separated by a filter membrane. CM induced neural differentiation in ES cells cultured on gelatin-coated dish. However the differentiation rate was lower than with direct coculture with Sertoli cells. Tuj III (green) and TH (red) double staining of ES cells when separated from Sertoli cells by a filter **(H)** and cultured in conditioned medium alone **(I).** Scale bar = 50um. **J-O.** The role of GDNF in Sertoli-induced dopaminergic neuron differentiation. **(J):** Immunostaining of GDNF in Sertoli cells. **(K):** GDNF protein was detected by Western blot of lysed Sertoli cells (lane 1) and in conditioned medium (lane 2). However, it was not detected in conditioned medium blocked by anti-GDNF antibody (lane 3). **(L):** In embryonic stem (ES) cells cocultured with conditioned medium derived from Sertoli cells, the TH+ cell percentage was reduced significantly when GDNF was blocked by antibody. TH staining of ES cells cultured on Sertoli cells **(M),** on Sertoli cells treated with extraneous GDNF **(N),** and on blocked conditioned medium **(O).** Scale bars =50um.

coated substrate after 3 weeks in culture. We found that GDNF increased the number of TH$^+$ cells in co-culture with Sertoli (Fig. 2 L, N) At the same time, we incubated the conditioned medium with GDNF-blocking antibodies and effectively removed GDNF as determined by Western blot (Fig. 2K, lane3). The number of TH$^+$ cells supported by anti-GDNF-treated conditioned medium was reduced to 35% ±6% (n= 6,000; Fig. 2L), which was significantly less than that induced by Sertoli cells (*p<.05; Fig. 2L), but still more than in colonies grown on gelatin alone. GDNF antibody inhibited the TH$^+$ neural induction activity of Sertoli cells, as shown by TH staining of ES/Sertoli cell co-cultures and ES cells cultured in conditioned medium blocked by GDNF antibody (Fig. 2 M-O).

Possible roles of Sertoli sells in the differentiation of ES cells into dopaminergic neurons were discussed. Sertoli cells have an active role in the promotion of neural differentiation of ES cells. The mechanism of dopaminergic neuron induction in co-cultures of ES cells with Sertoli cells remains to be understood. First, whether direct physical contact between ES cells and Sertoli cells was essential for the induction was tested through filter membrane to separate ES cells with Sertoli cells. The result showed that Sertoli cells were still able to induce significant neural differentiation of ES cells, indicating that Sertoli cells produce soluble inducing factors. However, Sertoli-conditioned medium could not elicit significant induction. It suggested two possibilities as to the molecular nature of neuron-inducing activity by Sertoli cells. One is that Sertoli cells secrete two different neuron inducing factors, a cell surface-anchored factor and a labile soluble factor. Another might be that the neuron-inducing activity is mediated by secreted factors. At present, we cannot exclude either possibility.

Some factors have been implicated in the regulation of dopaminergic differentiation [33], such as FGF8, Shh, interleukin (IL) 1, IL11, GDNF, and neutralizing antibodies of FGF8 and Shh. Among them, GDNF has the most potent neuroprotective and trophic effects on dopamine neurons in many model systems [34,35,36]. However, it is a large protein and has to be delivered directly to the brain rather than given peripherally. When successfully delivered, GDNF supports the survival and outgrowth of dopamine neurons following transplantation [37]. In addition, GDNF added to cell suspensions of embryonic ventral mesencephalic tissue improves the survival of dopamine neurons following grafting into the degenerative striatum [38]. Other studies have shown that intermittent injections of GDNF in the vicinity of intra-striatal nigral cell suspension grafts have similar effects on improving the survival and/or fiber outgrowth of transplanted dopamine neurons [39,40]. In a previous study [41], neurospheres modified to produce GDNF increased the survival of transplanted dopamine neurons in 6-OHDA-lesioned animals. GDNF is also capable of promoting differentiation of mesencephalic neurospheres towards the neuronal lineage, and more importantly, towards the dopaminergic development indicated by expression of NurrI and Ptx3. Buytaert-Hoefen et al. [42] proved that significant differentiation of dopaminergic neurons were not induced when cultured on PA6 stromal cells alone except for the presence of GDNF or striatal astrocytes. Sertoli cells secrete GDNF and promote the survival of transplanted dopaminergic neurons. In the present study, we showed that GDNF plays a role in dopaminergic neuron differentiation when primate ES cells were co-cultured with Sertoli cells. In our study, extraneous GDNF induced the differentiation of dopaminergic neuron. Sertoli-induced neural differentiation of ES cells was partly suppressed by a low-dose of anti-GDNF antibody. However, blocking GDNF did not completely inhibit the neural differentiation. We cannot be certain that GDNF activity was completely blocked, although it was not found by Western blot. Therefore, the diminished neuronal differentiation that occurred could have been in response to the remaining, unblocked GDNF. Alternatively, if all of GDNF was blocked, then one or more other factors were present in the conditioned medium and promoted differentiation at a reduced rate. If these factors exist, they are more effective in the presence of GDNF. This confirmed the conclusion of Buytaert-Hoefen et al. [42] that GDNF is required but not necessary for the induction of dopaminergic neurons.

From these results, we can conclude that Sertoli cells may stimulate dopaminergic differentiation by a complex combination of growth factors or other factors, including other unidentified components. Among these, GDNF plays some role, but not a decisive role. It is also possible that the supporting environment provided by Sertoli cells, or an interaction between Sertoli cells and primate ES cells, plays a role in their neuron inducing activity.

In addition, isolated Sertoli cells enable survival and function of co-grafted foreign dopaminergic neurons in rodent models of Parkinson's disease. They also promote regeneration of damaged striatal dopaminergic circuitry in those same Parkinson's disease models [43]. In our study, significant TH+ cells were found in the degenerative striatum when differentiated primate ES cells were co-transplanted with Sertoli cells. Moreover, 2-month survival of TH+ neurons derived from ES cells was observed. It is likely that the nutritive support of the Sertoli cells is responsible for this enhanced TH cell survival.

In common, dopaminergic neurons were generated from neural precursor cells amplified from EBs. One group [44] used a lengthy four-step method to produce TH+ neurons at an efficiency of approximately 7% of the Tuj III+ neurons. Kawasaki et al. [45] used the term stromal cell-derived inducing activity to describe the dopaminergic neuronal-inducing defect of PA6 cells. The stromal feeder-mediated neural induction had been demonstrated for mouse, primate, and human ES cells [46-48]. In contrast to the previous protocols, our methods does not require growth serum, the formation of EBs, selection of neural precursor cells, retinoic acid, growth factors, or other special treatment. Thus, our method is more suited to detailed analyses of differentiation and transplantation therapy.

3.2. Differentiation of primate ES cells into retinal cells induced by ES cell-derived pigmented cells

In the second study, retinal cells were induced from primate ES cells by co-culturing with ES-derived pigmented cells.

Photoreceptors are the primary sensory neurons residing in the outer nuclear layer (ONL) of the vertebrate retina. Photoreceptor degeneration is a common cause of human visual impairments resulting from light damage, genetic changes and aging. The unfortunate nonrenewable nature of photoreceptors has inspired that these degenerative diseases maybe treatable by transplantation of healthy fetal cells. Previous work has shown that freshly harvested retinal pigment epithelium (RPE) can be effective in rescuing photoreceptors in the

Royal College of Surgeons (RCS) rat, an animal model of indirect photoreceptor degeneration [49]. However, obtaining a sufficient number of suitable donor cells remains a problem.

The isolation of embryonic stem (ES) cells has drawn much attention, given their potential to generate all adult cell types. As ES cells continue to proliferate in an undifferentiated state in vitro, an unlimited stem cell source or its derivatives may be secured. It is also a potential benefit that ES cells may be genetically manipulated to permit the selective differentiation and/ or isolation of a specific cell type.

Recently, several laboratories have devised hetero chronic co-culture experiments to characterize the nature of the interactions necessary for the differentiation of retinal cells [50,51]. Early embryonic mouse cells (E12) were shown to differentiate into rod photoreceptor cells with a higher frequency when co-cultured with either postnatal rat retinal cells or with later staged embryonic retinal cells that were competent to generate rod photoreceptors. The results suggested that the differentiation of retinal progenitor cells as rod photoreceptors is influenced by locally diffusible signals in the extra cellular environment that are developmentally regulated during the period of retinal histogenesis.

Although the specific factors that promote differentiation of cells as rod photoreceptors are not known, several classes of molecules have been shown to play a role in the developing retina, for example, small peptide growth factors, Shh, taurine, epidermal growth factor (EGF) and fibroblast growth factor (FGF) [52-54]. The vitamin A derivative retinoic acid has been shown to influence cell fate in the developing nervous system. In particular, all-trans retinoic acid has been shown to alter cell fate decisions in the developing limb bud, hindbrain and inner ear [55,56]. In addition, several studies have demonstrated that all-trans retinoic acid and at least one of the nuclear retinoic acid receptors (RARa) are present in the developing retina (56). RA caused a dose-dependent, specific increase in the number of cells that developed as photoreceptors in culture throughout the period of retinal neurogenesis [52,53].

Retinal pigmented epithelium (RPE) is a neuroectodermal derivative essential for the survival of photoreceptors. It supplies nutrition and provides several trophic factors that help maintain the normal physiology within the neuro sensory retina and photoreceptors [57,58].

In most of studies, differentiation of the retinal progenitors into photoreceptors was infrequent in the absence of co-culture with embryonic retinal tissues [59,60]. Use of the fetal retina involves some ethical and practical consideration, and the cell supply is a problem. Osakada and colleagues [52,53] induced the generation of putative rod and cone photoreceptors from ES cells by stepwise treatments under defined culture conditions. However, the practical steps were complicated and time consuming. In this study, the monolayer of RPE derived from ES cells was used as an inducing feeder layer which could replicate the microenvironment of retina or sub-retinal to successfully induce photoreceptor cells. This is the first time that ES-derived cells are used to induce the differentiation of ES cells. Furthermore, retinoic acid was used to induce the differentiation of photoreceptors. To our knowledge, a few reports have produced photoreceptor cells in uncontaminated culture conditions except for Takahashi's group [52] Osakada [53] and lamba's [60,61,62,] research. The present study demonstrated the generation of photoreceptors from primate ES cells under conditions free of animal–derived substances.

During the study of ESC-Sertoli co-culture system, one unexpected finding was the appearance of epithelial cells with massive pigmentation from the second week and they grew at a constant rate. After monkey ES cells were cultured on Sertoli cells for 3 weeks, a patch of pigmented cells was mechanically isolated by using a tip after being loosened with trypsin and plated on a gelatin-coated dish without feeder cells in primate ES cell culture medium. The polygonal morphology with a compact cell-cell arrangement was reminiscent of the pigmented epithelium of the eye, and clearly distinct from pigmented melanocytes derived from neural crest (Fig3 A-I). In recent, transplantation of retinal pigment epithelium (RPE) has become a possible therapeutic approach for retinal degeneration. Meanwhile, RPE is a neural ectodermal derivative essential for the survival of photoreceptors. It serves as nutritional cells and provides several trophic factors that help maintain the normal physiology within the neural sensory retina and photoreceptors. Therefore, we investigated whether retinal cells could be induced by co-culturing ES cells together with RPE. At the same time, RA was treated in order to improve the differentiation efficiency. The results showed that after 10-day co-culture of ES cells and these RPE, some ES derivatives became immuno-positive for rhodopsin. RT-PCR analysis demonstrated expression of retina-related gene markers such as Pax6, CRX, IRBP, Rhodopsin, Rhodopsin kinase and Muschx10A. When RA was added, the distinct increase of photoreceptor specific proteins markers was found. Besides, the differentiation of bipolar, horizontal cells was demonstrated by protein and gene expression. RA treatment also altered more retinal cell differentiation (Fig3. J-M).

We demonstrated that pigment epithelial cells can be generated, enriched, and expanded from primate ES cells when ES cells were co-cultured with Sertoli cells. These ES-converted pigment epithelial cells showed development of several of the characteristics of RPE cells and were able to be used to induce the differentiation of retinal cells. For the clinical application, methods for purifying large numbers of lineage specific cells should be developed. In the present study, RPE cells could be easily identified under a dissecting microscope and selectively expanded into a uniform single cell layer.

The RPE cells contain melanin granules, have a characteristic polygonal morphology, and play some critical roles including (i) forming a barrier separating the retina from the blood vessels of the choroid coat; (ii) regulating nutritive substance transport required for retinal progenitors to differentiate into retinal neurons and the maintenance of retinal cells; (iii) regenerating visual pigments; (iv) digesting the shed parts of photoreceptor cells after having phagocytized them [63]. Therefore, we used ES cell- derived RPE cells to provide epigenetic retinal neurons, not only the efficient induction of photoreceptors, but also other retinal cell lineages, such as bipolar, and horizontal cells. It indicated that the secreted/diffusible factors from RPE or direct cell-cell contact were sufficient to induce retinal cells from ES cells.

A monolayer of ESC-derived RPE cells, an inducing feeder layer that replicates the retinal microenvironment and RA were used to successfully induce photoreceptor differentiation. To our knowledge, this is the first time that ESC-derived cells have been used to induce ESC differentiation. ES/RPE co-culture system can serve as a promising method for therapeutic application and basic research on retinal degeneration disease, although we are still far from an established in vitro or in vivo source of retinal cells.

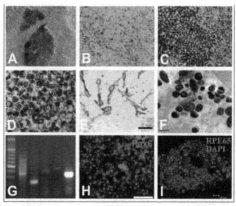

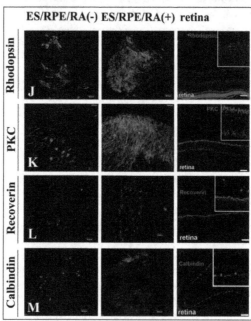

Figure 3. A-I. Analysis of pigmented epithelial cells derived from primate ES cells using LM (A-E), TEM (F), RT-PCR (G), immunofluorescence staining (H-I). (A) LM images showing pigmented cells present in the primate ESC colonies grown at a constant rate on Sertoli feeder cells for 2, 4, and 6 weeks (A,B and C, respectively). The polygonal morphology with a compact cell–cell arrangement (D) is similar to the pigmented epithelium of the eye and clearly distinct from pigmented melanocytes derived from the neural crest (E). (F) TEM images of primate ESC-derived pigmented cells displaying melanin granules. (G) Shown are the RT-PCR-amplified products of RPE cell-specific markers (C1): tyrosinase-related protein-2(Trp-2), RPE65, CRALBP, MertK. (H-I) Immunostaining of RPE cells derived from ES cells with

anti-Pax6 and RPE65 antibody is also shown. J-M. Analysis of differentiated retinal cells induced by ESC-derived RPE cells by immunofluorescence staining. Immunopositive ESC derivatives for retinal cell-specific markers are shown as follows: (J) ES cells were immunopositive for rhodopsin after a 21-day co-culture with RPE cells, and an increased frequency of rhodopsin-positive cells was estimated after RA treatment, and some of them developed into rosettes. The eyes of a db/db mouse (2 weeks) were used as a positive control to identify the positive immunofluorescence staining results and the specificity of retinal antibodies. (K) PKC-positive cells appeared as early as day 3 after starting co-cultures. A drastic increase was observed after RA treatment. Positive control with mouse eyes and PKC antibody is also shown. (L) Recoverin-positive cells appeared after a 10-day o-culture with RPE cells. Expression increased at a constant rate and after RA treatment. Positive control with mouse eyes and recoverin antibody is also shown. (D) After a 10-day co-culture with RPE cells, ES cells became immunopositive for calbindin. Immunopositive ESC derivatives for calbindin are shown at day 2. The number of calbindin-positive cells increased after RA treatment (D2). Positive control with mouse eyes and calbindin antibody is also shown. Scale bars = 50 lm.

3.3. Bone marrow stromal cells as an inducer for cardiomyocyte differentiation from mouse embryonic stem cells

In the third study, bone marrow stromal cells (BMSCs) were used as an inducer to induce cardiomyocyte differentiation from mouse ES cells.

Several studies reported that different feeder layers induced cardiomyocytes from ES cells [64-67]. It proved that the visceral-endoderm-like cell line, END-2 induced mouse P19EC, mouse and human ES cells to aggregate in co-culture and give rise to cultures containing beating areas. For mouse P19 EC cells, it has been demonstrated that a diffusible factor secreted by the END-2 cells is responsible for the induction of cardiomyocyte formation.

Like END-2 cells, various cell types of stem cells remain in a mature body. Among them, bone marrow stem cells (BMSCs) are unique because of rich functional products. A wide array of cytokines including vascular endothelial growth factor (VEGF), basic fibroblast growth factor (bFGF), and insulin growth factor-1 (IGF-1) were detected in the BMSC cultured medium by ELISA [68]. Furthermore, they secreted hepatocyte growth factor (HGF), and transforming growth factors (TGF-beta) [69], which are all potent cardiomyocyte growth and survival factors, or play an important role in proliferation and differentiation of stem cells [70]. IGF-1 can promote angiogenesis in infracted myocardium, reduce the degree of myocardial necrosis, maintain the myocardial structure, stimulate proliferation of cardiac fibroblast, and inhibit matrix degradation; thus preventing ventricular dilatation and reducing load capacity of the heart [71]. After binding to its receptor on ES cells, IGF-1 induces expression of a number of cardiac-specific transcription factors such as the zinc finger GATA proteins and Nkx-2.5, a co-activator of GATA-4. GATA- 4 and Nkx-2.5 are essential for heart development [72]. HGF is a multifunctional factor promoting cell mitosis. It can promote cell survival and regeneration, inhibit the apoptosis of stem cells, and increase the survival rate of transplanted cells. More importantly, HGF enhances growth and favors cell extracellular matrix interactions; the critical steps during myocardial regeneration after infarction. In the heart, high concentration and wide distribution of FGF has been identified from early embryonic stages. Basic FGF plays a vital role in the growth and differentiation of cardiac myocytes. FGF was found to induce DNA synthesis in adult rat myocytes, cells which were considered capable of regeneration [73]. Members of the

TGF-b superfamily play important roles in cardiac development during embryogenesis [74] as well as in various cardiac pathologies [75]. TGF-b1 has been shown to induce cardiac differentiation in vitro in embryonic explants and stem cells [76,77] as well as in adult bone marrow-derived cells [70]. Previous studies of non-conditional global VEGF or VEGF isoform gene deletion have demonstrated embryonic and early postnatal mortality associated with severe cardiac abnormalities and abnormal vascularization; thus establishing that systemic VEGF expression is essential normal myocardial development [78]. From these reports BMSCs are expected to function as inducer for cardiac differentiation from ES cells.

To confirm whether BMSCs are a real cardiac inducer to differentiate ES cells into cardiomyocytes, mouse embryoid bodies (EBs) were co-cultured with rat BMSCs. After about 10 days, areas of rhythmically contracting cells in more solid aggregates became evident with bundle-like structures formed along borders between EB outgrowth and BMSC layer. ESC-derived cardiomyocytes exhibited sarcomeric striations when stained with troponin I (Trop I), organized in separated bundles. Besides, the staining for connexin 43 was detected in cell–cell junctions, which demonstrated that ESC-derived cardiomyocytes were coupled by gap junction in culture (Fig4 A-F). In addition, an improved efficiency of cardiomyocyte differentiation from ESC-BMSC co-culture was found in the serum-free medium: 5-fold up-regulation in the number of beating area compared with the serum medium. Effective cardiac differentiation was also recognized in transfer filter assay and in condition medium obtained from BMSC culture. A clear increase in the expression of cardiac genes and TropI protein confirmed further cardiac differentiation by BMP4 and Retinoic Acid (RA) treatment (Fig4 G,H). These results demonstrate that BMSCs can induce cardiomyocyte differentiation from ES cells through soluble factors and enhance it with BMP4 or RA treatment. Serum-free ESC-BMSC co-culture represents a defined in vitro model for identifying the cardiomyocyte-inducing activity from BMSCs and, in addition, a straightforward experimental system for assessing clinical applications.

In our study, two experiments of separation from BMSCs by the filter and using CM without contact of BMSCs were performed. These results showed that both conditions were still able to induce significant cardiac differentiation (Fig4 I-M). As expected previously, these data have shown that it is due to varied soluble factors secreted by BMSCs, though effective soluble factors have to be determined in future. On the other hand, cardiomyocyte bundles were formed long the edge of EB outgrowth, which was a borderline with BMSC layer. These regular arrangements seemed to be associated with BMSC layer structures. Moreover, in fact, direct cell-to-cell interaction between BMSC and EBs was more effective to induce cardiac differentiation. It may be possible that the supporting environment provided by BMSCs or an interaction between BMSCs and EBs may play a role in their cardiac-inducing activity.

Compared with the inducing effects of low dose cytokines alone or with BMSCs alone, our co-culture with BMSCs supplemented with cytokines could increase the differentiation of cardiomyocytes, which indicated that BMSCs had the ability to promote the induction and proliferation of ESC-derived cardiomyocyte and the addition of low dose cytokines had a synergistic effect on this ability.

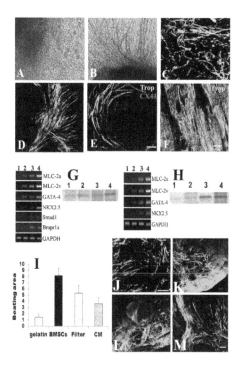

Figure 4. Characterization of cardiomyocyte induced by BMSC co-culture. (A,B) Morphology of serum or non-serum treated EB outgrowth on BMSC layer on day 14. (A) 20% FBS: Multi-angular and flattened cells spread out from EBs. (B) Absence of FBS: fiber-like cells extended radially and formed bundle-like structures each other. Scale Bars = 25um. (C-F) Beating areas stained for Trop I (green) and CX43 (Red). (C) In EBs formed in the presence of FBS, cardiomyocyte fibers are distributed disorderly. (D) Cardiomyocyte fibers are organized regular in EBs formed in the absent of FBS. Radial-morphological-like fibers surrounded or spread from EBs. Beating cells showed spindle, round and tri or multi-angular morphologies with characteristic organized in separated bundles. (E) CX43 staining among TropI-positive cardiomyocytes showed the presence of gap junctions. (F) The heart of C57BL/6 mice was used as a positive control to identify the positive immunofluorescence staining results and the specificity of retinal antibodies. Bars = 100um. **G-H** Examination of expression changes of cardiomyocytes from EBs after BMP4 and RA treatment. (G) Induction of cardiac-specific genes and BMP signaling molecules in EBs exposed to BMP4, as shown by RT-PCR. Lane1: undifferentiated ES cells; lane2: EB cultured on gelatin-coated dish, FBS(–); lane3: EB co-cultured with BMSCs, FBS(–); lane4: EB co-cultured with BMSCs, FBS(–), and treated with BMP4. The expression of cardiac markers and BMP signals were increased markedly by BMP4 treatment. TropI protein was also detected by Western of lysed EB on gelatin-coated dish (lane1), EB on gelatin-coated dish and treated with BMP4 (lane2), EB co-cultured with BMSCs (lane3); EB co-cultured with BMSCs and treated with BMP4 (lane4). Combined using BMP4 and BMSCs induced significant cardiac differentiation. (H) The effect of RA on the differentiation of cardiomyocytes. (D) RT-PCR analysis revealed that both early cardiac genes, MLC-2a and MLC-2v, were increased in RA-treated EBs. Lane1: undifferentiated ES cells; lane2: EB cultured on gelatin-coated dish, FBS(–); lane3: EB co-cultured with BMSCs, FBS(–); lane4: EB co-cultured with BMSCs, FBS(–), and treated with RA. TropI protein was detected by Western of lysed EB on gelatin-coated dish (lane1), EB on gelatin-coated dish and treated with RA (lane2), EB co-cultured with BMSCs (lane3); EB co-cultured with BMSCs and treated with RA (lane4). Combined using RA and BMSCs significantly induced cardiac differentiation. **I-M.** The physical and chemical role of BMSCs in cardiomyocyte induction. (I) BMSCs induced beating cardiomyocytes in co-cultured ES cells even when separated by a filter membrane. CM induced cardiac differentiation in ES cells cultured on gelatin-coated dish. However the differentiation rate was lower than with direct co-culture with BMSCs. (J-M) EB on gelatin-coated dish (J); EB co-cultured with BMSCs (K); TropI staining of ES cells when separated from BMSCs by a filter (L) and cultured in CM alone (M). Scale Bars = 50um.

4. Conclusion

Cell-to-cell interaction is important to differentiate varied cells or tissues from stem cells and/ or in embryogenesis. An important component to the stem cell microenvironment is the surrounding matrix, which includes numerous chemical and biophysical cues. The changing local molecular conditions through selecting specific co-culture system might thereby provide promising method to modulate stem cell differentiation. In our researches, we selected the different kinds of cells as a feeder cell to induce the specific differentiation of stem cells. The molecular basis of induction in co-culture system remains to be understood. We tested some factors that have been implicated in the regulation of differentiation, such as GDNF, bFGF, BMP4, or neutralizing antibodies of GDNF. So far, no significant effect factors on the induction were observed. Interestingly, as showed above, the differentiation efficiency of ES cells in co-culture system is as high as the efficiency in the multiple-step method with lots of growth factors treatment, or even higher than that. The possible explain for this is that supporting environment provided by co-culture basement cells, such as Sertoli, RPE or BMSCs, or an interaction between co-culture basement cells and ES cells, plays a role in their inducing activity.

In conclusion, we established a simple and effective system for the differentiation of specific cells from ES cells. Further study is warranted to establish selection methods, analyze cell functions, and transplanted for degeneration diseases. However, the co-culture system can serve as a promising method for therapeutic applications and basic research on degeneration diseases.

Acknowledgements

We thank Dr. Kametani Kiyokazo and Ms. Suzuki Kayo (Research Center for Instrumental Analysis of Shinshu University, Matsumoto, Japan) for excellent technical assistance.

Author details

Fengming Yue[1], Sakiko Shirasawa[2], Hinako Ichikawa[1], Susumu Yoshie[1], Akimi Mogi[1], Shoko Masuda[1], Mika Nagai[2], Tadayuki Yokohama[2], Tomotsune Daihachiro[1] and Katsunori Sasaki

1 Department of Histology and Embryology, Shinshu University School of Medicine, Matsu-moto, Nagano, Japan

2 Laboratory for Advanced Health Science, Bourbon Institutes of Health, Bourbon Corpora-tion, Matsumoto, Nagano, Japan

References

[1] "New Stem-Cell Procedure Doesn't Harm EmbryosCompany Claims". Fox News. (2006). Retrieved 2010-02-28.

[2] Wu, D. C, & Boyd, A. S. Wood KJ Embryonic stem cell transplantation: potential applicability in cell replacement therapy and regenerative medicine. Front Biosci (2007).

[3] David, A. Conner. Mouse Embryonic Stem (ES) Cell Culture. Current Protocols in Molecular Biology.

[4] Culture of Human Embryonic Stem Cells (hESC)"National Institutes of Health. Retrieved (2010).

[5] Chambers, I, Colby, D, Robertson, M, et al. Functional expression cloning of Nanog, a pluripotency sustaining factor in embryonic stem cells. Cell. (2003). , 113(5), 643-55.

[6] Eyckmans, J, Lin, G. L, & Chen, C. S. Adhesive and mechanical regulation of mesenchymal stem cell differentiation in human bone marrow and periosteum-derived progenitor cells. Biol Open. (2012). , 1(11), 1058-68.

[7] Xie, T, & Spradling, A. C. A niche maintaining germ line stem cells in the Drosophila ovary. Science (2000). , 290, 328-330.

[8] Abbott, A. Cell culture: biology's new dimension. Nature (2003).

[9] Zhang, s. Beyond the Petri dish. Nat Biotechnol (2004). , 22, 151-152.

[10] Cagnin, S, Cimetta, E, Guiducci, C, Martini, P, & Lanfranchi, G. Overview of Micro- and Nano-Technology Tools for Stem Cell Applications: Micropatterned and Microelectronic Devices. Sensors (Basel) (2012). , 12(11), 15947-15982.

[11] Hwang, N. S, Varghese, S, & Elisseeff, J. Controlled differentiation of stem cells. Adv Drug Del Rev (2008). , 60, 199-214.

[12] Chang, C. F, Lee, M. W, Kuo, P. Y, Wang, Y. J, Tu, Y. H, & Hung, S. C. Three-dimensional collagen fiber remodeling by mesenchymal stem cells requires the integrin-matrix interaction. J Biomed Mater Res A (2007). , 80, 466-474.

[13] Ichinose, S, Tagami, M, Muneta, T, Mukohyama, H, & Sekiya, I. Comparative sequential morphological analyses during in vitro chondrogenesis and osteogenesis of mesenchymal stem cells embedded in collagen gels. Med Mol Morphol. (2013). Jan 17 [Epub ahead of print]

[14] Battista, S, Guamieri, D, Borselli, C, Zeppetelli, S, Borzacchiello, A, Mayol, L, Gerbasio, D, Keene, D. R, Ambrosio, L, & Netti, P. A. The effect of matrix composition of 3D constructs on embryonic stem cell differentiation. Biomaterials (2005). , 26, 6194-6207.

[15] Dean, S. K, Yulyana, Y, Williams, G, Sidhu, K. S, & Tuch, B. E. Differentiation of encapsulated embryonic stem cells after transplantation. Transplantation (2006). , 82, 1175-1184.

[16] Wei-jun, S, Bao-yu, W, Xiang-he, S, Li-na, W, Yan-hua, L, Man-qian, Z, Ling-ling, T, & Zong-jin, L. Differentiation of Human Embryonic Stem Cells to Endothelial Cells via Improved Three-dimension Approach. Zhongguo Yi Xue Ke Xue Yuan Xue Bao. (2012). Dec 20;, 34(6), 539-44.

[17] Gerecht, S, Burdick, J. A, Ferreira, L. S, Townsend, S. A, Langer, R, & Vunjak-novakovic, G. Hyaluronic acid hydrogel for controlled self-renewal and differentiation of human embryonic stem cells. PNAS (2007). , 104, 11298-11303.

[18] Mohand-kaci, F, Assoul, N, Martelly, I, Allaire, E, & Zidi, M. Optimized Hyaluronic Acid-Hydrogel Design and Culture Conditions for Preservation of Mesenchymal Stem Cell Properties. Tissue Eng Part C Methods. (2012). Oct 25. [Epub ahead of print]

[19] Dawson, D, Mapili, G, Erickson, K, Taqvi, S, & Roy, K. Biomaterials for stem cell differentiation. Adv Drug Del Rev (2008). , 60, 215-228.

[20] Levenberg, S, Huang, N. F, Lavik, E, Rogers, A. B, Itskovitz-eldor, J, & Langer, R. Differentiation of human embryonic stem cells on three-dimensional polymer scaffolds.PNAS (2003). , 100, 12741-12746.

[21] Caplan, A. I. Adult mesenchymal stem cells for tissue engineering versus regenerative medicine. J Cell Physiol (2007). , 213, 341-347.

[22] Chen, R. R, & Mooney, D. J. Polymeric growth factor delivery strategies for tissue engineering. Pharm Res (2003). , 20, 1103-1112.

[23] Mcbeath, R, Pirone, D. M, Nelson, C. M, Bhadriraju, K, & Chen, C. S. Cell shape, cytoskeletal tension, and RhoA regulate stem cell lineage commitment. Develop Cell (2004). , 6, 483-495.

[24] Shirasawa, S, Yoshie, S, Yokoyama, T, Tomotsune, D, Yue, F, & Sasaki, K. A novel stepwise differentiation of functional pancreatic exocrine cells from embryonic stem cells. Stem Cells Dev (2011). , 20, 1071-1078.

[25] Sasaki, K, Ichikawa, H, Takei, S, No, H. S, Tomotsune, D, Kano, Y, Yokoyama, T, Shirasawa, S, Mogi, A, Yoshie, S, Sasaki, S, Yamada, S, Matsumoto, K, Mizuguchi, M, Yue, F, & Tanaka, Y. Hepatocyte differentiation from human ES cells using the simple embryoid body formation method and the staged-additional cocktail. ScientificWorldJournal. (2009). , 9, 884-890.

[26] Calza, L, Giuliani, A, & Fernandez, A. Neural stem cells and cholinergic neurons: Regulation by immunolesion and treatment with mitogens, retinoic acid, and nerve growth factor. Proc Natl Acad Sci USA (2003). , 100, 7325-7330.

[27] Bjorklund, A, & Lindvall, O. Cell replacement therapies for central nervous system disorders. Nat Neurosci (2000). , 3, 537-544.

[28] Rath, A, Klein, A, Papazoglou, A, Pruszak, J, Garciaa, J, Krause, M, Maciaczyk, J, Dunnett, S. B, & Nikkhah, G. Survival and Functional Restoration of Human Fetal Ventral Mesencephalon Following Transplantation in a Rat Model of Parkinson's Disease. Cell Transplant. (2012). Sep 7. [Epub ahead of print]

[29] Rosenthal, A. Auto transplants for Parkinson's disease? Neuron (1998). , 20, 169-172.

[30] Kim, J. H, Auerbach, J. M, Rodrigues-gomez, J. A, et al. Dopamine neuronsderived from embryonic stem cells function in an animal model of Parkinson's disease. Nature (2002). , 418, 50-56.

[31] Lescaudron, L, Naveilhan, P, & Neveu, I. The use of stem cells in regenerative medicine for Parkinson's and Huntington's diseases. Curr Med Chem. (2012). , 19(35), 6018-6035.

[32] Apostolides, C, Sanford, E, Hong, M, et al. Glial cell line-derived neurotrophic factor improves intrastriatal graft survival of stored dopaminergic cells. Neuroscience (1998). , 83, 363-372.

[33] Hynes, M, & Rosenthal, A. Specification of dopaminergic and serotonergic neurons in the vertebrate CNS. Curr Opin Neurobiol (1999). , 9, 26-36.

[34] Kirik, D, Georgievska, B, Rosenblad, C, et al. Delayed infusion of GDNF promotes recovery of motor function in the partial lesion model of Parkinson's disease. Eur J Neurosci (2001). , 13, 1589-1599.

[35] Rosenblad, C, Kirik, D, & Bjorklund, A. Sequential administration of GDNF into the substantia nigra and striatum promotes dopamine neuron survival and axonal sprouting but not striatal reinnervation or functional recovery in the partial 6-OH dopamine lesion model. Exp Neurol (2000). , 161, 503-516.

[36] Littrell, O. M, Granholm, A. C, Gerhardt, G. A, & Boger, H. A. Glial cell-line derived neurotrophic factor (GDNF) replacement attenuates motor impairments and nigrostriatal dopamine deficits in month-old mice with a partial deletion of GDNF. Pharmacol Biochem Behav. (2013). Jan 2. [Epub ahead of print], 12.

[37] Johansson, M, Friedemann, M, Hoffer, B, et al. Effects of glial cell line-derived neurotrophic factor on developing and mature ventral mesencephalic grafts in oculo. Exp Neurol (1995). , 134, 25-34.

[38] Apostolides, C, Sanford, E, Hong, M, et al. Glial cell line-derived neurotrophic factor improves intrastriatal graft survival of stored dopaminergic cells. Neuroscience (1998). , 83, 363-372.

[39] Yurek, D. M. Glial cell line-derived neurotrophic factor improves survival of dopaminergic neurons in transplants of fetal ventral mesencephalic tissue. Exp Neurol (1998). , 153, 195-202.

[40] Du, Y, Zhang, X, Tao, Q, Chen, S, & Le, W. Adeno-associated virus type 2 vector-mediated glial cell line-derived neurotrophic factor gene transfer induces neuroprotection and neuroregeneration in a ubiquitin-proteasome system impairment animal model of Parkinson's disease. Neurodegener Dis. (2013). , 11(3), 113-128.

[41] Roussa, E, & Krieglstein, K. GDNF promotes neuronal differentiation and dopaminergic development of mouse mesencephalic neurospheres. Neurosci Lett (2004). , 361, 52-55.

[42] Buytaert-hoefen, K. A, Alvarez, E, & Freed, C. R. Generation of tyrosine hydroxylase positive neurons from human embryonic stem cells after co-culture with cellular substrates and exposure to GDNF. Stem Cells (2004). , 22, 669-674.

[43] Emerich, D. F, Hemendinger, R, & Halberstadt, C. R. The testicular-derived Sertoli cell: cellular immunoscience to enable transplantation. Cell Transplant (2003). , 12, 335-349.

[44] Lee, S. H, Lumelsky, N, Studer, L, et al. Efficient generation of midbrain and hindbrain neurons from mouse embryonic stem cells. Nat Biotechnol (2000). , 18, 675-679.

[45] Kawasaki, H, Mizuseki, K, Nishikawa, S, et al. Induction of midbrain dopaminergic neurons from ES cells by stromal cell-derived inducing activity. Neuron (2000). , 28, 31-40.

[46] Kawasaki, H, Suemori, H, Mizuseki, K, et al. Generation of dopaminergic neurons and pigmented epithelia from primate ES cells by stromal cell-derived inducing activity. Proc Natl Acad Sci USA (2002). , 99, 1580-1585.

[47] Zeng, X, Cai, J, Chen, J, et al. Dopaminergic differentiation of human embryonic stem cells. Stem Cells (2004). , 22, 925-940.

[48] Swistowska, A. M. da Cruz, A.B., Han, Y., Swistowski, A., Liu, Y., Shin, S., Zhan, M., Rao, M.S., Zeng, X. Stage-specific role for shh in dopaminergic differentiation of human embryonic stem cells induced by stromal cells. Stem Cells Dev. (2010). , 19(1), 71-82.

[49] Lin, N, Fan, W, Sheedlo, H. J, et al. Photoreceptor repair in response to RPE transplants in RCS rats: outer segment regeneration. Curr Eye Res. (1996). , 15, 1069-1077.

[50] Reh, T. A. Cellular interactions determine neuronal phenotypes in rodent retinal cultures. J Neurobiol. (1992). , 23, 1067-1083.

[51] Mcusic, A. C, Lamba, D. A, & Reh, T. A. Guiding the morphogenesis of dissociated newborn mouse retinal cells and hES cell-derived retinal cells by soft lithography-patterned microchannel PLGA scaffolds. Biomaterials. (2012). , 33(5), 1396-1405.

[52] Osakada, F, Ikeda, H, Sasai, Y, & Takahashi, M. Stepwise differentiation of pluripotent stem cells into retinal cells. Nat Protoc. (2009). , 4, 811-824.

[53] Osakada, F, Ikeda, H, Mandai, M, et al. Toward the generation of rod and cone photoreceptors from mouse, monkey and human embryonic stem cells. Nat Biotechnol. (2008). , 2, 215-224.

[54] Hicks, D, & Courtois, Y. Fibroblast growth factor stimulates photoreceptor differentiation in vitro. J Neurosci. (1992). , 12, 2022-2033.

[55] Ruiz i Altaba AJessell TM. Retinoic acid modifies the pattern of cell differentiation in the central nervous system of neurula stage Xenopus embryos. Development. (1991). , 112, 945-958.

[56] Kelley, M. W, Xu, X. M, Wagner, M. A, et al. The developing organ of Corti contains retinoic acid and forms supernumerary hair cells in response to exogenous retinoic acid in culture. Development. (1993). , 119, 1041-1053.

[57] Kelley, M. W, Turner, J. K, & Reh, T. A. Retinoic acid promotes differentiation of photoreceptors in vitro. Development. (1994). , 120, 2091-2102.

[58] Klimanskaya, I, Hipp, J, & Rezai, K. A. Derivation and comparative assessment of retinal pigment epithelium from human embryonic stem cells using transcriptomics. Cloning Stem Cells. (2004). , 6, 217-245.

[59] Ikeda, H, Osakada, F, Watanabe, K, et al. Generation of Rx+/Pax6+ neural retinal precursors from embryonic stem cells. Proc Natl Acad Sci U S A. (2005). , 102, 11331-11336.

[60] Lamba, D. A, Karl, M. O, Ware, C. B, & Reh, T. A. Efficient generation of retinal progenitor cells from human embryonic stem cells. Proc Natl Acad Sci U S A. (2006). , 103(34), 12769-12774.

[61] La TorreA., Lamba, D.A., Jayabalu, A., Reh, T.A. Production and transplantation of retinal cells from human and mouse embryonic stem cells. Methods Mol Biol. (2012). , 884, 229-246.

[62] Lamba, D. A, Gust, J, & Reh, T. A. Transplantation of human embryonic stem cell-derived photoreceptors restores some visual function in Crx-deficient mice. Cell Stem Cell. (2009). , 4, 73-79.

[63] Marsh-armstrong, N, Mccaffery, P, Gilbert, W, et al. Retinoic acid is necessary for development of the ventral retina in zebrafish. Proc Natl Acad Sci U S A. (1994). , 91, 7286-7290.

[64] Mummery, C. L, & Van Achterberg, T. A. van den Eijnden-van Raaij, A.J., van Haaster, L., Willemse, A., de Laat, S. W., Piersma, A.H. Visceral-endoderm-like cell lines induce differentiation of murine embryonal carcinoma cells. Differentiation (1991). , 19.

[65] Shim, W. S, Jiang, S, & Wong, P. Ex vivo differentiation of human adult bone marrow stem cells into cardiomyocyte-like cells. Biochem. Biophys. Res. Commun. (2004). , 324, 481-488.

[66] Van den Eijnden-van RaaijA.J., van Achterberg, T.A., van der Kruijssen, C.M., Piersma, A.H., Huylebroeck, D., de Laat, S.W., Mummery, C.L. Differentiation of aggregated murine embryonal carcinoma cells is induced by a novel visceral endoderm-specific FGF-like factor and inhibited by activin A. Mech. Dev. (1991). , 19.

[67] Pal, R, Mamidi, M. K, Das, A. K, & Bhonde, R. Comparative analysis of cardiomyocyte differentiation from human embryonic stem cells under 3-D and 2-D culture conditions. J Biosci Bioeng. (2013). , 115(2), 200-206.

[68] Xu, M, Uemura, R, Dai, Y, Wang, Y, Pasha, Z, & Ashraf, M. In vitro and in vivo effects of bone marrow stem cells on cardiac structure and function. J Mol Cell Cardiol. (2007). , 42(2), 441-448.

[69] Soltan, M, Smiler, D, & Choi, J. H. Bone marrow: orchestrated cells, cytokines, and growth factors for bone regeneration. Implant Dent. (2009). , 18(2), 132-141.

[70] Li, Z, Gu, T. X, & Zhang, Y. H. Hepatocyte growth factor combined with insulin like growth factor-1 improves expression of GATA-4 in mesenchymal stem cells co-cultured with cardiomyocytes.Chin Med J (Engl). (2008). , 121(4), 336-340.

[71] Florini, J. R, Ewton, D. Z, & Magri, K. A. Hormones, growth factors, and myogenic differentiation. Annu. Rev. Physiol. (1991). , 53, 201-216.

[72] Pampusch, M. S, Kamanga-sollo, E, & White, M. E. Effect of recombinant porcine IGF-binding protein-3 on proliferation of embryonic porcine myogenic cell cultures in the presence and absence of IGF-I. J Endocrinol. (2003). , 176, 227-235.

[73] Speir, E, Tanner, V, Gonzalez, A. M, Farris, J, Baird, A, & Casscells, W. Acidic and basic fibroblast growth factors in adult rat heart myocytes. Localization, regulation in culture, and effects on DNA synthesis. Circ Res. (1992). , 71(2), 251-9.

[74] Valdimarsdottir, G, & Mummery, C. Functions of the TGF-b superfamily in human embryonic stem cells. Apmis (2005). , 113, 773-789.

[75] Sakata, Y, Chancey, A. L, Divakaran, V. G, Sekiguchi, K, Sivasubramanian, N, & Mann, D. L. Transforming growth factorbeta receptor antagonism attenuates myocardial fibrosis in mice with cardiac- restricted overexpression of tumor necrosis factor. Basic Res Cardiol (2008). , 103, 60-68.

[76] Bodmer, R. Heart development in Drosophila and its relationship to vertebrates. Trends. Cardiovasc. Med. (1995). , 5, 21-28.

[77] Garside, V. C, Chang, A. C, Karsan, A, & Hoodless, P. A. Co-ordinating Notch, BMP, and TGF-β signaling during heart valve development. Cell Mol Life Sci. (2012). Nov 16. [Epub ahead of print]

[78] Giordano, F. J, Gerber, H. P, & Williams, S. P. A cardiac myocyte vascular endothelial growth factor paracrine pathway is required to maintain cardiac function. Proc. Natl. Acad. Sci. U.S.A. (2001). , 98, 5780-5785.

Chapter 6

Oral and Maxillofacial Tissue Engineering with Adipose-Derived Stem Cells

Morikuni Tobita and Hiroshi Mizuno

Additional information is available at the end of the chapter

1. Introduction

Oral and maxillofacial tissues are a complex array of bone, cartilage, soft tissue, nerves and vasculature. Damage to these structures, even when minimal, usually leads to noticeable deformities. Therefore, the repair of large segmental bone defects of the jaw or mandible due to trauma, inflammation, or tumor surgery remains a major clinical problem. For many years, simple autogenic, allogenic, or xenogenic bone grafts, or combinations thereof, have been the mainstay for tissue replacement [1]. However, when large bone defects are present, advanced approaches such as free tissue transfer with microvascular reanastomosis of vascularized flaps from distant sites including the fibula, iliac crest, scapula, and radius are needed to repair or regenerate a functionally complex tissue such as maxillofacial tissue [2, 3]. While these procedures have proven to be reliable and effective, they require extended hospitalization, and a secondary donor site with the associated morbidity and complications. As an alternative to current surgical techniques or approaches, developments in tissue engineering using the gene therapy and stem cell biology strive to utilize cells, biomaterial scaffolds and cell signaling factors to regenerate large oral and maxillofacial tissues defect with precise replication of normal body contours. A tissue engineering approach offers several potential benefits, including a decrease in donor site morbidity, a decrease in technical sensitivity of the repair, and the ability to closely mimic the in vivo microenvironment in an attempt to recapitulate normal craniofacial development [1].

Mesenchymal stem cells (MSCs) derived from bone marrow have been used experimentally for tissue engineering applications [4-6]. MSCs can differentiate into several different cell types, such as those that produce bone, cartilage, tendon, and other connective tissues, as well as muscle, adipose, and dermal cells [7-10]. MSCs can be expanded in culture while maintaining their multipotency.

The concept of prefabricated bone engineering with MSCs for large bone defects may play a pivotal role in future therapies. However, bone marrow-derived MSCs have been reported to require selective sera lots and growth factor supplements for culture expansion [11]. Furthermore, traditional bone marrow procurement, particularly in volumes larger than a few milliliters may be painful, frequently requiring general or spinal anesthesia [12-14].

Bone marrow tissue provides the most universal and attractive source of MSCs; however, other tissues such as periosteal [15], muscle [16], synovial membrane [17] and adipose [18-20] tissues also appear to possess MSCs. Particularly, adipose tissue is an important source of stem cells because subcutaneous adipose tissue is an abundant and accessible source of both uncultured stromal vascular fraction (SVF) cells and cultured homogeneous adipose-derived stem cells (ASCs) (21). ASCs obtained from lipoaspirates have multilineage potential and will differentiate into adipogenic, chondrogenic, myogenic, osteogenic, and neurogenic cells [19, 22, 23]. Thus, ASCs have great potential for clinical applications such as the repair of damaged tissues and angiogenic therapy. Injection of human ASCs was recently shown to improve neovascularization in an ischemic hindlimb mouse model and osteoid matrix formation in immunotolerant mice [24-26]. Further, ASCs have been shown to increase the functional capacity of damaged skeletal muscle in vivo [27]. Therefore, these reports suggest that ASCs may also have the potential for use in large bone tissue engineering techniques such as prefabrication. Recently, prefabricated bone engineered with ASCs was reported both with in vivo studies in rat and a clinical human case. Thus, the use of ASCs in maxillofacial tissue reconstruction should be viewed favorably and these novel approaches may have advantages for tissue reconstruction.

In this chapter, the current approaches and the biomaterials used for repair of large bone defects are presented, and the novel approach of prefabricated bone engineering with MSCs and ASCs is introduced.

2. Current therapy for large bone reconstruction

Bone tissue is composed of heterogeneous cell types embedded in a three-dimensional mineralized extracellular matrix. The scaffolds for repair of large bone defects, including autogenous bone grafts or biomaterials, must provide the necessary support for cells to proliferate while maintaining their potential to differentiate, and must possess an architecture suitable for matching the final shape of the newly formed bone [28].

2.1. Autologous bone reconstruction

The current standard of care for repair of critical large bone defects consists of autogenous bone grafting using bone from the rib or iliac crest of the patient. An autologous bone graft is still the ideal material for the repair of craniofacial defects; however, the availability of autologous bone is limited and harvesting can be associated with complications [29]. Vascularized and avascular autogenous bone has a greater osteogenic capacity than any other bone replacement material, as revascularization attracts mesenchymal differentiation into osteogenic, chondrogenic and other cell types. Autogenous bone transplants possess an inherent biocompatibility and are therefore more easily incorporated without immunogenic responses [30]. However, the clinical use of autologous bone transplants is limited by considerable donor site morbidity, which increases with the amount of harvested bone. Bleeding, hematomas, infections, and chronic pain are common complications of autologous bone graft harvests [31, 32].

2.2. Allogenic/Xenogenic bone reconstruction

Demineralized bone matrix (DMB) is the de-cellularized and organic component of bone, and is a commercially available osteoinductive and osteoconductive biomaterial. DMB represents a concentrated source of bone morphogenetic proteins (BMPs) and has been used in numerous animals systems since its initial description in 1965 [33]. The widespread use of DMB in humans still remains restricted since the immunologic properties of donor DMB are unknown [34].

With the disadvantages of host morbidity and the limits in suitable harvesting sites and material for autologous grafts, the use of xenografts might be considered for large bone reconstructions, although the histocompatibility issues between the human recipient and animal donor preclude the use of bone xenografts [34]. However, bovine-derived DMB is currently used in oral and maxillofacial surgery [35].

2.3. Synthetic scaffolds for bone reconstruction

A wide variety of synthetic (alloplastic) scaffolds such as ceramics and polymers are used clinically for bone grafting [30]. Ceramics are crystalline, inorganic, nonmetallic minerals that are held together by ionic bonds and usually densified by sintering [36]. Ceramics such as hydroxyapatite and β-tricalcium phosphate (TCP) are currently in use clinically for bone tissue regeneration of large bone defects.

Various synthetic polymer scaffolds exhibit different structural, mechanical and degradation properties that make then suitable for bone tissue engineering [36]. Blending polymers of different molecular weights can achieve both optimal degradation rates and mechanical properties [37]. Some synthetic polymer scaffolds such as polycaprolactone (PCL) scaffold, polylactic acid (PLLA), polyglycolic acid (PGA) and polylactic-co-glycolic acid (PLGA) materials have been approved by the FDA for craniofacial applications or as absorbable sutures and bone pins/screws [36].

2.4. Gene therapy for bone reconstruction

The use of exogenous cytokines and growth factors, which are essential for bone regeneration, promotes cell adhesion, proliferation, migration and osteogenic differentiation [28]. Growth factors such as BMPs, fibroblast growth factors (FGFs), insulin-like growth factors (IGF), vascular endothelial growth factors (VEGF) and platelet-derived growth factors (PDGF) have been used in bone regeneration [28, 36].

Recently the use of combinations of growth factors, such as BMP-2 and NEL-like molecule-1 (NELL-1), was tested in rapid distraction osteogenesis in a rabbit model. The combined treatment produced significantly greater bone healing compared to single growth factor treatments after four weeks of treatment [38]. However, some reports have cautioned that the clinical use of BMPs and VEGF is in its infancy, and some risks may accompany their use. VEGF is commonly upregulated in various types of tumors to enhance their vascularization, and subcutaneous sarcomas were found in some rats administered recombinant human BMP-7 [39, 40], although no clinical relationship has been established between the use of these growth factors and tumor formation.

2.5. Prefabricated bone engineering for oral and maxillofacial tissue reconstruction

Prefabrication is an interesting area of oral and maxillofacial surgery and plastic and recon-structive surgery, because it represents a bridge between conventional reconstructive surgery and tissue engineering [41, 42]. The purpose of prefabrication is to build a tissue (muscle, bone, skin, or composite) with characteristics as similar as possible to those of the defect that is to be repaired [43]. Conventional osteomyocutaneous flaps do not always meet the requirements for repairing a composite defect. A prefabricated composite flap can be created according to the complex geometry of the defect. Prefabrication of multi-component flaps is a well estab-lished procedure in plastic and reconstructive surgery [41]. This concept is based on the revascularization phenomenon directly related to host tissue vascularity [44] and has signifi-cantly expanded the frontiers of reconstructive surgery.

Hirase et al. were the first to report the use of prefabricated myocutaneous and osteomyocu-taneous tissue in a rat model [45]. Flap prefabrication using conventional bone grafts allows for generation of new types of flaps independent of the vascular anatomy of the bone trans-plant. However, the donor site morbidity after harvesting of bone for grafting is still a problem. Recently, biomaterials, osteogenic cells and osteoinductive growth factors have been used for generation of vascularized bone tissues in combination with a vascular axis or vascularized flaps. An inflammatory wound healing response as a reaction to the surgical implantation induces vascularization of the scaffolds [31]. Induction of axial vascularization protected the porous biomaterials from bacterial infection and transfer of this vascularized hard tissue as a free flap has been demonstrated [46]. Prefabricated vascularized bone grafts have been used in a clinical setting for mandibular reconstruction following thorough in vivo evaluation in a pig model [47-49]. In these studies, granules of xenogenic bone minerals soaked with recombi-nant Osteogenic protein-1 were implanted into the latissimus dorsi muscle and the neo-tissue was subsequently transferred to sites of mandibular defects using microsurgical techniques.

3. Mesenchymal stem cells for oral and maxillofacial tissue reconstruction

3.1. Mesenchymal stem cells for bone engineering

The bone marrow is not only the site where hematopoiesis occurs in postnatal life, it is also a reservoir of pluripotent stem cells for mesenchymal tissues [50]. Plated at low densities, single precursor cells derived from bone marrow, and referred to as colony-forming units, give rise to distinct and heterogeneous colonies. These colonies have been shown to undergo osteogenic, chondrogenic and adipogenic differentiation [51].

Chang and colleagues showed that MSCs can produce ectopic bone generation in a mouse model [52]. A suspension of osteogenically induced MSCs was added to 2% alginate, which was then gelled by mixing with calcium sulfate. The gel was injected subcutaneously on the dorsal side of the experimental animals. Histological examination of the implants revealed signs of endochondrosis with woven bone deposition. The equilibrium modulus of the newly formed bone increased with time up to 678 kPa at 30 weeks, as determined by biomechanical analysis. This value is approximately 1.62% of native bovine cancellous bone. In another study [53] of large mandibular bone defect repair, dog MSCs cultured with ß-TCP to generate osteogenic cells were co-implanted with a titanium plate into a 30 mm segmental mandible defect. Biomechanical tests showed a significant difference between the experimental group (with cells) and the control group (without cells), highlighting the importance of the MSCs in bone formation. Pedicled bone flaps based on collagen I scaffolds, bone marrow stromal cells and a PTFE membrane have been successfully generated using the carotid artery and jugular vein or the saphenous bundle as a vascular axis in a mouse model [54]. The osteogenetic stimulus was supplied by the injection of mouse MSCs cultured in osteogenic medium inside the space delimited by the PTFE membrane. After only 4 weeks islands of bone tissue were present inside the membrane.

3.2. Clinical trials for bone engineering with mesenchymal stem cells

There is some clinical experience with bone reconstruction using expanded MSCs combined with scaffolds. Constructs of expanded autologous MSCs in macroporous hydroxyapatite were used in three patients with large segmental bone defects [55, 56].

Warnke and Terheyden have developed a two stage procedure for mandible reconstruction in humans [57]. This study used prefabrication in the latissimus dorsi muscle with the aim of reconstructing a 70 mm defect in the mandible of a man who underwent a tumor resection years previously. The entire construction of the mandible was built using blocks of Bio-Oss® and MSCs that had been cultured in the presence of BMP-7. The Bio-Oss® and MSCs were placed in a titanium cage, and implanted into the latissimus dorsi of the patient and maintained in situ for 7 weeks. Subsequently, this unit, together with the vascular bundle that supplied it, was removed and re-implanted in the mandible defect by fixation with titanium plates and microvascular sutures connecting the vasculature to the external carotid artery and the cephalic vein.

4. Adipose-derived stem cells for oral and maxillofacial tissue engineering

4.1. Characterization of adipose-derived stem cells

There is a general consensus that SVF cells are a heterogeneous population, and no specific ranges for each subpopulation have been agreed upon formally [21]. In contrast, the International Society for Cell Therapy has provided guidelines for the definition of MSCs, as follows. (1) MSCs must be plastic-adherent when maintained in standard culture conditions. (2) MSCs must express CD105, CD73 and CD90, and lack expression of CD45, CD34, CD14 or CD11b, CD79α or CD19 and HLA-DR surface antigens. (3) MSCs must differentiate into osteoblasts, adipocytes and chondroblasts in vitro [58].

SVF cells include preadipocytes, fibroblasts, vascular smooth muscle cells, endothelial cells (ECs), resident monocytes/macrophages, lymphocytes and ASCs [59]. Although the criteria to define SVF cells remain in contention, the heterogeneous SVF cell population includes putative ASCs (CD31-, CD34+/-, CD45-, CD90+, CD105-, CD146-), endothelial (progenitor) cells (CD31+, CD34+, CD45-, CD90+, CD105-, CD146+), vascular smooth muscle cells or pericytes (CD31-, CD34+/-, CD45-, CD90+, CD105-, CD146+), and hematopoietic cells (CD45+) in uncultured conditions [60]. Cultured ASCs show an extensive proliferative ability in an uncommitted state while retaining their multilineage differentiation potential. ASCs express the mesenchymal stem cell markers CD10, CD13, CD29, CD34, CD44, CD54, CD71, CD90, CD105, CD106, CD117, CD166 and STRO-1. They are negative for the hematopoietic lineage markers CD45, CD14, CD16, CD56, CD61, CD62E, CD104, and CD106 and for the EC markers CD31, CD144, and von Willebrand factor [20, 61, 62]. Morphologically, cultured ASCs are fibroblast-like and preserve their shape after expansion in vitro [20, 63]. The ASC specific surface markers CD29, CD90, and CD166 increase during culture [64]. In later passages, ASC cultures are homogeneous and exhibit fibroblastoid morphology. The composition of the subpopulations, therefore, may change during expansion [65, 66]. Therefore ASCs match the standard criteria for MSCs.

4.2. Differentiation potential of osteogenic cells in vitro and in vivo

Numerous studies have presented results that clearly show that ASCs can differentiate into osteoblasts [20, 59, 63, 67, 68]. ASCs exhibit a time-dependent expression of genes and proteins associated with the osteoblast phenotype, including ALP, Type I Collagen, OPN, ON, RUNX2, BMP-2, BMP-4 and BMP receptors I and II [20, 67, 69, 70]. Additionally, between 2 and 4 weeks of culture, mineralization of the extracellular matrix begins and proceeds via the activity of ALP, an enzyme that hydrolyzes phosphate esters making available inorganic phosphate to form hydroxyapatite [19, 20, 71].

Furthermore, recent reports have shown that ASCs co-cultured with ECs exhibit enhanced osteogenesis [72, 73]. ASCs exhibited increased secretion of alkaline phosphatase and osteocalcin, and an overall increase in osteogenesis in the co-cultured situation compare with other experimental groups. These interactions may be important to regenerate bone in large bone defects since angiogenesis plays a key role in regeneration of large amounts of tissue.

4.3. Fabricated bone engineering with adipose-derived stem cells

To make a functional prefabricated bone, three elements are required: scaffolds to provide a three-dimensional support, growth factors to stimulate neovascularization, and MSCs to give an osteoinductive stimulus. Okuda et al. have reported prefabrication of tissue engineered bone grafts using ASCs in a rat model [74]. ASCs and porous β-TCP as scaffold material were implanted into the superficial inferior epigastric artery flap. After prefabrication for eight weeks, the prefabricated flaps were elevated and the pedicles were clamped for 4 h; prefabricated tissue was harvested two weeks later. The osteogenic capacity of the prefabricated graft was not significantly different from non-prefabricated grafts examined after two weeks in a rat model. Furthermore, an analysis of angiogenesis suggested that the prefabricated model possessed significantly greater capillary density than the non-prefabricated model.

Recently, repair of a large bony defect using ASCs was clinically reported [75-77] (Table. 1). Mesima°ki and colleagues published a clinical case report of prefabricated bone tissue engineering [77]. The large bony defect was reconstructed with a microvascular flap using autologous ASCs, β-TCP and BMP-2, 36 months after a hemimaxillectomy due to a large keratocyst. After expansion of ASCs and cultivation with β-TCP and BMP-2 in vitro, a titanium cage filled with ASCs and β-TCP was inserted through a vertical incision into a pouch prepared in the patient's left rectus abdominis muscle. The rectus abdominis free flap was raised. Before severing the vascular supply to the muscle, the muscle pouch was carefully opened and the titanium cage was opened. After severing the vessels, the flap was placed in the maxillary defect; the inferior epigastric artery was anastomosed end-to-end to the facial artery and the vein end-to-end to the facial vein.

Clinical reports/trials with ASCs	Design	Results	Ref
Widespread calvarial defect	Autologous SVFs with fibrin glue	Success, follow-up: 3 months after operation	[75]
Large calvarial defect	Implant autologous cultured ASCs with β-TCP	No complications, follow-up: 3 months after operations	[76]
Maxillary reconstruction	Fabricated bone tissue using autologous cultured ASCs with β-TCP and BMP-2	Success, follow-up: 8 months after operations	[77]
Large osseous defect	Autologous ASCs with different scaffolds	Recruiting	NCT01218945 *
Avascular Necrosis of the Femoral Head	Autologous adipose tissue derived MSCs transplantation	Phase 1, 2	NCT01532076 *

Abbreviations: SVF; Stromal Vascular Fraction, ASCs; Adipose-derived Stem Cells, β-TCP; Beta-tricalcium phosphate, MSCs; mesenchymal stem cells, BMP; bone morphogenetic protein

(*Identifier on Clinical trials website: *http://clinicaltrials.gov/ct2/results?term=adipose+derived+cells+bone).

Table 1. Clinical reports/trials for large bony defect using adipose-derived stem cells

5. Future perspective

In the past decade, basic research characterizing ASCs shows that these cells have the potential to regenerate tissue defects such as large bone defects, and clinical studies have examined the potential use of ASCs to reconstruct oral and maxillofacial tissue. Although clinical studies have only just begun, the use of ASCs in the clinical setting is extremely promising because ASCs are a readily available, multipotent, and abundant cell type with the capability to undergo robust osteogenesis. However, further studies, including research to determine the mechanism of osteogenic differentiation and studies to evaluate the safety of ASC usage, will be necessary to realize the potential of ASCs in clinical regenerative medicine of the future.

Author details

Morikuni Tobita and Hiroshi Mizuno*

*Address all correspondence to: hmizuno@juntendo.ac.jp

Department of Plastic and Reconstructive Surgery, Juntendo University School of Medicine, Japan

References

[1] Ward BB, Brown SE, Krebsbach PH. Bioengineering strategies for regeneration of craniofacial bone: a review of emerging technologies. Oral Dis 2010;16(8):709-716.

[2] Disa JJ, Cordeiro PG. Mandible reconstruction with microvascular surgery. Semin Surg Oncol 2000;19(3):226-234.

[3] Emerick KS, Teknos TN. State-of-the-art mandible reconstruction using revascularized free-tissue transfer. Expert Rev Anticancer Ther 2007;7(12):1781-1788.

[4] Caplan AI. Mesenchymal stem cells. J Orthop Res 1991;9(5):641-650.

[5] Pittenger MF, Mackay AM, Beck SC, Jaiswal RK, Douglas R, Mosca JD, et al. Multilineage potential of adult human mesenchymal stem cells. Science 1999;284(5411): 143-147.

[6] Prockop DJ. Marrow stromal cells as stem cells for nonhematopoietic tissues. Science 1997;276(5309):71-74.

[7] Caplan AI. Adult mesenchymal stem cells for tissue engineering versus regenerative medicine. J Cell Physiol 2007;213(2):341-347.

[8] Chamberlain G, Fox J, Ashton B, Middleton J. Concise review: mesenchymal stem cells: their phenotype, differentiation capacity, immunological features, and potential for homing. Stem Cells 2007;25(11):2739-2749.

[9] Nixon AJ, Watts AE, Schnabel LV. Cell- and gene-based approaches to tendon regeneration. J Shoulder Elbow Surg 2012;21(2):278-294.

[10] Markowicz M, Koellensperger E, Neuss S, Koenigschulte S, Bindler C, Pallua N. Human bone marrow mesenchymal stem cells seeded on modified collagen improved dermal regeneration in vivo. Cell Transplant 2006;15(8-9):723-732.

[11] Donald P. Lennon SEH, Scott P. Bruder, Neelam Jaiswal and Arnold I. Caplan. Human and animal mesenchymal progenitor cells from bone marrow: Identification of serum for optimal selection and proliferation. In Vitro Cell Dev Biol 1996;32(10): 602-611.

[12] Auquier P, Macquart-Moulin G, Moatti JP, Blache JL, Novakovitch G, Blaise D, et al. Comparison of anxiety, pain and discomfort in two procedures of hematopoietic stem cell collection: leukacytapheresis and bone marrow harvest. Bone Marrow Transplant 1995;16(4):541-547.

[13] Nishimori M, Yamada Y, Hoshi K, Akiyama Y, Hoshi Y, Morishima Y, et al. Health-related quality of life of unrelated bone marrow donors in Japan. Blood 2002;99(6): 1995-2001.

[14] De Ugarte DA, Morizono K, Elbarbary A, Alfonso Z, Zuk PA, Zhu M, et al. Comparison of multi-lineage cells from human adipose tissue and bone marrow. Cells Tissues Organs 2003;174(3):101-109.

[15] Ball MD, Bonzani IC, Bovis MJ, Williams A, Stevens MM. Human periosteum is a source of cells for orthopaedic tissue engineering: a pilot study. Clin Orthop Relat Res 2011;469(11):3085-3093.

[16] Wu X, Wang S, Chen B, An X. Muscle-derived stem cells: isolation, characterization, differentiation, and application in cell and gene therapy. Cell Tissue Res. 2010;340(3): 549-567.

[17] Jo CH, Ahn HJ, Kim HJ, Seong SC, Lee MC. Surface characterization and chondrogenic differentiation of mesenchymal stromal cells derived from synovium. Cytotherapy 2007;9(4):316-327.

[18] Tobita M, Orbay H, Mizuno H. Adipose-derived stem cells: current findings and future perspectives. Discov Med 2011;11(57):160-170.

[19] Zuk PA, Zhu M, Mizuno H, Huang J, Futrell JW, Katz AJ, et al. Multilineage cells from human adipose tissue: implications for cell-based therapies. Tissue Eng 2001;7(2):211-228.

[20] Zuk PA, Zhu M, Ashjian P, De Ugarte DA, Huang JI, Mizuno H, et al. Human adipose tissue is a source of multipotent stem cells. Mol Biol Cell 2002;13(12):4279-4295.

[21] Gimble JM, Bunnell BA, Chiu ES, Guilak F. Concise review: Adipose-derived stromal vascular fraction cells and stem cells: let's not get lost in translation. Stem Cells 2011;29(5):749-754.

[22] Mizuno H, Zuk PA, Zhu M, Lorenz HP, Benhaim P, Hedrick MH. Myogenic differentiation by human processed lipoaspirate cells. Plast Reconstr Surg 2002;109(1): 199-209.

[23] Orbay H, Tobita M, Mizuno H. Mesenchymal stem cells isolated from adipose and other tissues: basic biological properties and clinical applications. Stem Cells Int 2012;2012:461718.

[24] Puissant B, Barreau C, Bourin P, Clavel C, Corre J, Bousquet C, et al. Immunomodulatory effect of human adipose tissue-derived adult stem cells: comparison with bone marrow mesenchymal stem cells. Br J Haematol 2005;129(1):118-129.

[25] Hicok KC, Du Laney TV, Zhou YS, Halvorsen YD, Hitt DC, Cooper LF, et al. Human adipose-derived adult stem cells produce osteoid in vivo. Tissue Eng 2004;10(3-4): 371-380.

[26] Miranville A, Heeschen C, Sengenes C, Curat CA, Busse R, Bouloumie A. Improvement of postnatal neovascularization by human adipose tissue-derived stem cells. Circulation 2004;110(3):349-355.

[27] Bacou F, el Andalousi RB, Daussin PA, Micallef JP, Levin JM, Chammas M, et al. Transplantation of adipose tissue-derived stromal cells increases mass and functional capacity of damaged skeletal muscle. Cell Transplant 2004;13(2):103-111.

[28] Zhang Z. Bone regeneration by stem cell and tissue engineering in oral and maxillofacial region. Front Med 2011;5(4):401-413.

[29] Kolk A, Handschel J, Drescher W, Rothamel D, Kloss F, Blessmann M, et al. Current trends and future perspectives of bone substitute materials - From space holders to innovative biomaterials. J Craniomaxillofac Surg 2012. DOI; 10.1016/j.jcms. 2012.01.002

[30] den Boer FC, Wippermann BW, Blokhuis TJ, Patka P, Bakker FC, Haarman HJ. Healing of segmental bone defects with granular porous hydroxyapatite augmented with recombinant human osteogenic protein-1 or autologous bone marrow. J Orthop Res 2003;21(3):521-528.

[31] Kneser U, Schaefer DJ, Polykandriotis E, Horch RE. Tissue engineering of bone: the reconstructive surgeon's point of view. J Cell Mol Med 2006;10(1):7-19.

[32] Arrington ED, Smith WJ, Chambers HG, Bucknell AL, Davino NA. Complications of iliac crest bone graft harvesting. Clin Orthop Relat Res 1996;(329):300-309.

[33] Urist MR. Bone: formation by autoinduction. Science 1965;150(3698):893-899.

[34] Zuk PA. Tissue engineering craniofacial defects with adult stem cells? Are we ready yet? Pediatr Res 2008;63(5):478-486.

[35] Browaeys H, Bouvry P, De Bruyn H. A literature review on biomaterials in sinus augmentation procedures. Clin Implant Dent Relat Res 2007;9(3):166-177.

[36] Bueno EM, Glowacki J. Cell-free and cell-based approaches for bone regeneration. Nat Rev Rheumatol 2009;5(12):685-697.

[37] Piskin E, Isoglu IA, Bolgen N, Vargel I, Griffiths S, Cavusoglu T, et al. In vivo performance of simvastatin-loaded electrospun spiral-wound polycaprolactone scaffolds in reconstruction of cranial bone defects in the rat model. J Biomed Mater Res A 2009;90(4):1137-1151.

[38] Zhu S, Song D, Jiang X, Zhou H, Hu J. Combined effects of recombinant human BMP-2 and Nell-1 on bone regeneration in rapid distraction osteogenesis of rabbit tibia. Injury 2011;42(12):1467-1473.

[39] Kirker-Head CA. Development and application of bone morphogenetic proteins for the enhancement of bone healing. J Orthopaed Traumatol 2005;6(1):1-9.

[40] Runyan CM, Taylor JA. Clinical applications of stem cells in craniofacial surgery. Facial Plast Surg 2010;26(5):385-395.

[41] Khouri RK, Upton J, Shaw WW. Principles of flap prefabrication. Clin Plast Surg 1992;19(4):763-771.

[42] Morrison WA, Penington AJ, Kumta SK, Callan P. Clinical applications and technical limitations of prefabricated flaps. Plast Reconstr Surg 1997;99(2):378-385.

[43] Di Bella C, Lucarelli E, Donati D. Historical review of bone prefabrication. Chir Organi Mov 2008;92(2):73-78.

[44] Khouri RK, Upton J, Shaw WW. Prefabrication of composite free flaps through staged microvascular transfer: an experimental and clinical study. Plast Reconstr Surg 1991;87(1):108-115.

[45] Hirase Y, Valauri FA, Buncke HJ. Prefabricated sensate myocutaneous and osteomyocutaneous free flaps: an experimental model. Preliminary report. Plast Reconstr Surg 1988;82(3):440-446.

[46] Bernard SL, Picha GJ. The use of coralline hydroxyapatite in a "biocomposite" free flap. Plast Reconstr Surg 1991;87(1):96-105.

[47] Terheyden H, Warnke P, Dunsche A, Jepsen S, Brenner W, Palmie S, et al. Mandibular reconstruction with prefabricated vascularized bone grafts using recombinant human osteogenic protein-1: an experimental study in miniature pigs. Part II: transplantation. Int J Oral Maxillofac Surg 2001;30(6):469-478.

[48] Terheyden H, Menzel C, Wang H, Springer IN, Rueger DR, Acil Y. Prefabrication of vascularized bone grafts using recombinant human osteogenic protein-1--part 3: dosage of rhOP-1, the use of external and internal scaffolds. Int J Oral Maxillofac Surg 2004;33(2):164-172.

[49] Terheyden H, Knak C, Jepsen S, Palmie S, Rueger DR. Mandibular reconstruction with a prefabricated vascularized bone graft using recombinant human osteogenic protein-1: an experimental study in miniature pigs. Part I: Prefabrication. Int J Oral Maxillofac Surg 2001;30(5):373-379.

[50] Cancedda R, Bianchi G, Derubeis A, Quarto R. Cell therapy for bone disease: a review of current status. Stem Cells 2003;21(5):610-619.

[51] Muraglia A, Cancedda R, Quarto R. Clonal mesenchymal progenitors from human bone marrow differentiate in vitro according to a hierarchical model. J Cell Sci 2000;113 (Pt 7):1161-1166.

[52] Chang SC, Tai CL, Chung HY, Lin TM, Jeng LB. Bone marrow mesenchymal stem cells form ectopic woven bone in vivo through endochondral bone formation. Artif Organs 2009;33(4):301-308.

[53] He Y, Zhang ZY, Zhu HG, Qiu W, Jiang X, Guo W. Experimental study on reconstruction of segmental mandible defects using tissue engineered bone combined bone marrow stromal cells with three-dimensional tricalcium phosphate. J Craniofac Surg 2007;18(4):800-805.

[54] Mankani MH, Krebsbach PH, Satomura K, Kuznetsov SA, Hoyt R, Robey PG. Pedicled bone flap formation using transplanted bone marrow stromal cells. Arch Surg 2001;136(3):263-270.

[55] Quarto R, Mastrogiacomo M, Cancedda R, Kutepov SM, Mukhachev V, Lavroukov A, et al. Repair of large bone defects with the use of autologous bone marrow stromal cells. N Engl J Med 2001;344(5):385-386.

[56] Marcacci M, Kon E, Moukhachev V, Lavroukov A, Kutepov S, Quarto R, et al. Stem cells associated with macroporous bioceramics for long bone repair: 6- to 7-year outcome of a pilot clinical study. Tissue Eng 2007;13(5):947-955.

[57] Warnke PH, Springer IN, Wiltfang J, Acil Y, Eufinger H, Wehmoller M, et al. Growth and transplantation of a custom vascularised bone graft in a man. Lancet 2004;364(9436):766-770.

[58] Dominici M, Le Blanc K, Mueller I, Slaper-Cortenbach I, Marini F, Krause D, et al. Minimal criteria for defining multipotent mesenchymal stromal cells. The International Society for Cellular Therapy position statement. Cytotherapy 2006;8(4): 315-317.

[59] Levi B, Longaker MT. Concise review: adipose-derived stromal cells for skeletal regenerative medicine. Stem Cells 2011;29(4):576-582.

[60] Mizuno H, Tobita M, Uysal AC. Concise review: Adipose-derived stem cells as a novel tool for future regenerative medicine. Stem Cells 2012;30(5):804-810.

[61] Musina RA, Bekchanova ES, Sukhikh GT. Comparison of mesenchymal stem cells obtained from different human tissues. Bull Exp Biol Med 2005;139(4):504-509.

[62] Romanov YA, Darevskaya AN, Merzlikina NV, Buravkova LB. Mesenchymal stem cells from human bone marrow and adipose tissue: isolation, characterization, and differentiation potentialities. Bull Exp Biol Med 2005;140(1):138-143.

[63] Arrigoni E, Lopa S, de Girolamo L, Stanco D, Brini AT. Isolation, characterization and osteogenic differentiation of adipose-derived stem cells: from small to large animal models. Cell Tissue Res 2009;338(3):401-411.

[64] Mitchell JB, McIntosh K, Zvonic S, Garrett S, Floyd ZE, Kloster A, et al. Immunophenotype of human adipose-derived cells: temporal changes in stromal-associated and stem cell-associated markers. Stem Cells 2006;24(2):376-385.

[65] Baer PC, Geiger H. Adipose-derived mesenchymal stromal/stem cells: tissue localization, characterization, and heterogeneity. Stem Cells Int 2012;2012:812693.

[66] Schellenberg A, Stiehl T, Horn P, Joussen S, Pallua N, Ho AD, et al. Population dynamics of mesenchymal stromal cells during culture expansion. Cytotherapy 2012;14(4):401-411.

[67] Rada T, Reis RL, Gomes ME. Adipose tissue-derived stem cells and their application in bone and cartilage tissue engineering. Tissue Eng Part B Rev 2009;15(2):113-125.

[68] Safwani WK, Makpol S, Sathapan S, Chua KH. Alteration of gene expression levels during osteogenic induction of human adipose derived stem cells in long-term culture. Cell Tissue Bank 2012. DOI; 10.1007/s10561-012-9309-1.

[69] Halvorsen YD, Franklin D, Bond AL, Hitt DC, Auchter C, Boskey AL, et al. Extracellular matrix mineralization and osteoblast gene expression by human adipose tissue-derived stromal cells. Tissue Eng 2001;7(6):729-741.

[70] Zhao Y, Lin H, Zhang J, Chen B, Sun W, Wang X, et al. Crosslinked three-dimensional demineralized bone matrix for the adipose-derived stromal cell proliferation and differentiation. Tissue Eng Part A 2009;15(1):13-21.

[71] Ciuffi S, Fabbri S, Zonefrati R, Galli G, Tanini A, Brandi ML. Subcutaneous adipocytes may become osteoblasts. Clin Cases Miner Bone Metab 2012;9(1):28-30.

[72] Zhao X, Liu L, Wang FK, Zhao DP, Dai XM, Han XS. Coculture of vascular endothelial cells and adipose-derived stem cells as a source for bone engineering. Ann Plast Surg 2012;69(1):91-98.

[73] Wang J, Ye Y, Tian H, Yang S, Jin X, Tong W, et al. In vitro osteogenesis of human adipose-derived stem cells by coculture with human umbilical vein endothelial cells. Biochem Biophys Res Commun 2011;412(1):143-149.

[74] Okuda T, Uysal AC, Tobita M, Hyakusoku H, Mizuno H. Prefabrication of tissue engineered bone grafts: an experimental study. Ann Plast Surg 2010;64(1):98-104.

[75] Lendeckel S, Jodicke A, Christophis P, Heidinger K, Wolff J, Fraser JK, et al. Autologous stem cells (adipose) and fibrin glue used to treat widespread traumatic calvarial defects: case report. J Craniomaxillofac Surg 2004;32(6):370-373.

[76] Thesleff T, Lehtimaki K, Niskakangas T, Mannerstrom B, Miettinen S, Suuronen R, et al. Cranioplasty with adipose-derived stem cells and biomaterial: a novel method for cranial reconstruction. Neurosurgery 2011;68(6):1535-1540.

[77] Mesimaki K, Lindroos B, Tornwall J, Mauno J, Lindqvist C, Kontio R, et al. Novel maxillary reconstruction with ectopic bone formation by GMP adipose stem cells. Int J Oral Maxillofac Surg 2009;38(3):201-209.

Chapter 7

Adipose Derived Stem Cells: Current State of the Art and Prospective Role in Regenerative Medicine and Tissue Engineering

Vincenzo Vindigni, Giorgio Giatsidis,
Francesco Reho , Erica Dalla Venezia ,
Marco Mammana and Bassetto Franco

Additional information is available at the end of the chapter

1. Introduction

1.1. Adipose tissue: The Good, the Bad, the Ugly

Excessive body fat has been socially recognized for ages as a symbol of wealth and prosperity. Clues of these concepts may be found in arts and literature. In addition, it has been substantially ignored by scientists, anatomists and physicians for many centuries. As a matter of fact only a minimal number of medical reports focused on "fat" have been historically handed down. Nowadays, however, adipose tissue has become a growing point of most interest for research-ers and physicians worldwide. Notably, societies and health care systems are facing a severe pandemic rise of obesity and of several associated co-morbidities such as cardiovascular disease, diabetes, metabolic disorders and cancer. Fat and misregulation of adipose-related pathways are recognized as key elements in each of these processes. Importantly, the role of adipose tissue has progressively evolved from being a passive energy store to representing an important endocrine organ that directly modulates metabolism and immunity towards an healthy phenotype or leading to pathologic processes. The investigation of the physiologic-pathologic attitudes of adipose tissue is currently among most relevant scientific targets of researchers, endocrinologists and bariatric surgeons. Beside, in the last fifteen years adipose tissue has been reappraised also for a different reason. In fact, nearly forty years after the identification of bone marrow stem cells, it has been gathering attention for the opportunity to obtain autologous pluripotent adipose-derived stromal stem cells (ADSCs). This population of cells has been extensively investigated and it currently holds out many hopes for prospective stem cell therapies for the repair and regeneration of various tissues and organs in a large number of different diseases. Thus, over the past years, this field has become a very active and attractive area of clinical and experimental research, providing significant outcomes and reaching important milestones. Today adipose tissue embodies an hot spot of regenerative medicine that may give rise to a new era of active stem cell therapy.

2. Purpose

2.1. Meeting the adipose tissue

Giving the increasing amount of experimental and clinical data regarding adipose tissue and ADSCs, in this chapter we are going to briefly review the concepts and the insights behind the role of adipose tissue in regenerative medicine and tissue engineering. In particular we are going to focus the attention on current cutting edge translational research from bench to bedside, including the investigation of biological properties of ADSCs, the state of art of their manipulation, the latest progresses in their clinical adoption, the development of bio-engineered products and the actual therapeutic prospective opportunities.

3. Basic science background

3.1. The outline and the anatomy of adipose tissue

Adipose tissue is a complex and multi-depot organ, constituted for one third by mature adipocytes and for the other two thirds by a combination of a large variety of other cells. [1] Among represented cell lines are included small blood vessels, nervous cells, fibroblasts and, importantly, adipocyte progenitor cells, also known as preadipocytes or Adipose Derived Stem Cells (ADSCs). Evolution has preserved in mammals two histologically different qualities of adipose tissue: white adipose tissue (WAT) and brown adipose tissue (BAT), which are composed by different types of mature adipocytes [Table 1]. In particular, white adipocytes are spherical, having a diameter ranging between 30 and 70 µm according to the amount of lipid depots, and lipids within the cells are organized in a single large "uni-locular" droplet, the size of which can exceed 50 µm. Thus, the lipid droplet occupies the vast majority of the whole intracellular space, pushing the remaining cytoplasm and nucleus into a thin marginal rim. On the other hand, brown adipocytes are polygonal with a centrally placed nucleus and their cellular size ranges from 20 to 40 µm. They accumulate lipids in smaller "multi-locular" droplets and they are rich of specific mitochondria, containing the protein UCP-1 which is responsible for uncoupling of oxidative phosporylation and production of heat. WAT and BAT are both innervated by noradrenergic fibers of the sympathetic nervous system. As for the vascularization of adipose tissue, white adipocytes are organized in collections of fat lobules, each supplied by a selective arteriole and surrounded by septae of connective tissue. An individual adipocyte is supplied by an adjacent capillary and it is associated to a glycoprotein layer, reticular fibrils, fibroblasts, mastocytes and macrophages. Compared to WAT, BAT provides a more extensive vascular tree, characterized by dense multiple capillaries. The relevant vascularization of the latter in combination with the presence of a significantly high number of mitochondria, account for the typical "brown" color. WAT and BAT have also different roles in energy metabolism. Primary function of white adipocytes is to store excess energy as lipid, which is then mobilized in response to metabolic needs. Brown adipocytes, on the other hand, use accumulated lipids primarily as a source of energy released in the form of heat. WAT can be found in several anatomically distinct and separate collections, or "depots." There are two major anatomic subdivisions of these depots, each showing unique anatomic, metabolic, endocrine, paracrine, and autocrine properties: intra-abdominal or visceral adipose tissue and subcutaneous adipose tissue. In addition, WAT can also be found in small amounts of fatty layers surrounding other organs, such as the heart, kidney and genitalia. Intra-peritoneal fat, composed of omental and mesenteric adipose tissue, comprises the vast majority of visceral fat. Importantly, subcutaneous adipose tissue shows different structural features in different anatomical districts. [2] In fact, fat depots in the abdominal area are characterized by the presence of large adipocytes, densely packed together and surrounded by a poor stromal (collagen) network. Instead, in more localized depots (such as throcanteric areas, the sovra-pubic area, arm pits, medial regions of the knees, tights, arms, pectoral and mammary areas) adipocytes present a smaller diameter, a more represented stromal component and a more extensive vascular network. BAT in newborns and children can be found in several body areas. However, while in other small mammals these depots persist during growth, in humans brown adipocytes undergo a morphologic transformation, rapidly accumulating lipids, becoming uni-locular and losing their typical ultrastructural and molecular properties, including mitochondria [Figure 1.]. As a consequence, there are no discrete collections of BAT that can be found in human adults.

	White Adipocyte	Brown Adipocyte
Shape	Spherical	Polygonal
Diameter	30-70 μm	20-40 μm
Ultra-structure	One large "unilocular" lipid droplet, cytoplasm and nucleus compressed into a thin visible rim	Multiple smaller "multilocular" droplets, high content of mitochondria, centrally placed nucleus
Innervation	Noradrenergic fibers, confined to capillary wall	Noradrenergic fibers, directly interfacing plasma membrane
Vascularization	Supplied by an adjacent capillary	Richer vascular tree, dense with multiple capillaries
Main function	Store excess energy as lipids	Thermogenesis
Localization	Visceral compartment (intraperitoneal, retroperitoneal, around organs) and subcutaneous compartment	Several areas in newborn, no discrete collections in adult. Probably isolated cells scattered between WAT depots

Table 1. Main differences between White and Brown adipocytes.

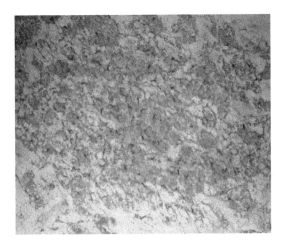

Figure 1. Monolayered culture of adipocytes in vitro with adipogenic medium.

3.2. The living image of adipose derived stem cells

The understanding of biochemical characteristics, molecular/cellular biology, immune-biological characteristics and phenotype of adipose tissue has significantly advanced in the last years. Adipose tissue has shown to consist mostly of cells of mesenchymal origin with few others endothelial cells, smooth muscle cells and pericytes, all showing low levels of cell senescence. Adipose tissue derives from the mesodermal layer of the embryo and develops both during pre-natal and post-natal growth. The microscopic location of the adipogenic progenitor cells in the adult is still controversial. [3] It remains to be proven whether the origin of the cells correlates with endothelial, pericytic or stromal compartments. A large number of surface antigens are in common with endothelial cells, suggesting a common origin. According to some researchers, adipogenic progenitor cells could be released directly by the bone marrow and distributed systemically by blood flow: experimental evidences of bone marrow derived-cells capable of differentiating into adipocytes in vivo have already been described but the contribution of these circulating cells to the overall growth and development of adipose tissue is still under investigation. Mesenchymal stem cells (MSC) were first described as immature cells in the bone marrow, capable to give rise to mesenchymal lineages such as osteoblasts, chondrocytes and adipocytes. [4] MSCs represent a small fraction of nucleated cells of human bone marrow (0.01%-0,0001%). MSCs are defined by three minimal criteria, as established by the International Society for Cellular Therapy in 2005: adherence to plastic dishes, specific surface antigen (CD73+, CD90+, CD105+, CD45-, CD34-, CD14 or CD11b-, CD79- or CD19-, HLA-DR) and in vitro capability to give rise to adipocytes, osteoblasts and chondrocytes. A similar protocol has been used for a long time to isolate adipose tissue progenitors: the resulting immature adherent cells were thus called pre-adipocytes. To obtain these cells fat pads are minced and digested with collagenase, separating an upper layer of floating mature adipocytes from a lower layer of pelleted stromal vascular fraction (SVF). [5] The SVF is an heterogeneous cell population of circulating blood cells, fibroblasts, pericytes, endothelial cells and pre-adipocytes. Pre-adipocytes may be isolated from the SVF by plating and washing. This cell population, adopting appropriate differentiating agents, can give rise to mature adipocytes, demonstrating their nature of adipose progenitors. Cell cultures have provided evidence of regenerative capacities in both the heterogeneous stromal vascular fraction (SVF) and in the more homogeneous adipose-derived stem cells (ADSCs). In 2002 pre-adipocytes were better characterized and they were demonstrated to show clear multi-potency potential: thus, they were named Adipose Derived Stem Cells (ADSCs). [6] In particular, ADSCs represent a mesodermal stem cell population with clonal mesodermal, ectodermal, and endodermal potentials capabilities that express multiple CD marker antigens similar to those of other mesenchymal stem cells as those residing in bone marrow. Several investigations have reported a differentiation into adipogenic, osteogenic, chondrogenic and myogenic lineages in vitro by means of specific culture media. In particular, the potential to differentiate into non-mesodermal lineages is exciting. The differentiation into neural precursors, which are of an ectodermal origin, has been described. In addition, evidence of differentiation into hepato-cytes, pancreatic islet cells, endothelial cells and other epithelial cells has been provided in different reports. By definition, a stem cell is characterized by the ability to self-renew and to differentiate along multiple lineage pathways. Since the self-renewal of ADSCs has not been fully established yet, it is accepted that some investigators may use the same acronym to mean "adipose-derived stromal cells", in agreement with the statement of the International Society for Cellular Therapy. Indeed, ADSCs present several differences from MSCs at genomic, proteomic and functional levels. For instance, during the earliest rounds of proliferation, ADSCs express the CD34 antigen: the frequency of these cells is much higher (100 to 500 folds higher) than that of MSCs in the bone marrow. In addition, MSCs are probably more committed towards osteoblastic and chondrogenic lineages than ADSCs. Thus, although numerous author use the same term "MSCs" both for cells derived from bone marrow and for those derived from adipose tissue, MSCs and ADSCs are probably two distinct cell populations. A more precise definition of ADSCs, based on their immune-phenotype and/or differentiation capabilities, has not been yet provided. Some authors believe that ADSCs are a heterogeneous group of progenitor cells with differences in their stem cell potential. Thus, ADSCs and SVFs cells represent an autologous alternative to pluri-potent embryonic stem cells with a multi-lineage differentiation potential, a significant therapeutic impact and a critical role in the rapidly expanding fields of tissue engineering and regenerative medicine. Significantly, further investigations are needed to better clarify these aspects. Importantly, the most important characteristics of ADSCs, with a possible interest for clinical applications, comprise their multi-potency, secretory functions and immune-modulatory capabilities.

3.2.1. Differentiation potential of ADSCs

ADSCs, like MSCs, have the ability to differentiate into mesodermal cells, such as adipocytes, fibroblasts, myocytes, osteocytes and chondrocytes, in a process called lineage-specific differentiation. The increasing evidence for the ability of ADSCs to differentiate into cells of non-mesodermal origin such as neurons, endocrine pancreatic cells, hepatocytes, endothelial cells and cardiac myocytes, is surprising. This process is called "cross-differentiation". Lineage-specific differentiation can be tracked at a molecular level by the expression of key transcription factors of mature tissues. The earlier stages of differentiation, named "allocation" or "commitment", that drive the ADSCs into the specialized lineage are not completely known yet. In vitro, the differentiation of multi-potent cells into a desirable cell phenotype can be obtained by appropriate culture conditions and stimulation with a cocktail of known differentiating agents [Table 2].

Type of differentiation	Stimulating factors
Adipogenic	Insulin; isobutylmethylxanthine (IBMX) ; dexamethasone; rosiglitazone; indomethacin.
Osteogenic	Dexamethasone; β-glycerophosphate; vitamin D3; bone morphogenetic protein (BMP-2)
Chondrogenic	insulin growth factor (IGF); BMPs; transforming growth factor-β (TGF-β)
Myogenic/cardiomyogenic	Dexamethasone; hydrocortisone; IL-3; IL-6
Vascular/endothelial	Specific environment
Neurogenic	Valproic acid; epidermal growth factor (EGF); fibroblast growth factor (FGF); nerve growth factor (NGF) and brain-derived neurotrophic factor (BDNF)
Tendinous	FGF; platelet derived growth factor (PDGF-BB); EGF; TGF-β; IGF-1; BMPs

Table 2. Experimental growth factors used for differentiation of ADSCs in different cell lineages.

- Adipogenic differentiation

ADSCs have an exceptional potential for differentiation into mature adipocytes, which is very promising in developing techniques for repairing soft-tissue defects. [7] Differentiation can be induced by a large variety of substances, including insulin, dexamethasone, rosiglitazone and indomethacin. During differentiation ADSCs, initially showing a fibroblast-like spindle or stellate shape, undergo morphologic changes with the appearance of one or more lipid vacuoles and they begin to express several genes and proteins characterizing the mature adipocyte, including leptin, peroxisome-proliferating activated receptor γ (PPARγ), glucose transporter type 4 (GLUT4) and glycerol-3-phosphate dehydrogenase (GPDH).

- Osteogenic differentiation

Osteogenic differentiation can be induced in vitro by supplementing the culture medium with dexamethasone, β-glycerophosphate and vitamin D3. The acquisition of the osteoblast phenotype is accompanied by expression of specific genes and proteins, including alkaline phosphatase, type I collagen, osteopontin, osteonectin, and Runx2. Osteogenic differentiation may also be obtained by transfection of osteogenic lineage-determining genes (BMP2 and Runx2): this approach has proved to be effective both in vitro and in vivo in a large number of reports. These experimental findings hold great promise for the use of ADSCs in bone regeneration.

• Chondrogenic differentiation

Insulin growth factor (IGF), bone morphogenetic proteins (BMPs), and transforming growth factor-β (TGF-β) have shown to induce chondrogenic differentiation of ADSCs when added to the culture medium. Chondrogenic differentiation occurs also by seeding ADSCs into poly-glycolic acid (PGA) scaffolds, as it was largely demonstrated in several other in vitro models and in vivo in nude mice.

• Differentiation into other lineages

Terminally differentiated myoblasts can be obtained in vitro, showing the ability to form multinucleated myotubules and to shrink/diastole under the influence of atropine. This property of ADSCs is of particular interest for the treatment of genetic muscular dystrophies: preclinical in vivo studies on animal models are currently ongoing. In addition, other studies have focused on the capability of ADSCs to differentiate into cardiomyocytes with a possible application in heart regeneration or repair after an ischemic injury. Furthermore, endothelial regeneration is another important field of research: ADSCs have shown to be able to differen-tiate into endothelial cells and to secrete several pro-angiogenic factors, like vascular endo-thelial growth factor (VEGF) and platelet-derived growth factor (PDGF). Differentiation into neuron-like cells has also been reported by different authors: ADSCs may acquire a neural-like morphology and they may express several proteins specific for the neuronal phenotype (Neuron Specific Enolase; Neuron Specific Nuclear Protein). Finally, some studies have explored the chance for ADSCs to differentiate into pancreatic islet cells, hepatocytes and epithelial cells with the purpose to find an alternative cellular therapy for diseases such as diabetes mellitus and liver disfunction: data and outcomes are however still preliminary and lacking of strong evidence.

3.2.2. ADSCs as a secretome

Importance of ADSCs does not only reside in their potential to differentiate in mature lineages. Similarly to the original adipose tissue from which they can be isolated, ADSCs have shown to act as a "secretome", accurately regulating proteins and growth factors secreted into the extracellular milieu and having a relevant impact on different organs and systems within the human body [Table 3.]. [8] Trophic effects of ADSCs include stimulation of angiogenesis, hematopoietic support, gene transfer and suppression of inflammation. Indeed ADSCs represent a source of several cytokine/soluble factors regulating the survival and differentia-tion of various endogenous cells/tissues. A large number of these molecules have been related to the regenerative attitude of ADSCs: among these, we may include hepatocyte growth factor (HGF), granulocyte and macrophage colony stimulating factors, interleukins (ILs) 6, 7, 8 and 11, tumor necrosis factor-alpha (TNF-alpha), vascular endothelial growth factor (VEGF), brain derived neurotrophic factor (BDNF), nerve growth factor (NGF), adipokines and others. Full characterization of the secretory profile of ADSCs, either by immune-enzymatic techniques (ELISA) or by mass spectrometry, is still object of investigation. Several adipokines such as adiponectin, angiotensin, cathepsin D, penetraxin, pregnancy zone protein and retinol binding protein, as well as stromal cell-derived growth factor (CXCL12) have been found in the conditioned media of ADSCs differentiating towards the adipocyte lineage. ADSCs secrete also oher different well characterized cytokines (GM-CSF, TGF-β, PGE2, IGF-1) and their release can be modulated by exposure to different agents, such as b-FGF and EGF or inflammatory stimula, like lipopolysaccharide (LPS). The role of these and other factors has been investigated by multiple studies regarding one or more possible applications of ADSCs in the field of regenerative medicine. Brain Derived Neurotrophic Factor (BDNF), Nerve Growth Factor (NGF), Glial Derived Neurotrophic Factor (GDNF) are thought to be important molecules secreted by ADSCs mediating neurotrophic effects and modulating in animal models of Parkinson Disease the recovery after hypoxic-ischemic injuries. Hepatocyte Growth Factor (HGF) and Vascular Endothelial Growth factor (VEGF) are the most important factors capable of inducing angiogenesis in areas that have undergone ischemic episodes and their importance is particularly relevant in wound healing. In cardiac regeneration, IGF-1 and VEGF mediate respectively an anti-apoptotic and angiogenic action, to which is attributed the capacity of ADSCs to have beneficial effects when transplanted/injected in different animal models of myocardial infarction/failure. In conclusion, most of ADSCs secreted factors act through mechanisms that mediate protection against cell death or, alternatively, induce cell migration and proliferation. Alternatively, they can indirectly act on the targeted cell populations: by promoting vascularization they can be indirectly linked to an increase of oxygen and nutrients in the affected areas, which may in turn promote local regenerative processes. Indeed, up to now most reports have focused on a limited set of known factors but it is expected that other molecules are responsible for the regenerative effects of ADSCs.

3.2.3. Immunomodulatory properties of ADSCs

The regenerative potential of ADSCs has been related also to their immune-modulatory abilities. ADSCs have been shown to be an immune-privileged site, preventing severe graft-versus-host response after transplantation procedures in vitro and in vivo. A concern of fundamental importance is the interplay between ADSCs and the host tissue, with particular focus on the immune system. Several studies have shown that ADSCs can be used either for autologous or allogenic cell transplants: this feature would be a major advantage for the employment of adipose tissue as a source for cell-based therapies. Furthermore ADSCs seem to act also as modulators of the immune system. The allogenic potential of these cells could be explained by the property of ADSCs to decrease the expression of hematopoietic markers and HLA-DR after subsequent passages. In addition, it has been observed that ADSCs only express HLA class I, but not HLA class II molecules: the latter can only be induced in ADSCs after incubation with IFN-γ. Furthermore, several experiments have proved that ADSCs do not stimulate lymphocyte proliferation and they do not elicit a response by Mixed Lymphocyte Reaction (MLR): in addition, they can also inhibit phyohemagglutinin (PHA)-stimulated lymphocyte proliferation. These immune-suppressive effects are likely mediated by soluble factors, among which PGE-2 seems to be the most important. Notably, the secretion of cytokines by ADSCs can be modulated not only by the inflammatory stimulus but also by the surface upon which they are seeded: thus the bio-scaffold/environment provided could be another mechanism to control the immune-modulatory properties of ADSCs.

Main properties of ADSCs	
Differentiation potential	*Into cells of mesodermal origin*: adipocytes, fibroblasts, myocytes, osteocytes, condrocyes
	Into cells of non-mesodermal origin: endothelial cells, neuronal-like cells, pancreatic islet cells, hepatocytes
Secretion of soluble factors (ADSCs "secretome")	Adiponectin, angiotensin, cathepsin D, penetraxin, pregnancy zone protein, retinol binding protein, CXCL12, HGF, GM-CSF, ILs 6 ,7, 8, 11, TNF-α, VEGF, BDNF, NGF, GDNF, IGF-1, TGF-β, FGF-2, PGE2,
Immunomodulatory capabilities	Allogenic cell transplant potential
	Lack of response by MLR,
	Inhibition of PHA-stimulated lymphocyte proliferation

Table 3. Synopsis of properties of ADSCs.

4. Manipulation of adipose tissue and ADSCs

4.1. Introduction

Human subcutaneous adipose tissue provides an ideal alternative source of autologous pluripotent stem cells showing several advantages compared with other sources. As a matter of fact it is ubiquitous and commonly easily obtainable in large quantity with minimal invasive harvesting procedures or methods (either liposuction aspirates or subcutaneous adipose tissue fragments), limited patient discomfort and minimal ethical considerations: it may be transplanted safely and efficaciously. The abundance of stem cells available enables the direct therapeutic adoption of primary cells without any need for culture expansion. Moreover, adipose tissue is also uniquely expandable: currently available procedures for cell isolation yield a high amount of stem cells with remarkable properties of stable proliferation and potential differentiation in vitro, being attractive candidates for clinical applications offering protocols that may provide alternative therapeutic solutions in cell-based therapies and tissue engineering to repair or regenerate damaged tissues and organs. The technologies for adipose tissue harvesting, processing, and transplantation have substantially evolved in recent years together with appropriate commercial development and with updated refinements and information regarding extraction, isolation, storage, options for cultures, growth and differentiation, cryopreservation and its effect on survival and proliferation of isolated ADSCs, also related to their adoption in tissue-engineered constructs involving biomaterials and scaffolds. Inconsistencies in literature regarding the handling of ADSCs require more extensive investigations and controls, in particular in the in vitro processing and differences between the regenerative properties of freshly-processed heterogeneous stromal vascular fraction cells and of culture-expanded relatively homogeneous ADSCs, or the related risk of complications and possible adverse events. There is a need for stronger evidence of the safety, reproducibility and quality of the ADSCs prior to a more extensive use in clinical applications. As a matter of fact, despite the clinical use of adipose tissue grafts and ADSCs worldwide has dramatically increased, questions concerning the safety and efficacy of these treatments are still opened and currently the use of isolated ADSCs for medical indications in a clinical setting has been approved only in selected cases and few countries.

4.2. Origins and delivery of adipose tissue grafts

Adipose tissue have been used for long time for reconstructive purposes through fat grafting or autologous fat transfer, a method according to which fat from the patient is removed from one area of the body ad reinserted into the desired recipient location. [9] Fat grafting has shown to be beneficial as a reconstructive and cosmetic procedure for patients with volume losses to soft tissues due to disease, trauma, congenital defects or aging. Even so, outcomes of these techniques are often unpredictable and rates of graft reabsorption may be disappointing. As a matter of fact, fat tissue is re-vascularized at the transplantation site within 48 hours from the surgical procedure, in the meantime being fed by diffused materials from surrounding free plasma. The survival rates of the graft are dependent on size of transplanted fat particles and on surface area from which these cells could re-establish their blood supply. In order to minimize reabsorption, studies have demonstrated the efficacy of less traumatic methods of harvesting, processing and injecting. Microinjection of fat by means of the "lipostructure technique" known also as Coleman's technique has been adopted by many plastic surgeons. [10] This technique distributes fat grafts in small aliquots by meticulous injection through multiple access sites, from which the graft fans out into various subcutaneous layers. The abundance of stem cells obtainable in many common procedures, such as liposuction and liposculture, enables their direct therapeutic adoption without any need for culture expansion. [11] Even so, precursor cells can be purified by a variety of processes and enzymatic techniques may be adopted to obtain an ADSC-rich stromal vascular fraction (SVF). This issues are currently investigated as adjuvants to free fat transfer in order to increase yield of graft retention (cell-assisted lipotransfer). The ADSCs contained in the stromal vascular fraction have been applied clinically as early as 2004 for the treatment of perianal fistulas in Crohn's disease. [12] However, it is worth pointing out that, even though harvesting and first processing steps overlap, fat grafts SVF cells and ADSCs represent three different therapeutic options. Fat grafts are obtained directly after centrifugation of lipoaspirates. They contain predominantly mature adipocytes and are poor in ADSCs. The stromal vascular fraction, as mentioned above, is obtained by digestion with collagenase of the lipoaspirate sample and a subsequent centrifugation step: its cellular composition is heterogeneous, being rich in ADSCs but containing also circulating blood cells, fibroblasts, pericytes and endothelial cells. The adoption of a pure ADSC population requires plating of the SVF and expansion of the stem cell population and thus, differently from the previous two options, ADSCs cannot be harvested and implanted in a one step-procedure. Even if all these approaches exploit to some extent the regenerative potential of adipose tissue they are quite different procedures having also different therapeutic indications. Thus, attention has to be paid in order to avoid confusion. As for harvesting of ADSCs, several factors related to the patient, such as Body Mass Index (BMI) and age, have been analyzed for their impact on cell viability and number. Results are controversial, there is no evidence of a strong correlation of BMI with stem cells viability, number or size. Instead, there seems to be a negative correlation between age and rates of pre-adipocytes proliferation or differentiation, with higher lipolitic activity in the younger population and lower levels of apoptosis. [13] The body region of the donor site is another important variable patient-dependent. The abdomen, according to some studies, seems to be the best harvest site, while medial thigh and knee seem to have the lowest levels of viability of ASDCs. [14] These differences have not been proved in other studies. Effects of infiltration of local anesthetics during harvesting have also been investigated: lidocaine and adrenaline seem to have no effects on adipocyte viability. The method of harvest can affect not only viability of ADSCs but also their level of adhesiveness to extracellular matrix proteins. Standard liposuction allows the harvest of larger volumes of adipose tissue but it might result in up to 90% rate of adipocyte rupture. For this reason this technique is not ideal for fat grafting, while it could be more appropriate for ADSCs harvesting. An equivalent damage to pre-adipocytes has been measured comparing syringe aspiration with fat surgical excision. It is accepted that a larger cannula diameter at harvest correlates with improved cell viability. Partial purification of lipoaspirate can be carried out in the operatory room. The first step is centrifugation, which separates harvested fat into three layers: infra-natant (lowest layer composed of blood, tissue fluid and local anesthetics), middle portion (mostly composed by fatty tissue) and supra-natant (least dense upper layer including lipids). Infra-natant components can be ejected from the base of the syringe, while supra-natant can be poured off and soaked up using absorbent materials. While this technique is the most practical and today commonly used for fat grafting, it may not produce the best fraction of ADSCs possible. Several studies have been conducted on this issue, revealing that gentle centrifugation produces the highest cell viability, while long periods of centrifugation lead to isolation of the most proliferative cell type. When comparing decantation, washing and centrifugation, stem cells concentration results greater in washed lipoaspirates and pellets contained at the bottom of the centrifuged samples contain the highest concentration of stem cells.

4.3. Origins and delivery of ADSCs

Embryonic stem cells have an enormous multilineage potential but many ethical and political issues accompany their use. Therefore researchers have directed their attention on pluripotent adult stem cells. Adult stem cells were initially thought to have the differentiation capacity limited to their tissue of origin, however, as already mentioned above, many studies have now demonstrated that stem cells have the capacity to differentiate into cells of mesodermal, endodermal and ectodermal origin. MSCs from the bone marrow show extensive proliferative capacity and a multilineage differentiation potential into several lineages, including osteoblasts, chondrocytes, adipocytes and myoblasts. However, pain, morbidity and low cell numbers upon harvest represent an obstacle to their extensive clinical application. The harvesting of adipose tissue, in comparison, is much less expensive than bone marrow. ADSCs can be isolated both from tissue samples and from lipoaspirate with less invasive procedures and are available in greater quantities (5 x 105 stem cells from 400 to 600 mg tissue). [15] ADSCs can be easily cultured and expanded, retaining their stem cell phenotypes and mesenchymal pluripotency still after several passages, features that make them an ideal source of stem cells for clinical applications.

• Isolation and culture of ADSCs

Since Rodbell's description of isolated pre-adipocytes from adipose tissue, a variety of methods have been developed. [16] Today, most laboratories use several common steps to process cells from adipose tissue. These methods include: washing, enzymatic digestion/mechanical disruption, centrifugal separation for isolation of cells which can be used directly, after cryopreservation, or after culture expansion for the generation of ADSCs. Still, despite the extensive use of ADSCs for research purposes, there is no any widely-accepted unique standard protocol for isolating and culturing these cells. For enzymatic digestion most laboratories use collagenases of different subtypes, trypsin, or a mixture of both, at various concentrations with an average incubation time of one hour, at 37°C, in constant shaking. The optimal centrifugation speed is considered to be around 1200g for 5 to 10 minutes. Some additional purification procedures can include filtration through nylon meshes and incubation with an erytrocyte-lysing buffer, usually Krebs Ringer Buffer (KRB) or NH4Cl. This procedure, however, seems to have a negative influence on the growth of ADSCs. Some investigators, after the identification of ADSCs surface immunophenotype, use immune-magnetic beads or flow cytometry to purify the stem cell population directly from the heterogeneous sample, using the CD34+ antigen. The most used culture medium are α-Modified Eagle's Medium (α-MEM), or Dulbecco's Modified Eagle's Medium (DMEM), after addition of fetal bovine/calf serum, (FBS/FCS), L-glutamine, penicillin and streptomycin.

• Cryopreservation of ADSCs

The development of simple but effective storage protocols for adult stem cells will greatly enhance their use and utility in tissue-engineering applications. [17] Cryopreservation is regarded as a promising technique and many studies have focused on this procedure. Other protocols investigated drying (anhydrobiosis) and freeze drying (lyophilization). The majority of in vitro studies agree that cryopreservation of adipocytes in liquid nitrogen, preferably using a set cooling and re-warming protocol, provides the lowest damage to cell viability. These results have been replicated in vivo (murine models) showing that grafts frozen in liquid nitrogen and stored at -35°C had a similar viability and histology compared to fresh tissue: in addition, this method obtained better results than freeze drying and immersion in glycerol. Recently, in order to increase the yield of adipose-derived stem cells post-thawing, the use of cryoprotective agents, such as dimethyl sulphoxide (DMSO) has been examined: samples frozen with DMSO achieved better outcomes than unprotected ones. Thus, cryoprotective agents are now considered as an essential part of any cryopreservation protocol aiming to provide appropriate conditions for the survival of ADSCs and adipocytes.

4.4. Safety concerns

Inconsistencies in literature regarding the handling of ADSCs require more extensive investigations and controls. In particular, a focus should be placed on in vitro processing as well as differences between the regenerative properties of freshly-processed heterogeneous adipose cells and those of culture-expanded relatively homogeneous ADSCs. Related risks of complications and possible adverse events like fat necrosis, seromas, oncological recurrences, should be accurately considered. In addition, adiponectin is implicated in the pathogenesis of insulin-resistant states, such as obesity and diabetes type 2. In particular, several studies reported that differentiated WAT cells and WAT resident progenitors may promote cancer growth and metastasis by means of a variety of different mechanisms (endocrine, paracrine, autocrine interactions). The main cellular component of WAT are adipocytes, the large cells accumulating tryglicerides in lipid droplets. In particular, in conditions like obesity, adipocytes in WAT may eventually became under oxygenated, leading to hypoxia, increased oxidative stress, recruitment of inflammatory leukocytes and eventually fibrosis. In recent experimental models, some adipokines showed to be able to promote tumor growth along with fatty acids released by adipocytes. High levels of adiponectin have been associated with the development of endometrial carcinoma and breast cancer. Leptin has been identified in regulation of cell proliferation and neo-vascularization in malignant and normal cells of different origins, including lung, gastric, colonic, kidney, leukemic, hematopoietic and epithelial cells. Notably, these molecules can enhance proliferation and survival of malignant cells and/or of tumor vasculature. So far, studies investigating the role of WAT in cancer have predominantly focused on pro-tumorigenic effect of ADSCs. In fact the increased proliferation and survivor of malignant cells may result from the engagement of perivascular ADSCs into angiogenesis and vascular maturation, resulting in improved tumor blood perfusion. Cytokines such as adiponectin, leptin, interleukin-6, and TNF alfa seem to be responsible for a chronic low-grade inflammation. Furthermore, mesenchymal cells are known to suppress the activation of T-killer cells: this finding suggests that also ADSCs may help tumors to evade the host immune response. Thus, adipocytes may be able to produce adipokines and several secretions which could potentially induce cancer reappearance by "fueling" dormant breast cancer cells in tumor bed true "tumor-stroma interaction": even so, up to now, especially for grafting of adipose tissue after breast cancer treatment, there is no strong clinical evidence or international agreement on this topic. [18-19] Depending on country, the safety of adipose tissue grafting is still a controversial issue. In 2009, the American Society of Plastic surgeons Fat Graft task Force concluded that no reliable studies could confirm definitely the oncologic safety of lipofilling in breast cancer patients. A more accurate point of view is provided by a large multicentric observational study on adipose tissue grafting in patients previously affected by breast cancer: considered parameters included the complication rate of the technique, the risk of modification of mammography and a rigorous long-term clinical/instrumental follow-up. [20] At the moment no studies on the effects of lipotransfer on human cancer breast cells in vivo are available. We cannot provide the definitive proof of the safety of lipofilling in terms of cancer recurrence or distant metastasis, but until then, should be performed in experienced hands, and a cautious oncologic follow-up protocol is advised.

5. Clinical use

5.1. The regenerative cells

The growing interest in this area of research has driven the adoption of adipose tissue and ADSCs in a wide number of clinical situations, medical fields and conditions for the repair and regeneration of acute and chronically damaged tissues, with an increasing number of translational efforts. Clinical trials have been advanced in order to investigate the therapeutic potential and applicability of these cells based on the induction of their properties similar to that observed in BMSCs. An extensive great knowledge concerning the harvesting, characterization and transplantation of ADSCs has been developed. Even so, current literature still lacks of strong evidence about the clinical potential of ADSCs and adipose tissue. In particular this may be due to the fact that human lipoaspirates may significantly differ in purity and molecular phenotype and that many reports have adopted heterogeneous populations of cells providing uncertain results. Remarkably, some problems still affect the correct interpretation of outcomes. One of the most significant issues limiting the interpretation of clinical progression is the lack of standardization in defining ADSCs, since both SVF and ADSCs may be used. [4] Another issue is whether ADSCs operate on tissue regeneration through direct transdifferentiation or paracrine mechanisms based on the secretion of numerous cytokines and growth factors. Thus, standardization of a method and improvement of current preclinical data may allow direct comparison of different results as well as a better definition of clinical potential of ADSCs. Current preclinical and clinical data of such cell-based therapies should include the osteogenic, chondrogenic, adipogenic, muscular, epithelial and neurogenic differentiation of progenitor, endothelial, and mesenchymal stem cells involved. Thus, skin, bone, cartilage, muscle, liver, kidney, cardiac, neural tissue, pancreas represent some of the most prominent clinical targets on which these therapies are focused. ADSCs are commonly adopted in clinical settings in surgical fields such as: cell-enriched lipotransfers, soft tissue augmentations and reconstructions of defects after trauma or oncologic surgery, healing of chronic wounds (phase 1 trials for the healing of recurrent Crohn's fistulae), skin regeneration and rejuvenation (repair of damages induced by aging or radiations), scar remodeling. In addition, they have been adopted in the treatment of cardiovascular disease, metabolic disease and encephalopathy (cerebral infarction) and a wide range of other surgical needs by orthopedic surgeons, oral and maxillofacial surgeons and cardiac surgeons. Indeed, the clinical application of adipose tissue relies on convincing results but the full therapeutic potential of ADSCs may still need further investigation.

5.1.1. The "Lipofilling technique"

Fat graft has been initially adopted to generate adipose tissue in the treatment of contour deformity or volumetric defects. The "lipofilling technique" has been used for many years and it has become rapidly popular especially in aesthetic surgery to improve cosmetic results in facial surgery. In fact it may be considered an ideal filler since it is totally biocompatible, readily available, inexpensive and it enables good aesthetic results. More variable are the application of fat injection in reconstructive surgical treatments. For example in breast reconstruction the indication of lipofilling include micromastia, tuberous breasts, Poland syndrome, post-lumpectomy deformity, post-mastectomy deformity, sequelae of post-radiotherapy (every anatomical region previously subjected to radiotherapy is subject to fat injection), refinement of secondary reconstructions after flap or prosthesis reconstruction and nipple reconstruction. In head and neck reconstructive surgeries it has been used to correct Treacher Collins syndrome o other cranio-synostosis. In burns, lipofilling has been adopted to improve the structural features of extracellular matrix in the treatment of burn sequaele, such as pathologic scars, with the aim to restore a more physiologic skin architecture. The lipofilling is also a valuable option to enhance volumes in facial hypotrophies, for example in patients affected by HIV-related lipo-distrophy. In addition, fat injection has proved to be very useful to improve local vascularization and trophism in chronic ulcers, especially vascular or post-traumatic ulcers.

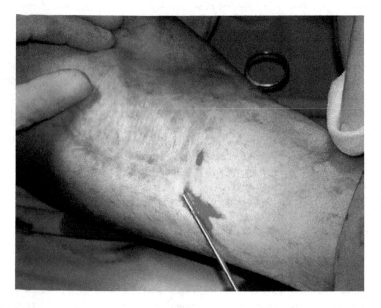

Figure 2. Injection of autologous adipose tissue ("lipofilling technique") in a scar.

5.1.2. Clinical trials with ADSCs

Most of clinical trials on humans are based on previous experiments on animal models. The evidence of the ability of ADSCs to differentiate into cells of non-mesodermal origin has been tested in some models in treatment of several diseases. The ADSC-derived hepatocytes transplanted into nude mice restored liver function and freshly isolated ADSCs could differentiated in to hepatocytes after intrasplenic transplantation into nude mice in vivo, supporting their application in clinical setting. [21] However clinical trials are still mostly lacking of promising results. [4] A recent study showed that the direct injection of ADSCs could restore blood flow in a mouse ischemic hindlimb model, as confirmed by clinical data. [22] The myogenic differentiation of ADSCs may be used in the treatment of muscular diseases such as Duchenne dystrophy and for regenerative cell therapy in heart failure. [23] Other novel potential clinical uses of ADSCs include the treatment of Alzheimer disease, of multiple sclerosis due to the anti-inflammatory effect of ADSCs, of neurogenic bladder and other neurologic disorders. A preliminary study showed that peri-urethral injection of autologous ADSCs acts positively in stress urinary after prostatectomy. Regarding current clinical applications of ADSCs, apart from a phase III trial on the treatment of Crohn's fistula, most clinical trials are in phase I. Beside the use in breast reconstruction, trials are in progress to treat acute myocardial infarction and chronic myocardial ischemia by intracoronary injection of SVF. Other trials are focused on the treatment of cirrhosis and of diabetes I or II. [4] Another trial adopted ADSCs (after purification and expansion) for the management of fistulas associated or not to Crohn's disease: results demonstrated an efficient control of inflammation and an improvement of healing process, most likely due to paracrine action that cells differentiation. Another trial investigated the restoration of volumes in hypotrophic scars after subcutaneous injection of ADSCs. Only two trials have studied the effect of ADSCs on chronic critical limb ischemia: the first adopting intra-muscular injection, the second by intravenous injection in diabetic patients. The literature regarding different clinical trials [Table 4.]demonstrates that ADSCs-based therapies are a concrete opportunity but despite these results, molecular, cellular e biological features of these cells are still uncertain and it is also unclear if regenerative therapy is related to their differentiation potential or paracrine activity: indeed, more appropriate in vivo investigations are necessary.

Pathology	Operating methods	Condition
Stress urinary after prostatectomy	peri-urethral injection of autologous ADSCs	Report of three initial cases
Crohn's fistula	injection into rectal mucosa of autologous of ADSCs with fibrin glue	Phase III
Cirrhosis	intrahepatic arterial administration of autologous SVF	Phase I
Diabetes I	intravenous injection of autologous SVF	Phase I/II
Diabetes II	autologous SVF	Phase I/II
Hypotrophic scars	subcutaneous injection of ADSCs	Phase III
Chronic critical limb ischemia	intra-muscular injection of ADSCs	Phase I
Chronic critical limb ischemia in diabetic patients	intravenous injection of ADSCs	Phase I/II
Myocardial infarction	intracoronary injection of SVF	Phase II/III
Multiple sclerosis	intravenous injection of autologous ADSCs	Phase I/II
Reumathoid arthritis	intrarticular injection of autologous ADSCs	Phase III

Table 4. Clinical trials using adipose-derived stem cells (ADSCs) or stromal vascular fraction (SVF).

6. Tissue engineering

6.1. Adipose derived bio-products

In the past decade, preclinical and translational efforts have established the future basis for the application of ADSCs from the bench to the bedside. Significantly, ADSCs have been widely used in tissue engineering, organ repair and gene therapy. These multipotent cells, have shown a remarkable plasticity and the ability to differentiate towards different cell lineages with similar yet enhanced properties (their multipotency and proliferative efficiency) in comparison to bone marrow-derived mesenchymal stem cells. [3,6-7,21-24,26] Moreover, ADSCs also show adjuvant angiogenic properties likely related to the secretion of vascular endothelial growth factor. [21] In vitro studies have rapidly increased during the last decade, resembling the need to optimize the variables of the differentiation process cells towards the desired lineage. The efficient use of biomaterials, delivery vehicles and bioreactors has promoted the development of a large variety of novel tissue engineered products for repair and regeneration of various tissues and organs. The use of suitable animal models in an extensive preclinical literature has also established the basis for successful stem cell-based therapies that may implement current therapeutic solutions for several diseases. Thus, a focus of most interest for the scientific community is posed today in the production of safe and reliable cell delivery vehicles/ scaffolds useful in applying ADSCs as a therapy as well as in the development of novel suitable in vivo animal models. A large variety of bioengineered products have been developed by means of selected differentiating cultures of ADSCs. [Table 5] Preclinical studies have experimentally reported the adoption of ADSCs in order to develop cells of mesodermal origin as well as cells of non-mesodermal lineage such as neural o neural-like cells for repair of neural traumatic injuries, fibroblast for reconstruction of soft tissue defects, tenocytes or regenerated tendon constructs for optimal musculoskeletal system reconstruction, osteoblasts for bone tissue replacement, chondrogenic lineages and cartilage substitutes for implantation, skeletal muscle cells and subsequent myotube-like formation depicting myogenic differentiation in vivo in muscular dystrophy model. Other reported lineages and engineered tissues that may be obtain through selective differentiation include hepatocytes, pancreatic endocrine cells, cardiomyocytes and vascular endothelial cells. [24] Most relevant transcription factors involved in differentiation into adipocytes, chondrocytes, myocytes and osteocytes are well-known. However, in addition to specific differentiation factors, tridimensional biomaterials are essential to address differentiation of ADSCs to the required cell type and to use them for tissue-engineering purposes. Among investigated effective scaffolds and matrices we may include: type I collagen, hyaluronic, poly lactic-co-glycolic acid (PLGA) and silk fibroin-chitosan. [26] Moreover, the combination with specific growth factors determines the overall outcome of the applied biopolymer.

Tissue	Cell type	Gene	Scaffold	Result
Bone	human ADSCs	BMP-2	-	heal critical sized femoral defects in a nude mouse model
	ADSCs	BMP-2	collagen sponge	increase bone induction in SCID mice
	Autologous SVF	-	bone graft	treat calvarial defects in human
	Autologous ADSCs	-	β-tricalcium phosphate-filled titanium scaffold	create neo-maxilla in human
Cartilage	ADSCs	-	polyglycolic acid scaffolds	exhibit in vitro chondrogenic characteristics
	ADSCs	-	-	improve outcome measures in osteoarthritis in dogs
Endothelia	ADSCs	-	porous polycaprolactone (PCL) scaffold	endothelial differentiation
Tendon	ADSCs	-	decellularized human tendon	recellularize
Nerve	ADSCs	-	hyaluronan membrane and fibrin meshes	differentiate in glial-like and neuronal-like cells

Table 5. Synopsis of current approaches in ADSCs and tissue engineering.

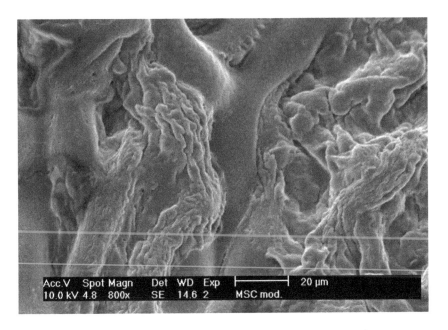

Figure 3. Electron microscopy scanning of ADSCs cultured on a Hyaluronic acid-based biomaterial.

6.1.1. Bio-engineered bone

There is still a clinical need to generate bone for the repair of large osseous defects, since current strategies are based on non-vascularized bone grafts, suitable only for small defects. As an alternative, progenitor cells might be implanted on biomaterials and differentiated in vivo supporting reconstruction of large bone losses. Osteo-inductive factors include vitamin D3, β-glicerophosphate, acid ascorbic and Bone Morphogenic Proteins (BMPs). [7] Treating ADSCs with recombinant BMP-2 has shown to stimulate osteogenic differentiation: [27] human ADSCs overexpressing BMP-2 could heal critical sized femoral defects in a nude mouse model. Similarly, ADSCs exposed to BMP-2 adenoviral transfection and seeded in collagen sponges increased bone induction in SCID mice. [27-28] These results suggest that transfected stem cells can replace the exogenous addition of growth factors when transplanted in a bio-engineered scaffold. The use of scaffolds is critical in repair of structural tissues such as bone. Demineralized bone matrix, collagen, PLGA, hydroxyapatite and β-tricalcium phosphate scaffolds were reported to be suitable for ADSC-derived osteochondral tissue engineering. Most of clinical trials of osteogenesis in ADSCs rely on murine studies and human trials are based on very limited reports. The first human case involved transplantation of SVF together with bone graft to treat calvarial defects [29] and in another case a neo-maxilla has been created using a β-tricalcium phosphate-filled titanium scaffold associated to cultured ADSCs. [30] Thus, ADSCs-based osteogenesis is possible, however, more adequate evidence is needed in the clinical setting.

6.1.2. Bio-engineered cartilage

ADSCs might be used to generate cartilage for clinical use in the treatment of degenerative joints. The list of potentially useful growth factors for cartilage repair comprises TGFβ, IGF-1, FGFs, EGF and BMPs, transcription factors as SOX9 and signal transduction molecules such as SMADs. Several in vitro studies have shown the chondrogenic differentiation of ADSCs and this feature is confirmed by their ability to generate cartilage in a variety of experimental models. ADSCs seeded into polyglycolic acid (PGA) scaffolds exhibited in vitro chondrogenic characteristics and they could synthesized cartilage extracellular matrix. [23] The great potential of ADSCs in cartilage tissue engineering was also demonstrated in different studies in vivo. Moreover ADSCs have been used recently for treatment of osteoarthritis in dogs [32] and rheumatoid arthritis in human. [33] However, given the lack of evidence, it seems likely that the symptomatic benefits seen in these trials may relate to the anti-inflammatory properties of ADSCs rather than to a real chondrogenic differentiation.

6.1.3. ADSCs and vascular/endothelial tissue engineering

The vascularization of regenerated tissues is an important field of research since it allow the survival of tissue and the differentiated cells. [24] It has been reported that human ADSCs have the potential for endothelial differentiation and they can participate in blood vessel formation by means of the secretion of several pro-angiogenic factors, like vascular endothelial growth factor (VEGF) and platelet-derived growth factor (PDGF). [23] This feature makes these cells suitable for regenerative cell therapy, treatment of ischemic disorders and construction of vascularized grafts in one-step procedure, as it has already been performed in many experiments on animal models. [22] Furthermore, as reminded, the angiogenetic properties of ADSCs have been already investigated in several clinical trials to treat various diseases.

6.1.4. Bio-engineered tendon

Tendon tissue engineering is relatively unexplored due to the difficulty to maintain in vitro preservation of tenocyte phenotype: only recently research has demonstrated the fundamental role of in vitro mechanical stimuli in maintaining the phenotype of tendinous tissues. [34] The main growth factors inducing tendon differentiation include fibroblast growth factor (FGF), platelet-derived growth factor-BB (PDGF-BB), epidermal growth factor (EGF), insulin-like growth factor (IGF)-1 and members of the transforming growth factor-β (TGF-β)/bone morphogenetic proteins (BMPs) family. Several in vivo and in vitro studies have showed the ability of ADSCs to differentiate in tenocytes under specific stimuli and under biomechanical force. [34] Furthermore, recent experiments have focused on the possibility of re-cellularize by means of seeded ADSCs a decellularized human tendon. [35] Thus, an integration of ADSCs, growth factors, mechanical stimuli and biopolymers may provide a solution for the treatment of difficult tendon injuries

6.1.5. ADSCs and neuronal tissue-engineering

Incubation of ADSCs under neuro-inductive conditions (culture medium containing EGF, FGF, NGF and BDNF) has shown the potential to form neurospheres expressing neurospecific markers, including nestin, βIII tubulin, S100 and glial fibrillar acidic protein (GFAP). [36] Moreover, seeding of these neurospheres in different scaffolds (hyaluronan based membranes and fibrin glue meshes) demonstrated further differentiation in glial-like and neuronal-like cells. [37] Although these are only preliminary researches, these promising results are of significant clinical interest. ADSCs-induced neural cells may provide beneficial therapeutic effects in treatment of injuries occurring to both the peripheral and central nervous systems such as in the treatment of neurodegenerative states, including Parkinson's disease, Hungtinton's disease, multiple sclerosis and Alzheimer's disease.

7. Prospectives

Regenerative medicine is an evolving field of research and therapeutics in which adipose tissue and ADSCs hold great promise for translational research and future clinical applications in many fields of tissue regeneration with a wide range of potential clinical implications. In the past decade, preclinical data from in vitro studies and pre-clinical animal models has been provided on the reproducibility, safety and efficacy of ADSCs in tissue regeneration or tissue engineering, supporting their use in clinical applications and establishing the basis for a translational application in the bedside: consistently, recent preliminary clinical trials have confirmed positive outcomes. The enhancing effect of ADSCs on autologous repair might enable better clinical outcomes and play a relevant role in healing acute and chronic tissue damage. Thus, more accurate information regarding optimal management and methods to promote differentiation lineages (among which differentiation factors, cell scaffolds, cell culture conditions) are strongly required. Further translational research, adequate clinical investigation and novel strategies should be promoted and designed to overcome current limitations, encourage future therapeutic implementation and face challenges posed by regenerative medicine.

Acknowledgements

Authors acknowledge their colleagues of the Clinic of Plastic Surgery of the University of Padua and of related laboratories for their kind support in the critical review of current clinical and preclinical experimental literature.

Author details

Vincenzo Vindigni, Giorgio Giatsidis, Francesco Reho , Erica Dalla Venezia ,
Marco Mammana and Bassetto Franco

*Address all correspondence to: giorgio.giatsidis@gmail.com

Clinic of Plastic Surgery, Department of Surgery, University of Padova, Padova, Italy

References

[1] Avram, A. S, Avram, M. M, & James, W. D. Subcutaneous fat in normal and diseased states: 2. Anatomy and physiology of white and brown adipose tissue. J Am Acad Dermatol. (2005). , 53(4), 671-83.

[2] Sbarbati, A, Accorsi, D, Benati, D, Marchetti, L, Orsini, G, Rigotti, G, & Panettiere, P. Subcutaneous adipose tissue classification. Eur J Histochem. (2010).

[3] Gimble, J. M, Katz, A. J, & Bunnell, B. A. Adipose-derived stem cells for regenerative medicine. Circ Res. (2007). , 100(9), 1249-1260.

[4] Casteilla, L, Planat-benard, V, Laharrague, P, & Cousin, B. Adipose-derived stromal cells: Their identity and uses in clinical trials, an update. World J Stem Cells. (2011). , 3(4), 25-33.

[5] Hausman, D. B, Park, H. J, & Hausman, G. J. Isolation and culture of preadipocytes from rodent white adipose tissue. Methods Mol Biol. (2008). , 456, 201-219.

[6] Zuk, P. A, Zhu, M, Ashjian, P, De Ugarte, D. A, Huang, J. I, Mizuno, H, Alfonso, Z. C, Fraser, J. K, Benhaim, P, & Hedrick, M. H. Human adipose tissue is a source of multipotent stem cells. Mol Biol Cell. (2002). , 13(12), 4279-4295.

[7] Witkowska-zimny, M, & Walenko, K. Stem cells from adipose tissue. Cell Mol Biol Lett. (2011). , 16(2), 236-257.

[8] Salgado, A. J, Reis, R. L, Sousa, N. J, & Gimble, J. M. Adipose tissue derived stem cells secretome: soluble factors and their roles in regenerative medicine. Curr Stem Cell Res Ther. (2010). , 5(2), 103-110.

[9] Tabit, C. J, Slack, G. C, Fan, K, Wan, D. C, & Bradley, J. P. Fat grafting versus adipose-derived stem cell therapy: distinguishing indications, techniques, and outcomes. Aesthetic Plast Surg. (2012). , 36(3), 704-713.

[10] Coleman, S. R. Structural fat grafting: more than a permanent filler. Plast Reconstr Surg. (2006). Suppl):108S-120S.

[11] Wilson, A, Butler, P. E, & Seifalian, A. M. Adipose-derived stem cells for clinical applications: a review. Cell Prolif. (2011). , 44(1), 86-98.

[12] García-olmo, D, García-arranz, M, Herreros, D, Pascual, I, Peiro, C, & Rodríguez-montes, J. A. A phase I clinical trial of the treatment of Crohn's fistula by adipose mesenchymal stem cell transplantation. Dis Colon Rectum. (2005). , 48(7), 1416-1423.

[13] Schipper, B. M, Marra, K. G, Zhang, W, Donnenberg, A. D, & Rubin, J. P. Regional anatomic and age effects on cell function of human adipose-derived stem cells. Ann Plast Surg. (2008). , 60(5), 538-44.

[14] Padoin, A. V, Braga-silva, J, Martins, P, Rezende, K, Rezende, A. R, Grechi, B, Gehlen, D, & Machado, D. C. Sources of processed lipoaspirate cells: influence of donor site on cell concentration. Plast Reconstr Surg. (2008). , 122(2), 614-618.

[15] Zhu, Y, Liu, T, Song, K, Fan, X, Ma, X, & Cui, Z. Adipose-derived stem cell: a better stem cell than BMSC. Cell Biochem Funct. (2008). , 26(6), 664-675.

[16] Rodbell, M. The metabolism of isolated fat cells. IV. Regulation of release of protein by lipolytic hormones and insulin. J Biol Chem. (1966). , 241, 3909-3917.

[17] Carvalho, P. P, Wu, X, Yu, G, Dias, I. R, Gomes, M. E, Reis, R. L, & Gimble, J. M. The effect of storage time on adipose-derived stem cell recovery from human lipoaspirates. Cells Tissues Organs. (2011). , 194(6), 494-500.

[18] Petit, J Y, Botteri, E, Lohsiriwat, V, et al. Locoregional recurrence risk after lipofilling in breast cancer patients. Ann.Oncol. (2012). , 23(3), 582-588.

[19] Petit, J Y, Clough, K, Sarfati, I, et al. Lipofilling in breast cancer patients: from surgical technique to oncologic point of view. Plast.Reconstr.Surg. (2010). , 126(5), 262-263.

[20] Petit, J Y, Lohsiriwat, V, Clough, K B, et al. The oncologic outcome and immediate surgical complications of lipofilling in breast cancer patients: a multicenter study--

Milan-Paris-Lyon experience of 646 lipofilling procedures. Plast Reconstr Surg. (2011)., 128(2), 341-346.

[21] Utsunomiya, T, Shimada, M, Imura, S, Morine, Y, Ikemoto, T, Mori, H, Hanaoka, J, Iwahashi, S, Saito, Y, & Iwaguro, H. Human adipose-derived stem cells: potential clinical applications in surgery. Surg Today. (2011)., 41(1), 18-23.

[22] Nakagami, H, Morishita, R, Maeda, K, Kikuchi, Y, et al. Adipose tissue-derived stromal cells as a novel option for regenerative cell therapy. J Atheroscler Thromb. (2006)., 13, 77-81.

[23] Locke, M, Feisst, V, & Dunbar, P. R. Concise review: human adipose-derived stem cells: separating promise from clinical need. Stem Cells. (2011)., 29(3), 404-411.

Chapter 8

Is the Articular Cartilage Regeneration Approachable Through Mesenchymal Stem Cells Therapies?

José M. López-Puerta, Plácido Zamora-Navas,
Silvia Claros, Gustavo A. Rico-Llanos, Inés Avedillo,
José A. Andrades and José Becerra

Additional information is available at the end of the chapter

1. Introduction

Today great hope is set on regenerative medicine in all medical fields. Leland Kaiser introduced the term "Regenerative Medicine" in 1992. He forecasted that a "new branch of medicine will develop that attempts to change the course of chronic diseases and in many instances will regenerate tired and failing organ systems" (Kaiser, 1992). Since then, scientists all over the world try to develop cell-based approaches to regenerate damaged tissues, or even substitute whole organs (Ehnert et al., 2009).

Degenerative disease of articular cartilage (AC), generically known as osteoarthritis (OA), is an irreversible evolution process towards terminal articular failure. Due to its high prevalence on population and its socioeconomic impact, this condition is of great concern, and this way more resources and effort are dedicated to the research on its development. Cartilage tissue engineering seeks to combine cells, biomaterial scaffolds, and bioactive signals to create functional tissue replacements to treat cartilage injuries or osteoarthritis (Song et al., 2004).

Cartilage degenerative disease, OA, is the end stage of several conditions such as trauma, inflammatory diseases, overweight etc. The fatalistic theory that states that it is impossible to recover the cartilage once it has been damaged leads to the assumption that the progression to any form of OA is unavoidable (Fig. 1). The annual incidence of young adults suffering any cartilage injury in UK is 10000 and this figure is continuously increasing (NICE, 2008).

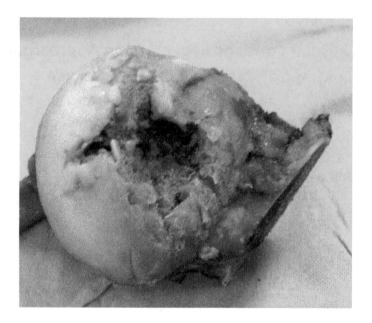

Figure 1. Osteochondral injury in a femoral head from a surgical intervention in our hospital

The new patient does not accept a reduction in his demands and quality of life because of the OA as the culmination of an articular injury during sport activity. On the other hand, a higher risk for developing degenerative disease and obesity, mainly knee arthritis, has been correlated. The symptomatic cohort of pain, swelling, range of motion diminution and loss of quality life can only be partially recovered by a total joint replacement (Fig. 2).

Unfortunately, joint replacement is neither a procedure free of complication nor a forever-realistic solution. It is expected that by the year 2030 the number of total hip or knee replacement implanted annually will be respectively 1.8 and 7 times the current figures (Kurtz et al., 2007). It is doubted that such an economic impact could be ever be afforded. Finding an alternative option to manage these lesions will be a challenge and this must be closer to achieve an almost AC tissue able to bear the requirements of an active long period of life.

AC is a quite simple structure with scarce cellularity within an extracellular matrix (ECM). However, in spite of this simplicity, its structure and performance is very complex.

The ability of the AC to heal these injuries on its own is almost none. The lack of blood supply is the main handicap this tissue has at the time of healing. Without vessels the preliminary inflammatory step of the healing process is not possible. To start with, the dead tissue needs to be removed and the flood of new cells from the vascular stream is essential for this.

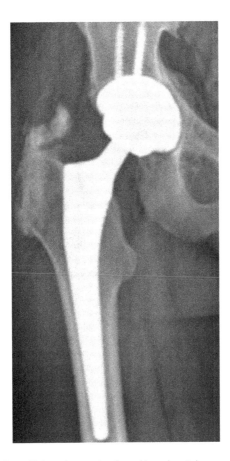

Figure 2. Treatment of a OA by total joint replacement performed in our hospital

Furthermore, the cell mediators will not appear as the granulocytes are not present and the degranulation of these is its source. Secondly, the chondrocytes are well-differentiated cells with a limited capacity to produce ECM. This is sufficient to cover the necessities of a still cartilage turnover but not to cope with the healing of a traumatic defect.

In any case, if the trauma produces a lesion that breaches the subchondral plate, it allows access to the vascular network and the final produced tissue is made of collagen type I, more resistant to tension, instead of type II, more resistant to compression.

1.1. How can this be sorted out?

Several attempts have been made in order to repair the traumatic defect and to achieve a regeneration of the original injured cartilage.

A first group of interventions can be described as "marrow stimulating techniques". Drilling the defect beyond the subchondral plate is its essential and allowing a repair promoted by the bleeding from the subchondral bone creating a "super clot" its rationale (Mithoefer et al., 2005). The star cells here are the mesenchymal stem cells (MSCs) emerging with the hematoma and its subsequent proliferation and differentiation. Unfortunately, the final result is the promotion of a fibrous tissue not durable in time (Steret et al., 2004). Pridie et al. promoted this concept in 1959. Abrasion arthroplasty (Steret et al., 2004), microfracture (Steadman et al., 2003), or Autologous Matrix Induced Chondrogenesis (Gille et al., 2010) have been more recently developed with the same rationale.

In essence, previous treatments have attempted to promote the healing of the damaged reminding nature. That is to say, allowing the flood of blood from the inner areas of the subjacent bone. Unfortunately, this will promote a scar tissue that in the long run will be lost and the joint degenerative process will be stated (Kreuz et al., 2006).

In a second group of interventions, it is proposed the articular defect to be covered by a "replacement technique". In these, the defect is reshaped to a standard cylindrical way and substituted with a plug of osteochondral graft harvested from a non-weight bearing donor site. Using this technique two handicaps can be appreciated: the limited available graft and the morbidity of the donor site. Additionally, the differences in characteristics between the donor and the receiver areas may impede a complete integration. This may be the reason why the clinical results have not been in accordance with the initial enthusiasm (Mishima et al., 2008). Both, auto- and fresh allograft (Gross et al., 2002) have been attempted with the name of mosaicplasty. With the aim of avoiding the donor site morbidity, synthetic reabsorbable scaffolds have been used to fill up the osteochondral defect. A "toast and butter" cylinder, engineered mimicking components, bone and cartilage. In contrast with the graft, this scaffold will have osteoconductive properties instead and eventually resorb in 12 months. The pseudo-cartilage now created will be poorly incorporated and the biomechanics will fail (Yasen et al., 2012).

The third group of proposed interventions are cellular-based. The aim in this alternative option is producing a regeneration of the cartilage mediated by the own patient chondrocytes. This is a two-stage procedure. During the preliminary intervention a biopsy from the cartilage is obtained and then the chondrocytes are isolated and cultured till the number of cells is about fifty folds. For the second intervention, *ex vivo* expanded chondrocytes are implanted in the damaged area. This procedure has evolved with the aim of getting a watertight seal environment in order to receive the chondrocytes and avoid the leakage. First, it was attempted a sheet of periosteum, then a collagen gel and a collagen membrane has been developed. But, are the delivered chondrocytes, the MSCs coming from the subchondral bone or the cells evading from the layer of periosteum the source for promoting the repaired tissue?. In spite of the rationale of this techniques, the autologous chondrocytes implant has not finally reached the expected results, the final tissue obtained was fibrous instead of AC (Tins et al., 2005) and hence, the OA is once more the undesirable expected long-term result (Hunziker, 2002; Temenoff et al., 2000).

2. Therapeutic interventions without active biologics

2.1. Bone marrow stimulation

First approaches to heal cartilage by *in situ* regeneration date back to 1959. Pridie technique was directed to BM cells recruitment to be used in cartilage defects by drilling small holes into the subchondral BM space underlying the damaged cartilage regions. It was improved later on by reducing the size of the perforations and being then called microfracture technique which is now a frequently performed and well-studied procedure (Steadman et al., 1999). This technique is based on the mechanism of mesengenesis or capacity of the non-differentiated mesenchymal cells in choosing a determined phenotype as a response to inducing or GFs. A non-differentiated cell from the BM can be promoted to different cell types such as osteoblasts, with a later maturing to osteocytes, chondroblasts and chondrocytes, but also to endothelial cells, mesothelial cells, fibroblasts or adipocytes. It is a cell signalling process of local cytokines on local cells. In order to achieve all this, the surgical technique is based on drilling the subchondral plate to get bleeding and a superclot that will become a scaffold and supply cells and proteins, starting this way the physiological cascade of the chondrogenic cell differentiation. Other alternative techniques of BM stimulation to regenerate cartilage would be abrasion chondroplasty and in case the articular surface remained untouched, the retrograde stimulation technique. Cartilage defects are repaired only with fibrous tissue or fibrocartilage when using these methods, probably because the number of chondroprogenitors recruited from the BM is too small to promote the hyaline cartilage repair and results are often followed by degeneration of the repair tissue. This was used as an explanation for the observations of other studies that good short term results may be followed by deterioration starting about 18 months after surgery.

Clinical observations and theoretical considerations pointed towards several possible limitations of marrow stimulation techniques. The non-adhesive properties of the cartilage surface and the softness and shrinking of the superclot can lead to only partial defect filling and facilitate an early loss of repair tissue from the cartilage lesion. To avoid this, the treatment has been recently advanced into a matrix-supported technique in which the performed defect was stabilized in an additional way with a biomaterial. The microfractured lesion is covered with a collagen type I/III scaffold and it is called autologous matrix induced chondrogenesis (AMIC) (Kramer et al., 2006; Steinwachs et al., 2008). This technique has been developed to allow the treatment of larger defects by microfracturing and it is used as alternative treatment to autologous chondrocytes transplantation (ACT).

2.2. Autologous osteochondral transplantation: Mosaicplasty

Autologous osteochondral mosaicplasty, sometimes known as osteoarticular transfer system, OATS, is an effective method for the resurfacing of osteochondral defects of the knee. The technique consists in transplantation of many osteocondral autologous plugs obtained from the periphery of the femoral condyle articular surface, which supports less weight and transferring them to create a durable resurfaced area in the defect (Fig. 3). The procedure shows some advantages regarding other repair techniques, such as the viable hyaline cartilage transplantation, a relatively short rehabilitation period and the possibility of carrying out the procedure in one only operation.

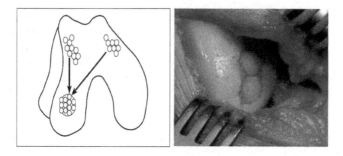

Figure 3. In mosaicplasty cylindrical osteochondral plugs are harvested from nonload-bearing sites in the affected joint and pressed into place within the osteochondral defect, creating an autograft "mosaic" to fill the lesion

However, the OATS limitations are the donor-site morbidity and a limited availability of grafts that can be obtained from the femoropatellar joint or the area adjacent to the intercondylar fossa. Other possible limitations are differences in bearing, thickness and mechanical proper-ties between the donor's and the receiver's cartilages, as well as the graft sinking into the surface due to the support of weight after surgery. Besides, the lack of filling and the possible dead space between cylindrical grafts can limit the repair quality and integrity. Lane et al. transplanted autologous osteochondral grafts into sheep knee joints and reported the lack of integration of the cartilage, which determined the persistence of gaps through the full thickness in all the specimens (Mishima et al., 2008).

2.3. Alogenic osteochondral transplantation

Osteochondral allograft transplantation is a procedure for cartilage resurfacing which involves the transplantation into the defect a cadaveric graft composed of viable, intact AC and its underlying subchondral bone. It is a well known resource, especially for tumour surgery. The defect size, its location and its depth are crucial factors for the suitability of the donor graft. Advantages of using osteochondral allografts are the possibility if achieving a precise archi-tecture of the surface, the immediate transplantation of viable hyaline cartilage in a one-time procedure, the possibility to repair large defects, even half-condyles and the donor-site lack of morbidity. Gross et al. have reported results from fresh allografts in 123 patients with good clinical results in 95% of the patients after five years (Gross et al., 2002). There are different possible allografts. Fresh osteochondral allografts are generally used because both freezing and cryopreservation have proved to reduce the chondrocytes viability. Traditionally grafts have been obtained, kept in lactated Ringer's solution at 4 °C and then transplanted in a week. Another alternative for allografts conservation and implantation is cryopreservation, which involves freezing at a controlled speed of specimens within a nutrients rich medium, a cryoprotector agent (glycerol or dymethil sulfoxide), to minimize the cells freezing and keep their viability; finally, there is the possibility of fresh-frozen allografts, with the advantages of lower immunogenic capacity and less transmission of diseases but with lower chondrocyte viability.

2.4. Soft tissues transplantation

Two main theories support the practicing of covering the cartilage defects with soft tissues, such as perichondrium or periosteum. On one hand, the defect has to be covered mechanically and on the other, we know about the presence of pluripotential stem cells in the perichondrium and the periosteum cambium layer. The different factors able to promote these cells differentiation into active chondrocytes still remain unknown.

3. Therapeutic interventions with active biologics

3.1. Autologous chondrocytes implant

The clinical use of the autologous chondrocytes implant (ACI) technique was first reported by Brittberg et al. in 1994, following animal studies which had shown its effectiveness (Grande et al., 1989). In this method, chondrocytes are obtained from a biopsy taken from a non-weight bearing part of the patients cartilage, and are expanded *in vitro*, followed by the injection of a suspension of chondrocytes into cartilage defects, covered with autologous periosteal flap (Fig. 4). This technique premises are based on the capacity of adhesiveness of the cells to certain surfaces, they spread on them and proliferate producing their specific ECM. Although clinical results of the original ACI looked promising (Minas, 2001; Peterson et al., 2000), this procedure has some potential disadvantages, such as leakage of transplanted cells, invasive surgical method, hypertrophy of periosteum (Haddo et al., 2005; Kreuz et al., 2009) and loss of chondrogenic phenotype of expanded chondrocytes in monolayer culture (Benya & Shaffer, 1982). Second generation ACI, named membrane autologous chondrocyte implantation (MACI), has a similar procedure, but a collagen type I and III membrane instead of periosteum. This technique was introduced to improve the ACI problems, and biomaterials such as collagen type I gel (Ochi et al., 2002), hyaluronan-based scaffold (Manfredini et al., 2007) and collagen type I/III membrane (Bartlett et al., 2005) were applied to secure cells in the defect area, to restore chondrogenic phenotype by way of three dimensional cultures (Gigante et al., 2007]) and to replace the periosteum as defect coverage. This is the way MACI technique is created *a posteriori*, by implanting autologous chondrocytes in three dimensional matrices of collagen types I and III, or hyaluronic acid.

At present, only two prospective studies comparing the original and second generation ACI are available (Bartlett et al., 2005; Manfredini et al., 2007) and both studies show no significant differences in the short term clinical results. As for the first generation ACI, the newly regenerated cartilage often consists of fibrous tissue (Horas et al., 2003; Tins et al., 2005), possibly due to the limited number of chondrocytes and their low proliferation potential. Bone overgrowth that causes thinning of the regenerated cartilage and the violation of the tidemark are also of concern. Moreover, this method still sacrifices healthy cartilage. Thus, these aspects

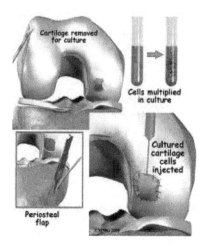

Figure 4. In autologous chondrocytes implantation (ACI) a chondral biopsy is taken from a donor site at the time of clinical examination to be treated with enzymes in the laboratory to obtain chondrocytes cultures that are re-injected under the periosteal flap

limit ACI in the treatment of large defects and may increase the long-term risk of osteoarthritis development.

3.2. Are Mesenchymal Stem Cells what we need?

Stem cells are of particular interest in Regenerative Medicine. They inhere several unique characteristics that distinguish them from other cell types. Besides autograft transplantation and ACI, current therapeutic concepts of cartilage defects include the recruitment of MSCs. Tissue engineering (TE) based on cell and genetic therapy offers some of the most promising strategies of tissue repair, including AC repair. It is the science able to create alive tissue to replace, repair or strengthen ill tissue. Thus, the TE refers to a wide variety of techniques.

The process for using MSCs to produce cartilage tissue comprises four elements: cells, inductor factors, scaffold to deliver the cells and vascular supply to the host area.

From the previous experiences we have learned that we need:

• To minimize the risk and inconveniences of the donor site. In this case, MSCs are easily available from bone marrow, synovial membrane, adipose tissue, etc. So then, we can get a variable number of cells from a different tissue, partially avoiding the donor site secondary complication (Winter et al., 2003). In ACI, this extra procedure adds a risk for infection, inflammatory changes in the joint, pain and rises up the final cost of the treatment (Hunziker, 2002)

• To achieve a minimum number of cells. MSCs have a high proliferation and differentiation potential. In any case, MSCs coming from different tissue have an uneven chondrogenic differentiation capacity and it must be related to the special cytokines, growth factor and induction molecules composition of the medium (Claros et al., 2012; Hennig et al., 2007). To induce the differentiation of predifferentiated cells, MSCs, is a more controlled way of driving the process to a cartilage final effector. One of the cons of chondrocyte transplantation is the dedifferentiation process that these cells suffer when they are treated *in vitro* and the limited ability to redifferentiate them (Benz et al., 2002). On the contrary, MSCs are very stable and they do not suffer this dedifferentiation (Najadnik et al., 2010) process and have a high differentiation capacity.

Up to now, MSCs have been used to treat osteochondral defects in two different ways. We have the option of implanting the MSCs once expanded. It is of concern in this case the lack of control on the growth after transplantation and how much exhausted the cells will result after the expansion and how it will influence on the aging of the new induced tissue. The clinical results after implantation of these expanded MSCs have been analysed and were substantially the same compared with those obtained after any marrow stimulating techniques (Wakitani et al., 2002; López-Puerta, 2013). A second option is to implant the MSCs after the induced differentiation to a chondrocyte phenotype. In these circumstances, to assure the stability of the achieved phenotype is of concern as this lineage is able to go on with the complete chondral process and ends in producing final stages of hypertrophy and calcification (Pelttari et al., 2006; Andrades et al., 2010; López-Puerta, 2013). In any case, the final challenge will be to produce a stable cellular lineage that produces an AC tissue that works under compression forces without losing its initial characteristics as time goes by.

Beside the characteristics of MSCs exposed before, these cells have self-renewal potential as well as multilineage differentiation potential (Becerra et al., 2011), including chondrogenesis (Johnstone et al., 1998; Pittenger et al., 1999; Prockop 1997; Sacchetti et al., 2007). MSCs chondrogenesis was first reported by Ashton et al. (1980) and the first ones to describe a defined medium for *in vitro* chondrogenesis of MSCs were Johnstone et al. (1998), who used micromass culture with TGF-β and dexamethasone. Sekiya et al. (2001, 2005) reported that addition to bone BMPs enhanced chondrogenesis under the conditions employed by Johnstone et al. (1998). Nowadays, the micromass culture is widely used to evaluate chondrogenic potential of MSCs *in vitro*. However, this *in vitro* chondrogenesis does not mimic cartilage formation during development. During micromass culture, MSCs increase expressions of both collagen type II (chondrocytes marker) and X (hypertrophic chondrocytes marker) (Barry et al., 2001; Ichinose et al., 2005). Other cytokines such as IGF (Pei et al., 2008) and parathyroid hormone-related peptide (PTHrP) had been tried for better differentiation cocktails, but it is still difficult to obtain *in vitro* MSC-based cartilage formation comparative to native cartilage tissue.

To initiate any regeneration based on MSCs activity, the cells first have to be recruited to the site of damage (Fig. 5). Second step is adhesion to a local matrix followed by activation and extensive proliferation to provide the necessary high numbers of chondroprogenitor cells to build up new tissue. In stem 3, the cells need to switch from expansion to chondrogenic matrix production by induction of chondrogenesis to build up the shock absorbance and gliding characteristics for proper tissue function. The seamless integration with neighbouring cartilage and bone tissue depends on successful crosstalk between new and old tissue, and an instructional capability to guide neighbouring cells. For durable cartilage regeneration, the tissue eventually needs to regenerate a tidemark, adapt to biomechanical loading and build up a balanced tissue homeostasis. We are going to summarize these steps including talking points taken from our annual meetings in NACRE (New Approaches for Cartilage Regeneration; CIBER-BBN, Spain) consortium, in order to propose strategies for the Regenerative Medicine of AC (Becerra et al., 2010; Andrades et al., in press)

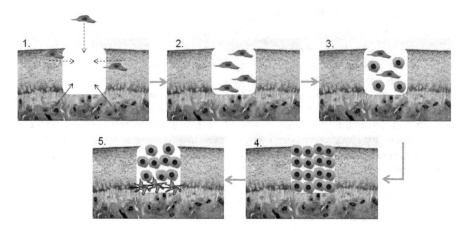

Figure 5. Principal mechanisms for *in vivo* cartilage regeneration. 1) MSCs recruitment from the surrounding tissues such as synovial fluid/membrane, neighbors cartilage, or subchondral bone; 2) MSCs retention by local adhesion, and proliferation; 3) MSCs are induced to chondrogenic differentiation by local factors; 4) chondroblasts and chondrocytes arranged according to the cartilage zones pattern and biomechanical loading; 5) integration of repair tissue interaction with cartilage and subchondral bone

3.2.1. Recruitment of MSCs

Cell migration is a prerequisite for development from conception to adulthood and plays a major role in regeneration of all tissues. Even articular chondrocytes, which are encased in a dense matrix throughout their life, can show cell motility when transferred *in vitro*. A number of studies demonstrated that chondrocytes migrate under the action of different stimuli on or within planar and 3D matrices. Attracting factors include bone morphogentic proteins (BMPs) (Frenkel et al., 1996), insulin-like growth factor-one (IGF-1), transforming growth factor-beta (TGF-β), fibronectin (Andrades et al., 2003: Chang et al., 2003), plateled-derived growth factor (PDGF) (Fujita et al., 2004), fibroblast growth factor (FGF) (Hidaka et al., 2006), fibrin and collagen type I (Kirilak et al., 2006).

But, what are the best factors to attract more MSCs to a cartilage lesion? Recent work has established that MSCs are not largely distinct from chondrocytes regarding the panel of factors capable to attract the cells *in vitro*. All tested factors were further effective in stimulating the migration of MSCs but not fibroblasts (Ozaki et al, 2007). Factors contained in a natural blood clot are highly chemoattractive for MSCs; augmentation of a clot-stabilizing matrix with a potent chemoattractive factor like PDGF may be an attractive way to further enhance cell numbers early after microfracturing.

In this sense, a quick release kinetics within hours and days from the biomaterial is desired for this first step of healing. Unfortunately, no 3D *in vitro* model in a biomatrix has yet been applied to test chemoattraction of human MSCs under more natural conditions and no adequate animal model has been used to dissect the factor requirement of progenitor cell recruitment from bone marrow into cartilage defects. Most likely, the presence of synovial fluid and the joint loading initiated pumping mechanism will strongly affect attraction and retention of MSCs. A search for superior factor combinations to enhance and speed up MSC attraction, and the best retention matrix to keep cells local, thus, is an important topic for upcoming studies.

3.2.2. Multiplication of MSCs

Proliferation of MSCs is the second important step to rapidly enhance the cell numbers in the repair tissue. As the replicative lifespan of MSCs is, however, not unlimited and telomerase activity is absent or low (Parsch et al., 2004) this can only ground on the sufficient attraction of initial MSCs numbers to the defect. During embryonal development proliferative chondro-progenitors are densely packed and condensed to an area in which cartilage tissue is forming. The high cell numbers may be needed to deposit the vast amount of ECM characterizing this tissue. Low cellularity of AC is rather a late phenomenon during tissue formation and may have developed in adaptation to its biomechanical competence and the extremely slow turnover of its ECM. Proteoglycan turnover in cartilage is up to 25 years and collagen half-life was estimated to range from several decades up to 400 years (Eyre et al., 2006). Based on the assumption that embryonal traits should best be recapitulated during tissue regeneration, early defect filling tissue should contain densely packed proliferating chondroprogenitors. This would mean that rather hundreds of millions of new cells are needed per cm^3 during this step in the defect to allow for optimal chondrogenesis and rapid ECM production. At a later phase, cell numbers could decline to a density of 5-10 million cells per gram tissue, when homeostasis is the left over task for the cells in the fully regenerated tissue.

These points towards an outstanding need for highly efficient transient induction of prolifer-ation, a typical feature ascribed to adult stem cells. Growth requirements of human MSCs are distinct from those of other species (Kuznetsov et al., 1996) and many factors have been identified as potent mitogens, being PDGF-BB, EGF and TGF-β have been regarded as the most important amongst them (Kuznetsov et al., 1997). As they induced the migration of MSCs and have at the same time the potency to enhance their proliferation, the migration and prolifera-tion steps of MSCs can take place simultaneously *in vivo*. However, whilst nutrients and oxygen are almost unlimited in tissue culture, a rapid supply of cells with O_2 and nutrients may be more restricted in a cartilage defect and depend on the distance to and conditions found within the subchondral bone. Histology of early human cartilage repair tissue demonstrates that indeed cartilage differentiation initiates in contact with subchondral bone (Steck et al., 2009) whilst upper regions remain fibrous for quite a long time and may need to mature over years (Brun et al., 2008). Furthermore, earliest chondrogenesis is often seen in areas where active remodeling of the subchondral bone plate occurs and, thus, enhanced nutrition and a higher anabolic rate of the cells can take place. Beside strong mitogenic factors used for augmentation of a clot-stabilizing biomaterial, the access to optimal nutrition in the course of tissue remodeling may indeed be a limiting aspect of cartilage regeneration techniques. Enhanced remodeling of microfractured compared with unopened subchondral bone areas is likely, but quantitative and localization-dependent studies have so far not been reported. The stimuli mentioned here could be obtained by direct administration of recombining growth factors in the culture media or via transfer of the respective genes. Thus, the possibility of considering genetic therapy as an applicable measure for the treatment of cartilaginous lesions arises.

4. The recapitulation of AC morphogenesis through MSCs differentiation

In spite of therapeutic strategies mentioned, which offer the patient a temporary relief of symptoms, they do not resolved, in the medium or long term, the disease that affects the joint. In most cases, fibrocartilage is generated that does not provide the necessary structural integrity and this often results in the subsequent replacement of the damaged joint (Mahmoudifar and Doran, 2012).

The main problem with these strategies is that only tries to restore the biomechanical characteristics of tissue but not its physiology. That is why the goal of current research in AC regeneration with MSCs is moving to methods that attempt to recapitulate the morphogenesis of the tissue. The challenge is to develop strategies that will cover the widest possible range of intervening factors including: the dynamics of genes and proteins that control and participate in the chondrogenic process, their spatiotemporal patterns of expression, variations in culture conditions, biomaterials functionalized with effector molecules inducers of chondrogenesis and the inclusion of differentiation enhancers using genetic engineering and others.

4.1. Novel genes and protein: The path to recapitulating AC morphogenesis

As previously mentioned, the AC's ECM is composed mainly of collagen type II fibers and proteoglycans with strong negative charges, aggrecan being the most abundant of them (Han et al, 2011). That is why the detection of both proteins and their corresponding genes has been classically used as markers of chondrogenesis in numerous studies *in vitro* and *in vivo*. However, most modern regenerative strategies should aim at obtaining a more complete and organized ECM that achieves the greatest similarity with the ECM on the original AC. With this objective, have been identified dozens of genes that play a fundamental role in the formation and maintenance of AC, which are potential targets for research in the design of regenerative strategies (Quintana et al., 2009; Bobick et al., 2009; Mahmoudifar and Doran, 2012).

4.1.1. Proteoglycan 4 (PRG4): Biological function and its relationship to OA

A good example is the proteoglycan 4 (PRG4), also known as "superficial zone protein" (SZP) and "lubricin". It is a proteoglycan specifically synthesized by chondrocytes located at the surface of AC and by synoviocytes. Their functions are the lubrication of articular joints, elastic absorption and energy dissipation of synovial fluid (Jay et al., 2007).

It has been shown that mutant mice $Prg4^{-/-}$ have normal joints at birth and during the newborn period but older mice exhibit accumulation of proteinaceous deposits on the cartilage surface, disappearance of the surface zone of flattened chondrocytes, synoviocyte hyperplasia, calcification of structures flanking the ankle joints and, consequently, a total failure of the joint (Coles et al., 2010). These data are consistent with OA degeneration, and have also been observed in veterinary cases of sheep with early OA which has been shown a downregulation of the expression of *PRG4* (Young et al., 2006). In a human clinical example, a case study reported in 2004 a 10 year old boy with Camptodactyly-Arthropathy-Coxa vara-Pericarditis syndrome (CACP) which arises as a result of truncating mutations of this gene. Clinical manifestations of CACP include congenital or early-onset camptodactyly, noninflammatory arthropathy with synovial hyperplasia and progressive coxa vara deformity, all symptoms related with the cartilage's physiology (Choi et al., 2004).

All these studies show that PRG4 is closely related to morphogenesis, maintenance and functioning of the AC as well as defects in its expression are related to the development of OA. That is why in recent years has aroused interest in the field of *in vitro* studies as a potential aim in developing AC regenerative strategies.

4.1.2. PRG4: An in vitro, in vivo and clinical marker of chondrogenesis

Several studies show that this protein participates in the chondrogenic process and that its expression can be induced on *in vitro* chondrogenesis experiments. Recently, has been found an increase in *PRG4* gene expression in cells derived from infrapattelar fat pad (IFP) in response to treatment with TGF-β1 and BMP-7, demonstrating that the *in vitro* induction of this gene expression is possible. Furthermore, it served to demonstrate the suitability of the source cell used (Lee et al., 2008). However, the same research group in a similar characteristics experiment but using human embryonic stem cells (hESC) was able to induce chondrogenesis but failed inducing PRG4 expression, concluding that the induction conditions should be optimized. PRG4 use as a marker allowed the discrimination of both experiments (Nakagawa et al., 2009). It has also been observed that in rat skeletal muscle-derived mesenchymal stem/ progenitor cells (MDMSCs) treated with TGF-β1 and BMP-7, PRG4 increased in a time-dependent manner on days 3, 7 and 10. As early as day 3, there was a three-fold increase of the PRG4 detected by ELISA analysis. This was confirmed by immunochemical localization of PRG4 as early as day 3 after treatment with TGF-β1. Even, the mRNA expression of PRG4 was enhanced by the two factors, along or in combination. This work demonstrates that is possible induce *in vitro* not only the increased of PRG4 gene expression, but also the accumulation of the protein in the medium (Andrades et al., 2012).

In clinical setting, there are also studies related with PRG4. Patients with OA tend to form small cartilaginous deposits in the exposed subchondral bone. The histological study of aggregates of patients undergoing total knee replacement, reveals that these aggregates were fibrocartilaginous, positive staining for glucosaminoglycan Safranin-O and type II collagen expression but, more interestingly, of PRG4. In those aggregates embedded in the bone, the staining was positive for the entire surface while in which protruded to the surface, the PRG4 was detected only in the edge surface as would be observed in normal cartilage. This *in vivo* observation is an excellent example of the cell's genetic response to the environment. Osteo-chondroprecursors contact with the synovial fluid and physicochemical stimuli inherent to the articular surface is able to modify the spatial distribution patterns of PRG4 expression and thus, the tissue architecture. These results are an invitation to test culture conditions that attempt to emulate not only the biochemical environment, but also mimic the biophysical characteristics of the physiological niche (Zhang et al., 2007) (Fig. 6).

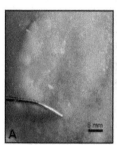 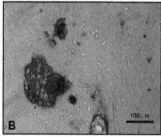 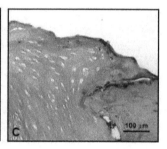

Figure 6. A) Probe pointing to a white spot on the exposed bone surface of an osteoarthritic femoral condyle obtained at the time of total knee arthroplasty. B) Immunohistochemistry for PRG4 to subsurface chondrocyte aggregate in subchondral bone staining fully for PRG4; and C) fibrocartilaginous deposit protruding through the joint surface containing PRG4 in a zone just below the surface. *From the same authors, published by Journal of orthopaedic research: official publication of the Orthopaedic Research Society 25(7): 873–883. Copyright 2007*

It has also been demonstrated the possibility of reversing the decline in the expression of PRG4 in cartilage chondrocytes culture from OA patients. In this study, cartilage explants were obtained from healthy and OA patients and performed monolayer cultures and encapsulated in poly (ethylene glycol) diacrylate scaffold (PEG-DA). The OA cartilage explants have weaker inmunolabeling of PRG4 than healthy cartilage explants. However, the difference was reduced significantly between these 2 samples when were cultured in PEG-DA hydrogels. OA chondrocytes regain the ability to express PRG4 at levels virtually identical to those obtained in chondrocytes from normal cartilage demonstrating the importance of culture conditions in the condrogenic induction (Musumeci et al., 2011).

All these evidences indicate that the inclusion of proteins as PRG4 in experimental designs offers advantages such as:

1. The inclusion of more highly specific markers that allow a better understanding of chondrogenic potential of cell sources, bioactive scaffolds and treatments applied.

2. Implant design that better mimic the characteristics of the AC and try to emulate not only the composition but also tissue architecture.

3.   The ability to understand more deeply the dynamics of diseases that affect the AC like OA, in order to raise regenerative strategies that offer to patients, medium and long term solutions.

4.2. Genetic engineering: Enhance of chondrogenic potencial beyond biochemical signals and functionalized scaffolds

4.2.1. SOX9: The key regulator of the chondrogenic process

Given the low regenerative capacity of the AC, it is vital find ways to increase the chondrogenic potential of bioimplants designed. Today, not only can enhance the biochemical environment biomaterials and implants, but genetic engineering can increase the potential of MSCs used, changing their gene expression patterns from "inside". For this, it is important to consider transcription factors and their intracellular signaling cascades. Perhaps the most studied of these factors is SOX9, considered the key regulator of the chondrogenic process (Bi et al., 1999). The expression of SOX9 is upregulated by members of the FGFs, TGF-βs and BMPs, all of them widely used chondroinducers. In turn, SOX9 is responsible for regulating SOX5, SOX6 and activating the expression of collagens type II, VI, IX and XI, the proteoglycans Aggrecan, Byglican and Perlecan and important binding proteins as COMP (Quintana et al., 2009) (Fig. 7).

On the other hand, during skeletogenesis, SOX9 is responsible for the osteochondroprogenitors differentiation into chondroblasts and not into osteoblasts to direct and indirect repression of RUNX2 (the main regulator of osteogenic differentiation) favoring the endochondral ossification (Zhou et al., 2006).

4.2.2. Transfection of SOX9 as an activator of chodrogenesis

The application of these regulatory genes on regenerative design strategies could be useful to increase both specificity and efficiency of the bioimplants. This opens the possibility of using not only functionalized biocompatible scaffolds, but also cells previously treated to have a higher chondrogenic potential. In a recent study, human MSCs are transfected with a nonviral vector plasmid complexed with SOX9 cDNA in order to induce chondrogenesis. Micromass culture and transplantation into nude mice of control and transfected cells were made. Both procedures showed increased levels of mRNA for COL2A1, Aggrecan and COMP; increased GAG content; alcian blue staining positive and detection of type II collagen and Aggrecan by immunofluorescence, all of the cells transfected with respect to control. Similar results were achieved using a viral vector transfection of SOX9 (Fig. 8). Additionally, this group demonstrated that transfection of the gene, in addition to inducing chondrogenesis, reduces the levels of markers of hypertrophy, osteogenesis and adipogenesis, thereby inhibiting the possibility that the human MSCs to differentiate into these mesenchymal lineages (Venkatesan et al., 2012).

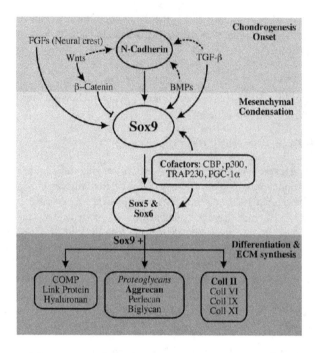

Figure 7. Upstream and downstream regulation of Sox9. From the same authors, published by Tissue engineering. Part B, Reviews 15(1): 29–41. Copyright 2009

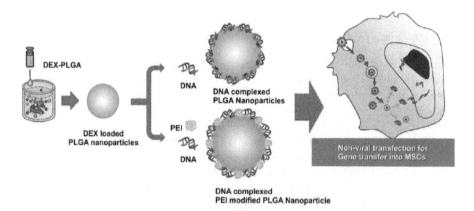

Figure 8. Schematic diagram of SOX9 gene transfection using a modified and non-modified biodegradable nanoparticles, an example of Non-viral transfection. During hMSCs transfection, nanoparticles interact with the negatively charged lipid bilayers and are influxed into endosomes and destabilized, resulting in the release of the transfected genes into the cytosol. *From the same authors, published by Biomaterials 32(1): 268–278. Copyright 2011*

The possibility of genetically engineering the different types of MSCs used in cartilage regeneration is a promising tool for increasing chondrogenic capacity and, consequently, improving future regeneration bioimplants. A deepest and detailed knowledge of gene regulation involved in the process and their possible clinical utilities will lead the way of successful recapitulation of AC morphogenesis through MSCs differentiation.

5. Commercial and industrial translations in tissue engineering

Applications for TE and biomaterials were originally limited to prosthetic devices and surgical manipulation of tissues but now include development of biomaterial scaffolds, bone/cartilage engineering, tissue-engineered blood vessels and wound healing, among other fields.

As an industry, it could significantly contribute to economic growth if products are successfully commercialized. However, to date, relatively few products have reached the market owing to a variety of barriers, including a lack of funding and regulatory hurdles. Policy interventions, including increased translational government funding, adaptation of policies, and regulatory clarity, would likely improve the general outcomes for the regenerative medicine industry.

The technical challenges of TE are, of course, intellectually and scientifically interesting and can add substantial and previously unattainable knowledge to our understanding of biological systems (Mansbridge et al., 2006). TE models of biological systems can even provide insight into pathologic processes. However, perhaps the major attraction of academic researchers and industrial organizations to this field is the potential of the technology to be readily converted to clinical applications. For this to happen, the technology almost always will be transferred from an academic environment to an industrial organization that will lead the comprehensive translational studies and convert scientific observations into a manufactured product.

As s technology, TE has been shown to be feasible *in vitro* and *in vivo*, but the true demonstration of the potential value of the technology is in its clinical applications. Although the field is still in its infancy, there are already tissue-engineered products on the market, addressing previously unmet clinical needs in wound care and in orthopedics and demonstrating that the attractiveness and motivation of the field is justified. Perhaps one of the next major challenges is demonstration that the technology can lead to commercially feasible products, with manageable investment, product development costs, and time to market and, finally, a revenue generation that justifies the expense. The close connection between new technology, clinically effective treatment, and commercially feasible product is obvious and is no better demonstrated than in TE. All three of these areas, each complex in itself, must be aligned and achieved before TE can be regarded as successful.

5.1. Product development pathway

To appreciate the challenge of developing a tissue-engineered product, it is useful to first understand in general terms the various processes that must be completed (Fig. 9). The development of a product through to approval, manufacture, and marketing is complex, and most companies (within and outside health care) use a staged process to ensure efficient and effective product development. The general scheme that applies for health care products (devices, biologics, or drugs) is outlined in the figure. These stages encompass all the activities that are required to develop a product through to the market. This integrated product development process can be customized to be appropriate for the development of products addressing repair and regeneration.

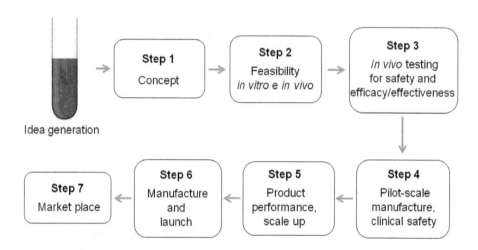

Figure 9. The general product development pathway used to develop tissue-engineered products

Patient protection for an individual product is a critical feature of product development. Developing new patents is costly, the outcome is uncertain, and it must occur near the beginning of product development. The limited time for patent protection (usually 10 years from initial submission) requires that the product development pathway be followed in an efficient manner; otherwise, patent protection will be lost by the time profitability arrives.

Acknowledgements

Laboratory of Bioengineering and Tissue Regeneration-University of Málaga (LABRET-UMA) is supported by grants from the Spanish (PI10/02529, and Red de Terapia Celular, RD06/00100014), and the Andalusian Governments (PI-0729-2010, and PAID BIO217). CIBER-BBN is an initiative funded by the VI National R&D&I Plan 2008-2011, *Iniciativa Ingenio 2010, Consolider Program, CIBER Actions* and financed by the Instituto de Salud Carlos III (Ministry of Economy and Competitiveness) with assistance from the *European Regional Development Fund.*

The authors have written this chapter in collaboration with Dr. Avedillo, Scientific Director of the company Innovaxis Biopharmaceuticals Ltd., with which we have established an agreement regarding patent number WO 2012001124 A1, referenced below.

Author details

José M. López-Puerta[1,2], Plácido Zamora-Navas[2,3], Silvia Claros[2,4], Gustavo A. Rico-Llanos[2,4], Inés Avedillo[5], José A. Andrades[2,4] and José Becerra[2,4]

1 Department of Orthopaedic Surgery and Traumatology, Universitary Hospital Virgen del Rocío, Sevilla, Spain

2 Networking Biomedical Research Center in Bioengineering, Biomaterials and Nanomedicine (CIBER-BBN), University of Málaga, Málaga, Spain

3 Department of Orthopaedic Surgery and Traumatology, Universitary Hospital Virgen de la Victoria, Málaga, Spain

4 Laboratory of Bioengineering and Tissue Regeneration (LABRET-UMA), Department of Cell Biology, Genetics and Physiology. Faculty of Sciences, University of Málaga, Málaga, Spain

5 Innovaxis Biopharmaceuticals Ltd., Technological Park of Jerez, Jerez de la Frontera, Spain

References

[1] Andrades, J.A.; Han, B.; Nimni, M.E.; Ertl, D.C.; Simpkins, R.J.; Arrabal, M.P. & Becerra, J. (2003) A modified rhTGF-beta1 and rhBMP-2 are effective in initiating a chondroosseous differentiation pathway in bone marrow cells cultured in vitro. *Connective Tissue Research*, 44(3-4), 188-197.

[2] Andrades, J.A.; López-Puerta, J.M.; Claros, S.; Rico-Llanos, G.; & Becerra, J. Articular cartilage regeneration using autologous mesenchymal stem cells and a biphasic collagen scaffold. *Osteoarthritis and Cartilage* (in press).

[3] Andrades, J.A.; López-Puerta, J.M.; Cuenca-López, M.D.; Jiménez-Palomo, P. & Becerra, J. (2010). Mesenchymal stem cells and a composed membrane for osteocondral wound treatment. *Patent application* nº 201031016, international publication number WO 2012001124 A1, 29 pages.

[4] Andrades, J.A.; Motaung, S.C.; Jiménez-Palomo, P.; Claros, S.; López-Puerta, J.M.; Becerra, J.; Schmid, T.M., et al. (2012). Induction of superficial zone protein (SZP)/lubricin/PRG 4 in muscle-derived mesenchymal stem/progenitor cells by transforming

growth factor-β1 and bone morphogenetic protein-7. *Arthritis research & therapy*, 14(2), R72.

[5] Becerra J.; Andrades J.A.; Guerado, E.; Zamora-Navas, P.; López-Puerta, J.M. & Reddi, A.H. (2010). Articular cartilage: structure and regeneration. *Tissue Engineering Part B Review*, 16(6), 617-627.

[6] Becerra J.; Santos-Ruiz, L.; Andrades, J.A. & Marí-Beffa, M. (2011). The stem cell niche should be a key issue for cell therapy in regenerative medicine. *Stem Cell Review*, 7, 248-255.

[7] Beiser, I. H., & Kanat, I. O. (1990). Subchondral bone drilling: a treatment for cartilage defects. *The Journal of foot surgery*, 29(6), 595-601.

[8] Benz K, Breit S, Lukoschek M, Mau M, Richter W (2002). Molecular analysis of expansion, differentiation, and growth factor treatment of human chondrocytes identifies differentiation markers and growth-related genes. Biochem Biophys Res Commun, 293:284-292.

[9] Bi, W., Deng, J. M., Zhang, Z., Behringer, R. R., & de Crombrugghe, B. (1999). Sox9 is required for cartilage formation. *Nature genetics*, 22(1), 85-89.

[10] Bobick, B. E., Chen, F. H., Le, A. M., & Tuan, R. S. (2009). Regulation of the chondrogenic phenotype in culture. *Birth defects research*. Part C, Embryo today: reviews, 87(4), 351-371.

[11] Brittberg, M., Lindahl, A., Nilsson, A., Ohlsson, C., Isaksson, O., & Peterson, L. (1994). Treatment of deep cartilage defects in the knee with autologous chondrocyte transplantation. *New England Journal of Medicine*, 331(14), 889-895.

[12] Choi, B.-R., Lim, Y.-H., Joo, K.-B., Paik, S. S., Kim, N. S., Lee, J., & Yoo, D.-H. (2004). Camptodactyly, Arthropathy, Coxa vara, Pericarditis (CACP) Syndrome: A Case Report. *Journal of Korean Medical Science*, 19(6), 907-910.

[13] Claros, S.; Rodríguez-Losada, N.; Cruz, E.; Guerado, E.; Becerra, J.; & Andrades, J.A. (2012). Characterization of adult/progenitor cell populations from bone marrow in a three-dimensional collagen gel culture system. *Cell Transplant*, 21(9): 2021-2032.

[14] Coles, J. M., Zhang, L., Blum, J. J., Warman, M. L., Jay, G. D., Guilak, F., & Zauscher, S. (2010). Loss of Cartilage Structure, Stiffness, and Frictional Properties in Mice Lacking PRG4. *Arthritis and Rheumatism*, 62(6), 1666-1674.

[15] Ehnert S, Glanemann M, Schmitt A. (2009). The possible use of stem cells in regenerative medicine: dream or reality?. Langenbeck's Archives of Surgery, 394(6): 985-997.

[16] Gille J, Kunow J, Boisch L, Behrens P, Bos I, Hoffmann C, Köller W, Russlies M, Kurz B. (2010). Cell-laden and cell-free matrix-induced chondrogenesis versus microfracture for the treatment of articular cartilage defects: a histological and biomechanical. Cartilage, 1: 29-42.

[17] Gross, AE, Aubin P, Cheah, HK, Davis AM, (2002). Ghazavi MT A fresh osteochondral allograft alternative. J Arthroplasty, 17 (4 suppl 1): 50-3.

[18] Han, L., Grodzinsky, A. J., & Ortiz, C. (2011). Nanomechanics of the Cartilage Extracellular Matrix. *Annual review of materials research*, 41, 133–168.

[19] Hennig T, Lorenz H, Thiel A, Goetzke K, Dickhut A, Geiser F, Richter W. (2007). Reduced chondrogenic potential of adipose tissue derived stromal cells correlates with an altered TGFbeta receptor and BMP profile and is overcome by BMP-6. J Cell Physiol, 211:682–691.

[20] Hunziker EB (2002). Articular cartilage repair: basic science and clinical progress. A review of the current status and prospects. Osteoarthritis Cartilage, 10:432–463.

[21] Jay, G. D., Harris, D. A., & Cha, C. J. (2001). Boundary lubrication by lubricin is mediated by O-linked beta(1-3) Gal-GalNAc oligosaccharides. *Glycoconjugate journal*, 18(10), 807–815.

[22] Jay, G. D., Torres, J. R., Warman, M. L., Laderer, M. C., & Breuer, K. S. (2007). The role of lubricin in the mechanical behavior of synovial fluid. *Proceedings of the National Academy of Sciences of the United States of America*, 104(15), 6194–6199.

[23] Kaiser LR. (1992). The future of multihospital systems. Topics in Health Care Financing, 18(4): 32-45.

[24] Kreuz PC, Steinwachs MR, Erggelet C, Krause SJ, Konrad G, Uhl M, Südkamp N. (2006). Results after microfracture of full-thickness chondral defects in different compartments in the knee. Osteoarthritis Cartilage, 14: 1119-1125.

[25] Kurtz S, Ong K, Lau E, Mowat F, Halpern M. (2007). Projections of primary and revision hip and knee arthroplasty in the United States from 2005 to 2030. J Bone Joint Surg, 89-A: 780-5.

[26] Mishima Y, Lotz M. (2008). Chemotaxis of human articular chondrocytes and mesenchymal stem cells. Journal of Orthopaedic Research, 26: 1407–12.

[27] Lee, S. Y., Nakagawa, T., & Reddi, A. H. (2008). Induction of chondrogenesis and expression of superficial zone protein (SZP)/lubricin by mesenchymal progenitors in the infrapatellar fat pad of the knee joint treated with TGF-β1 and BMP-7. *Biochemical and Biophysical Research Communications*, 376(1), 148–153.

[28] López-Puerta JM. (2013). Mesenchymal stem cells and a biphasic biomaterial as cell therapy application for articular cartilage regeneration in the knee. Doctoral Thesis, 1-209.

[29] Mahmoudifar, N., & Doran, P. M. (2012). Chondrogenesis and cartilage tissue engineering: the longer road to technology development. *Trends in Biotechnology*, 30(3), 166-76.

[30] Mansbridge J. (2006). Commercial considerations in tissue engineering. J Anat, 209:527-532.

[31] Mithoefer K, Williams RJ, Warren RF, Potter HG, Spock CR, Jones EC, Wickiewicz TL, Marx RG. (2005). The microfracture technique for the treatment of articular carti-lage lesions in the knee : a prospective cohort study. J Bone Joint Surg, 87-A: 1911-1920.

[32] Nakagawa, T., Lee, S. Y., & Reddi, A. H. (2009). Induction of chondrogenesis from human embryonic stem cells without embryoid body formation by bone morphoge-netic protein 7 and transforming growth factor beta1. *Arthritis and Rheumatism*, 60(12), 3686–3692.

[33] National Institute of Health and Clinical Excellence 2008 Technology Appraisal 89 (2010). The use of autologous chondrocyte implantation for the treatment of cartilage defects in knee joints. www.nice.org.uk

[34] Nejadnik H, Hui JH, Feng Choong EP, Tai BC, Lee EH. Autologous bone marrow-derived mesenchymal stem cells versus autologous chondrocyte implantation: an ob-servational cohort study. Am J Sports Med, 38:1110–1116.

[35] Pelttari K, Winter A, Steck E, Goetzke K, Henning T, Ochs BG, Aigner T, Richter W. (2006). Premature induction of hypertrophy during in vitro chondrogenesis of hu-man mesenchymal stem cells correlates with calcification and vascular invasion after ectopic transplantation in SCID mice. Arthritis Rheum, 54: 3254–3266.

[36] Quintana, L., zur Nieden, N. I., & Semino, C. E. (2009). Morphogenetic and regulato-ry mechanisms during developmental chondrogenesis: new paradigms for cartilage tissue engineering. *Tissue engineering*. Part B, Reviews, 15(1), 29–41.

[37] Rhee, D. K., Marcelino, J., Baker, M., Gong, Y., Smits, P., Lefebvre, V., Jay, G. D., et al. (2005). The secreted glycoprotein lubricin protects cartilage surfaces and inhibits synovial cell overgrowth. *The Journal of clinical investigation*, 115(3), 622–631.

[38] Richter W (2003). Cartilage-like gene expression in differentiated human stem cell spheroids: a comparison of bone marrow-derived and adipose tissue-derived stromal cells. Arthritis Rheum, 48:418–429.

[39] Robert, H., Bahuaud, J., Kerdiles, N., Passuti, N., Capelli, M., Pujol, J.-P., Hartman, D., et al. (2007). Treatment of deep cartilage defects in the knee with autologous chondrocyte transplantation: a review of 28 cases. *Revue de chirurgie orthopédique et réparatrice de l'appareil moteur*, 93(7), 701–709.

[40] Song L, Baksh D, Tuan RS. (2004). Mesenchymal stem cell-based cartilage tissue engi-neering: cells, scaffold and biology. Cytotherapy, 6: 596.

[41] Steadman JR, Briggs KK, Rodrigo JJ, Kocher MS, Gil TJ, Rodkey WG. (2003). Out-comes of microfracture for traumatic chondral defects of the knee : average 11-year follow-up. Arthroscopy, 19: 477-484.

[42] Steadman JR, Rodkey WG, & Rodrigo JJ. (2001). Microfracture: surgical technique and rehabilitation to treat chondral defects. *Clinical orthopaedics and related research*, (391 Suppl), S362–369.

[43] Sterett WI, Steadman JR. (2004). Chondral resurfacing and high tibial osteotomy in the varus knee. Am J Sports Med, 32: 1243-1249.

[44] Temenoff JS, Mikos AG. (2000). Review: tissue engineering for regeneration of articular cartilage. Biomaterials, 21: 431–440.

[45] Tins, B.J, McCall IW, Takahashi T, Cassar-Pullicino V, Roberts S, Ashton B, Richardson J. (2005). Autologous chondrocyte implantation in knee joint: MR imaging and histologic features at 1-year follow-up. Radiology, 234:501–8.

[46] Venkatesan, J. K., Ekici, M., Madry, H., Schmitt, G., Kohn, D., & Cucchiarini, M. (2012). SOX9 gene transfer via safe, stable, replication-defective recombinant adeno-associated virus vectors as a novel, powerful tool to enhance the chondrogenic potential of human mesenchymal stem cells. *Stem cell research & therapy*, 3(3), 22.

[47] Wakitani S, Imoto K, Yamamoto T, Saito M, Murata N, Yoneda M. (2002). Human autologous culture expanded bone marrow mesenchymal cell transplantation for repair of cartilage defects in osteoarthritic knees. Osteoarthritis Cartilage, 10:199–206.

[48] Williams, R. J., 3rd, & Harnly, H. W. (2007). Microfracture: indications, technique, and results. *Instructional course lectures*, 56, 419–428.

[49] Winter A, Breit S, Parsch D, Benz K, Steck E, Hauner H, Weber RM, Ewerbeck V, Richter W. (2003). Cartilage-like gene expression in differentiated human stem cell spheroids: a comparison of bone marrow-derived and adipose tissue-derived stromal cells. Arthritis Rheum, 48:418–429.

[50] Yasen SK, Melton JTK, Wilson AJ. (2012). Treatment of focal chondral lesions in the knee using the TRUFTT plug : A case series. J Bone Joint Surg, 94-B (Supp XXIX): 9.

[51] Young, A. A., McLennan, S., Smith, M. M., Smith, S. M., Cake, M. A., Read, R. A., Melrose, J., et al. (2006). Proteoglycan 4 downregulation in a sheep meniscectomy model of early osteoarthritis. *Arthritis Research & Therapy*, 8(2), R41.

[52] Zhang, D., Johnson, L. J., Hsu, H.-P., & Spector, M. (2007). Cartilaginous deposits in subchondral bone in regions of exposed bone in osteoarthritis of the human knee: histomorphometric study of PRG4 distribution in osteoarthritic cartilage. *Journal of orthopaedic research: official publication of the Orthopaedic Research Society*, 25(7), 873–883.

Chapter 9

Regulatory Issues in the Therapeutic Use of Stem Cells

Bridget M. Deasy, Jordan E. Anderson and
Shannon Zelina

Additional information is available at the end of the chapter

1. Introduction

1.1. Stem cell tourism

Advances in stem cell research and media publicity of stem cell potential have raised the hopes of patients with severe disabilities and conditions which lack a cure. While stem-cell-based therapies are the clinical standard of care for a few conditions, such as leukemia and more recently for some burns and corneal disorders, stem cell tourism continues to rise worldwide.

Unfortunately, clinics around the world are exploiting patients' hopes by offering supposed stem cell therapies, without credible scientific rationale, oversight or patient protections. Occurring particularly in Asia and South America, treatments which are illegal in most counties are being offered for what are often considered incurable conditions, such as brain tumors, congestive heart failure or chronic obstructive pulmonary disease. In addition, countless other conditions are listed as candidates by these clinics including eye disease or orthopedic injuries or disease. In response to this, the International Society for Stem Cell Research (ISSCR) released "The *Guidelines for the Clinical Translation of Stem Cells*" which called for rigorous standards in the development of stem cell therapies and outlining what needs to be accomplished to move stem cells from promising research to proven treatments[1]. The goal of ISSCR in shining this light on the dangers of stem cell tourism is to ensure that the promise of stem cell research is delivered to patients in a safe, effective and fair manner. A number of professional organizations have also published guidance documents for the responsible conduct in translational stem cell research.

The general public receives information regarding stem cell potential from mainstream media and does not fully understand the risks associated with unproven treatments. In the most desperate situations, patients may see no other options, or may view the years of continuing research as an obstacle to their potential cure. Yet, untested treatments can be dangerous and years of preclinical and clinical research are required to determine which novel stem-cell based therapies are effective and safe. In one example, brain tumors were discovered in a 9-year old boy who travelled to Russia to receive stem cell treatments to his brain; later it was found that the tumors were the result of cells from at least 2 different donors [2]. Even carefully planned and approved studies can go wrong and have unfortunate results, as in the fatal gene therapy case of Jesse Gelsinger, who received experimental therapy at University of Pennsylvania[3, 4].

Lau et al reported on the clinics around the world that are exploiting patients' hopes by professing to have effective stem cell therapies for seriously ill patients. These therapies often carry a hefty pricetag. However, they occur in counties which have limited oversight and allow treatment to occur in the absence of credible scientific rationale, transparency, oversight, or patient protections [5].

Comprehensive government regulations exist in the US, and several other countries. Below, we describe the U.S. and other government regulations associated with the use of human stem cell and tissues in regenerative medicine.

2. Cell Products must follow FDA regulatory guidelines

2.1. FDA's risk-based approach

To protect the public from risks associated with cell therapies and demonstrate the effectiveness of treatments, the U.S. FDA and other professional societies such as the ISSCR, and the United States Pharmacopia (USP), have established guidelines for therapies using human cellular and tissue-based products (HCT/Ps). The FDA has statutory authority to prevent the spread of communicable diseases granted under Section 361 of the Public Health Service Act (PHS Act, 42 U.S.C. § 264). HCT/Ps are regulated through a risk-based approach outlined predominantly in 21 C.F.R. Part 1271. Some HCT/Ps are regulated solely under Part 1271 while other HCT/Ps are regulated under both Part 1271 and FDA's Federal Food, Drug, and Cosmetic Act (FDCA, premarket and post- market regulation of medical devices and drugs), & section 351 of the PHS Act for biological products. FDA's regulation focuses on three general areas: 1) limiting the risk of transmission of communicable disease from donors to recipients; 2) establishing manufacturing practices that minimize the risk of contamination; 3) requiring an appropriate demonstration of safety and effectiveness for cells and tissues that present greater risks due to their processing or their use [6, 7].

Stem cell therapies show excellent promise for many types of treatments. However, scientific, manufacturing and safety challenges exist. Once the optimal stem cell type is identified for a given treatment (Table 1), there is a requirement to demonstrate the product's safety and efficacy in a clinical setting. Cell therapies must overcome several challenges before they can be considered safe for human use. First, most cell therapies will require large numbers of cells. Large cell doses are obtained by increasing cell harvest yields and by increasing ex vivo expansion yields. As cell cultures are expanded over long time periods, they show signs of aging that may be similar to human aging [8, 9]. Lengthy expansion periods can result in ineffective cellular products[10]. Cells may also be manipulated in other manufacturing steps that include cell-selection processes, genetic modifications, or encapsulation with another biological device. Cells that undergo ex vivo manipulation may lose potency, or acquire infectious contaminants, or become transformed / tumorogenic due to the cell culture conditions [11, 12]. Finally, the cells themselves may pose a risk, simply due to the novelty of the therapy and unknowns associated with their behavior in the body.

	Embryonic Stem Cells	Adult iPS	Adult BM-MSCs	Adult Adipose MSC
Ethical concerns	[56-60]	[61-67]		
Tumorogenic	[68-72]	[59, 73-75]		[76-79]
Scale-Up challenge	[80-83]		[84-86]	[87]
Genetically unstable	[88, 89]	[34, 39, 90-94]		[95]
Immunogenic difficulties	[96, 97]	[37, 98]		

Table 1. Scientific and Manufacturing Challenges in Stem Cell Sourcing (*numbers refer to literature references)* Several stem cell types are studied for their potential use in regenerative medicine, including, but not limited to, embryonic stem cells [20-27], inducible pluripotent stem cells [28-41], bone-marrow stem cells [42-46] and adipose-derived stem cells [47-55]. However, there are challenges with all stem cell types. A major concern with clinical application of iPSCs is their tendency to form tumors and cause cancer. Both ESC and iPSCs form teratoma in vivo, a major obstacle to stem-cell based regenerative medicine by the FDA. Also they are ethically controversial since they require genetic engineering using oncogenes. More recently, proteins have been used to generate piPSCs but the conversion efficiency us quite low. Adult derived BM-MSCs or adipose MSC are limited by their expandability.

In 1993, the US FDA began establishing regulatory and guidance documentation for cell therapies with the issuance of Application of Current Statutory Authority to Human Somatic Cell-therapy and Gene-therapy Products [13] which provided a biologics regulatory framework for the use of HCT/Ps. Table 2 provides a list of other key regulatory and guidance documents. The tiered risk-based approach means that products which present a lower perceived risk will be less regulated, while products with a larger perceived risk will undergo more extensive controls and examination. Both will require the cell products to be manufactured following Good Manufacturing Practices (GMP), and Good Tissue Practices (GTP). Additional regulatory requirements will depend on whether the cell product is minimally manipulated or more-than-minimally manipulated.

Guidance for Industry: Guidance for human somatic cell therapy and gene therapy		1998
GMPs	GMP	2001
Suitability determination for donors of HCT/Ps; proposed rule		1999
Current good tissue practice for manufacturers of HCT/Ps; inspection and enforcement; proposed rule	GTP	2001
Human cells, tissues and cellular and tissue-based products (HCT/Ps); establishment registration and listing; final rule		2001
Good clinical practice, GCP, ICH E6	GCP	1996
Validation of procedures for processing of human tissues intended for transplantation: final guidance		2002
Guidance for Industry: Eligibility Determination for Donors of Human Cells, Tissues, and Cellular and Tissue-Based Products		2007
Guidance for Industry Potency Tests for Cellular and Gene Therapy Products		2011

Table 2. Key US FDA Regulatory and Guidance Documents. Over the past 15 years, the FDA has provided several guidance documents for HCT/Ps. A few products such as Genezyme's *Carticel* received approval prior to the issuance of these documents and has been grandfathered in. Many of these guidance documents are issued by CBER, the center within FDA that regulates biological products for human use following applicable federal laws, including the Public Health Service Act and the Federal Food, Drug and Cosmetic Act.

Minimal manipulation is defined by the FDA for cells or nonstructural tissue as processing that does not alter relevant biological characteristics of cells or tissues. HCT/Ps that meet 1271 criteria for regulation solely under section 361 of the PHS Act and the regulations in Part 1271 are called "361 HCT/Ps", and are not subject to any premarket review requirements. The Center for Biologics Evaluation and Research (CBER) has jurisdiction over 361 HCT/Ps.

According to 21 CFR 1271.10, minimal manipulation criteria include:

1. The HCT/P is minimally manipulated;

2. The HCT/P is intended for homologous use only, as reflected by the labeling, advertising, or other indications of the manufacturer's objective intent;

3. The manufacture of the HCT/P does not involve the combination of the cell or tissues with another article, except for water, crystalloids, or a sterilizing, preserving, or storage agent, provided that the addition of water, crystalloids, or the sterilizing, preserving, or storage agent does not raise new clinical safety concerns with respect to the HCT/P; and

4. Either:

i. The HCT/P does not have a systemic effect and is not dependent upon the metabolic activity of living cells for its primary function; or

ii. The HCT/P has a systemic effect or is dependent upon the metabolic activity of living cells for its primary function, and:

a. is for autologous use;

b. is for allogeneic use in a first-degree or second-degree blood relative; or

c. is for reproductive use.

For cells, minimal manipulation means processing that does not alter the relevant biological characteristics of cells or tissues. Examples of products regulated as 361 HCT/Ps include bone marrow or blood transplants and organ transplants.

HCT/Ps that do not meet one or more of the four major criteria, are considered more-than-minimally- manipulated HCT/P. FDA has stated that density-gradient separation, cell selection, centrifugation, and cryopreservation constitute minimal manipulation. All processes that manipulate the cell / tissue product such as cell activation, encapsulation, ex vivo expansion, and gene modifications are considered more-than-minimal manipulations. Most advanced cellular therapies meet criteria for the more-than minimally manipulated category [14]. Finally, it is possible to request an informal jurisdictional determination on the level of manipulation from the Tissue Reference Group (TRG), or submit a formal Request for Designation (RFD) from the Office of Combination Products (OCP). Figure 1 is a schematic of regulatory pathway assessment to determine which guidelines apply to a given HCT/Ps product.

2.2. Manufacturing of HCT/Ps requires GTPs

For HCT/Ps that do not meet the criteria established in Section 1271.10, FDA premarket review is required; this includes obtaining FDA license, approval, or clearance.

All steps in the manufacturing of HCT/Ps will require compliance with Current Good Tissue Practice (cGTPs). cGTPs cover manufacturing facilities and processes. The manufacturing process can be broadly described as 1) procurement of HCT/Ps (donor screening and testing, product recovery), 2) processing of HCT/Ps (tissue or cell recovery /isolation, product handling, product labeling), 3) storage (e.g. cryopreservation), and 4) distribution. Many of these steps are common to GTPs and GMPs with the goal of safe and effective products via well-controlled processes and thorough supporting documentation. Requirements for standard operating procedures (SOPs), labeling controls, and storage requirements also exist.

2.2.1. Procurement

Therapies with HCT/Ps will require a determination of donor eligibility. For the FDA, donor eligibility is determined based on donor screening and testing for relevant communicable disease agents and diseases, and is required for all donors of cells or tissue used in HCT/Ps, with some exceptions listed in C.F.R. Part 1271.90.

As part of clinical or industry compliance with donor testing requirements, procedures to process, store, label, and package cell products also are needed. Hospitals and companies involved in cell/tissue therapeutics manufacturing must establish quality programs which consist of a comprehensive system for manufacturing and tracking HCT/Ps. The quality program must follow CGTP requirements, and be designed to prevent, detect, and correct deficiencies that may lead to circumstances that increase the risk of introduction, transmission, or spread of communicable diseases.[6, 7]

2.2.2. Processing

The implementation of a Quality Assurance (QA) program includes principles of good manufacturing practice (GMP) and a quality control (QC) system. A QC system is required to ensure safety and efficacy of cell applications. GMP regulations apply to all phases of cell/tissue collection, processing and expansion, and storage. GMP quality practices are required for HCT/Ps to be used for clinical procedures and INDs. A compliant quality program for record and process control is a critical part of a QC system.

A compliant material control program is essential for FDA licensure. During review of new license applications, clinics and companies are asked to provide detailed descriptions of the manufacturing process and documentation of source country for all materials of animal origin. Additionally, for FDA-regulated products intended for administration to humans, companies must minimize any chance that BSE could be introduced into products during the manufacturing process and ensure that all materials are used as intended in the processing and are contamination free. Subsequently, a program for control of materials used in the process is necessary to meet FDA compliance and product safety.

2.2.3. Storage

If the HCT/P product involves cryopreservation, then compliance requires that the process includes an understanding of the shelf-life and how the freezing & storage process affects the HCT/Ps to complete the quality testing program. Banked cells should be stored under conditions shown to be suitable for long-term stability. Cell/tissue stability under the freezing and storage conditions should be validated using cell recovery or viability data. It is expected that establishment of a stability program for a banking process will lead to the development of quality products over a long term storage period and provide confidence that they will be effective in clinical applications.

2.2.4. Distribution testing

For the lot release of patient's cells/tissues for clinical use, standards for in-process and final product quality must be established. Specifically for FDA licensure, companies must submit their facility controls, process controls, and product standards designed with scientific principles to ensure the safety and effectiveness of all HCT/Ps products. This again is based on SOPs and controls for adherence to the cGTP, Current Good Manufacturing Practice (cGMP) and 21 CFR 1271 requirements. Product lot release specifications ensure that all products are produced in a safe and consistent manner and should be effective in clinical applications. In order to meet HCT/Ps regulations, product lot release specification should include testing for cell phenotype to confirm purity, potency, and identity.

The application for licensure requires that companies demonstrate that the HCT/P product standards and procedures are based on good science, and thorough and extensive data. A comprehensive product characterization program is needed to understand the products and how they may be clinically beneficial. During the application process, the FDA may request that the hospital or company applicant expand on a concept or further explain the rationale/ approach or provide additional data. FDA premarket review and licensing is considered a lengthy and arduous process, however new products applicants may benefit by the recent approvals of several cell-based products (Table 3).

Product (Company)	Condition	Cell Type	Approval
Carticel (Genzyme BioSurgery)	Articular cartilage damage in the knee	Autologous chondrocytes (adult/ differentiated)	US FDA approval 1997 (grandfathered in)
Apligraf(Organogenisis)	Diabetic foot ulcers and venous leg ulcers	Neonatal foreskin allogeneic keratinocytes and fibroblasts in bovine collagen scaffold	US FDA approval 1998
Provenge (Dendreon)	Asypmptomatic or hormone refractory prostate cancer	Autologous dendritic cells (adult/ differentiated)	US FDA approval 2010
Gintuit (Organogenesis)	Asypmptomatic or hormone refractory prostate cancer	Autologous dendritic cells (adult/ differentiated)	US FDA approval 2010
La Viv (Fibrocell Science inc)	Moderate to severe nasolabial fold wrinkles	Autologous fibroblasts (adult/ differentiated)	US FDA approval 2012
ChondroCelect* (TiGenix)	Single symptomatic cartilage defects in the knee	Autologous chondrocytes (adult/ differentiated)	EMEA approval 2009
Prochymal (Osiris)	Graft vs. host disease in children who are refractory to steroid therapy post-BMT	Allogeneic mesenchymal stem cells from donor bone marrow	Health Canada/New Zealand grant conditional approval 2012
Hearti-cellgram-AMI (FCB-Pharmicell)	Heart repair post-myocardial infarction	Autologous bone marrow-derived mesenchymal stem cells	Korean approval 2011
Cartistem (Medipost)	Traumatic and degenerative osteoarthritis	Allogeneic mesenchymal stem cells from donor umbilical cord blood	Korean approval 2012
Cupistem (Anterogen)	Anal fistula in Crohn's Disease	Autologous fat-derived 'stem cells'	Korean approval 2012

Table 3. Approved Cell Therapy Products by the U.S. FDA and non-3rd World Countries. Several cell products have received US approval[99] and are in current use for a number of patients. Most US approved products are for autologous use, only Apilgrafs foreskin cells are used allogeneically. Osiris recently received conditional approval for allogeneic use of mesenchymal stem cells in pediatric graft-vs-host disease.

3. Non-U.S. regulatory systems

The European Union, Australia and Canada and other countries have established similar regulatory systems for the use of post-natal human HCT/Ps.

The European Medicines Agency (EMEA) is the regulating body with authorization and supervision of cell therapy products and other "advanced therapy medicinal products" [15]. As of January 2011, the EMA's Committee for Advanced Therapies (CAT) recognized the potential of stem cell therapies and released a reflection paper to work in conjunction with the *Guideline on Human Cell-based Medicinal Products* (EMEA/CHMP/410869/2006) for the Marketing Authorization Application (MA). Both the reflection paper and the guidance detail the quality and manufacturing, non-clinical, and clinical aspects required for MA approval. The quality and manufacturing considerations include starting and raw materials, manufacturing process, quality control, validation of the manufacturing process, development pharmaceutics, traceability and biovigilance, and comparability. Pharmacology and toxicology are the non-clinical development aspects to be considered. From a clinical development standpoint, general aspects, pharmacodynamics, pharmacokinetics, dose finding studies, clinical efficacy, clinical safety,pharmacovigilance, and risk management plans are necessary for approval.

In Australia, HCT/Ps or products (biologicals) are regulated by the Therapeutic Goods Administration (TGA) which is the Australian equivalent to the FDA. Similar to the FDA approach, the TGA's regulatory framework for biological imposes varying levels of regulation on the therapy or product depending on risk, extent of manipulation, and whether the intended use of the biological is its *usual biological function[16]*. In order to gain approval a treatment that used a biological, and the biologicals intended use was not its normal function, a hospital or company would be required to submit substantial evidence that the particular therapy or product is safe, effective and of high quality.

In order for a stem cell therapy to be approved by Health Canada it must meet the regulations as stated in the Safety of Human Cells, Tissues and Organs for Transplantation Regulations (CTO Regulations[17]). The CTO Regulations detail requirements to ensure safety in processing; storage; record keeping; distribution; importation; error, accident and adverse reaction investigation and reporting. Requirements for donor screening, testing, and suitability assessment are described in the processing regulations as well as the testing and measurements performed on the products after retrieval or in preparation for use, preservation, or packaging[17].

Health Canada, the FDA equivalent in Canada, is the first approving body in the world to approve a manufactured stem cell based drug intended to treat a systemic disease -acute Graft versus Host Disease (aGvHD) [18]. Osiris Therapeutics of Columbia, Maryland developed Prochymal [remestemcel-L, adult human mesenchymal stem cells (hMSCs) for intravenous infusion], a liquid cell suspension of ex vivo cultured adult MSCs derived from the bone marrow of healthy adult donors. Prochymal is the first stem cell therapy approved for clinical use in patients, specifically pediatric patients. Health Canada required Osiris to continue a Risk Management Plan to demonstrate that the benefits of Prochymal continue to outweigh risk, the addition of post-market studies, and maintenance of a treated patient registry for approval[19].

Table 3 provides a list of cell therapy products that have received U.S. FDA approval or other government approval. Despite extensive stem cell research over the past 15 years, most cell products are not stem cell derived. Only Osiris' BM-MSC product and 3 Korean products are stem cell based products.

4. Conclusions

This report examines the different processes involved in HCT/Ps manufacturing and high-lights the guidelines that must be followed to obtain FDA or other country specific regulatory approval. Ex vivo expansion, cell selection or gene modification will likely be necessary for most advanced cell and tissue therapies. These modifications increase the risk associated with the treatment and render the product to be regulated under a higher risk category of more-than-minimally-manipulated product. Key to biomanufacturing is the implementation of a QA/QC program including a quality control system and GMP principles which apply to all phases of manufacturing.

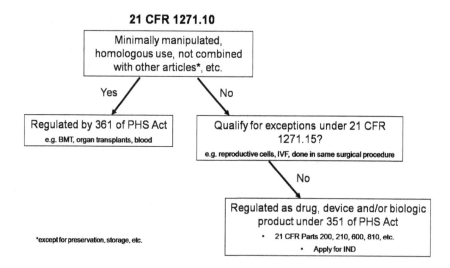

Figure 1. Regulatory Pathway Assessment If an HCT/Ps product is minimally manipulated it is regulated as a "361 HCT/Ps", and it is not subject to any premarket review requirements. However, if the HCT/Ps is more-than-minimally manipulated, and does not qualify for exemptions under 21 CFR 1271.15, it will be regulated as drug, device and/or biologic product under 351 of the PHS Act.

Many counties actively regulate the use of stem cell products, however, there are still a number of areas around the world that have little regulations and unregulated treatments pose risk to patients and the careful development of the field. The current challenge to deliver safe cell and tissue therapies and curb unregulated treatments may soon apply to gene therapy and other innovative technologies. Early government regulation and active education by a number of professional organizations should reduce the spread of medical tourism and aid in the development of safe and effective treatments in the field of regenerative medicine.

Author details

Bridget M. Deasy[1,2*], Jordan E. Anderson[3] and Shannon Zelina[1]

*Address all correspondence to: deasybm@gmail.com

1 CellStock, Pittsburgh, PA, USA

2 McGowan Institute for Regenerative Medicine, University of Pittsburgh, Pittsburgh, PA, USA

3 Dept. of Biomedical Engineering, School of Engineering, University of Connecticut, Storrs, CT, USA

References

[1] ISSCR, *Guidelines for the Clinical Translation of Stem Cells.* International Society for Stem Cell Research, 2008.

[2] Amariglio, N., et al., *Donor-derived brain tumor following neural stem cell transplantation in an ataxia telangiectasia patient.* PLoS Med, 2009. 6(2): p. e1000029.

[3] Liang, B.A. and T. Mackey, *Confronting conflict: addressing institutional conflicts of interest in academic medical centers.* Am J Law Med, 2010. 36(1): p. 136-87.

[4] Wilson, R.F., *The death of Jesse Gelsinger: new evidence of the influence of money and prestige in human research.* Am J Law Med, 2010. 36(2-3): p. 295-325.

[5] Lau, D., et al., *Stem cell clinics online: the direct-to-consumer portrayal of stem cell medicine.* Cell Stem Cell, 2008. 3(6): p. 591-4.

[6] National Academies (U.S.). Committee on Ranking FDA Product Categories Based on Health Consequences Phase II. and National Research Council (U.S.), *A risk-characterization framework for decision-making at the Food and Drug Administration.* 2011, Washington, D.C.: National Academies Press. xiv, 192 p.

[7]   US Food and Drug Administration. Guidance for Industry. Current Good Tissue Practice (CGTP) and Additional Requirements for Manufacturers of Human Cells, Tissues, and Cellular and Tissue-Based Products (HCT/Ps). 2011.

[8]   Carlson, M.E. and I.M. Conboy, Loss of stem cell regenerative capacity within aged niches. Aging Cell, 2007. 6(3): p. 371-82.

[9]   Gazit, R., I.L. Weissman, and D.J. Rossi, Hematopoietic stem cells and the aging hematopoietic system. Semin Hematol, 2008. 45(4): p. 218-24.

[10] Deasy, B.M., et al., Long-term self-renewal of postnatal muscle-derived stem cells. Mol Biol Cell, 2005. 16(7): p. 3323-33.

[11] Kirouac, D.C. and P.W. Zandstra, The systematic production of cells for cell therapies. Cell Stem Cell, 2008. 3(4): p. 369-81.

[12] Parenteau, N.L., Commercial development of cell-based therapeutics: strategic considerations along the drug to tissue spectrum. Regen Med, 2009. 4(4): p. 601-11.

[13] US Food and Drug Administration. Application of current statutory authority to human somatic cell-therapy and gene-therapy products, in Fed Reg 58:53248-51. 1993.

[14] Burger, S.R., Current regulatory issues in cell and tissue therapy. Cytotherapy, 2003. 5(4): p. 289-98.

[15] Schussler-Lenz, M. and C.K. Schneider, [Clinical trials with advanced therapy medicinal products]. Bundesgesundheitsblatt Gesundheitsforschung Gesundheitsschutz, 2010. 53(1): p. 68-74.

[16] Wall, D.M. and H.M. Prince, Regulation of cellular therapies: the Australian perspective. Cytotherapy, 2003. 5(4): p. 284-8.

[17] HealthCanada, GUIDANCE DOCUMENT FOR CELL, TISSUE AND ORGAN ESTABLISHMENTS.Safety of Human Cells, Tissues and Organs for Transplantation, Health Products and Food Branch Guidance Document, Editor. 2009, Minister of Health.

[18] Pollack, A., A Stem-Cell-Based Drug Gets Approval in Canada, in The New York Times. 2012: New York.

[19] HealthCanada, Notice of Decision for Prochymal, in Control Number 150026, Office of Regulatory Affairs Biologics and Genetic Therapies Directorate, Editor. 2012, http://www.hc-sc.gc.ca/dhp-mps/prodpharma/sbd-smd/drug-med/nd_ad_2012_prochymal_150026-eng.php.

[20] Rada-Iglesias, A. and J. Wysocka, Epigenomics of human embryonic stem cells and induced pluripotent stem cells: insights into pluripotency and implications for disease. Genome Med, 2011. 3(6): p. 36.

[21] Sumer, H., J. Liu, and P.J. Verma, Cellular reprogramming of somatic cells. Indian J Exp Biol, 2011. 49(6): p. 409-15.

[22] Han, J. and K.S. Sidhu, *Current concepts in reprogramming somatic cells to pluripotent state*. Curr Stem Cell Res Ther, 2008. 3(1): p. 66-74.

[23] Do, J.T., D.W. Han, and H.R. Scholer, *Reprogramming somatic gene activity by fusion with pluripotent cells*. Stem Cell Rev, 2006. 2(4): p. 257-64.

[24] Zeng, X. and M.S. Rao, *Human embryonic stem cells: long term stability, absence of senescence and a potential cell source for neural replacement*. Neuroscience, 2007. 145(4): p. 1348-58.

[25] Atkinson, S. and L. Armstrong, *Epigenetics in embryonic stem cells: regulation of pluripotency and differentiation*. Cell Tissue Res, 2008. 331(1): p. 23-9.

[26] Tavakoli, T., et al., *Self-renewal and differentiation capabilities are variable between human embryonic stem cell lines I3, I6 and BG01V*. BMC Cell Biol, 2009. 10: p. 44.

[27] Bhattacharya, B., S. Puri, and R.K. Puri, *A review of gene expression profiling of human embryonic stem cell lines and their differentiated progeny*. Curr Stem Cell Res Ther, 2009. 4(2): p. 98-106.

[28] Guenther, M.G., et al., *Chromatin structure and gene expression programs of human embryonic and induced pluripotent stem cells*. Cell Stem Cell, 2010. 7(2): p. 249-57.

[29] Yu, J., et al., *Induced pluripotent stem cell lines derived from human somatic cells*. Science, 2007. 318(5858): p. 1917-20.

[30] Shafa, M., R. Krawetz, and D.E. Rancourt, *Returning to the stem state: epigenetics of recapitulating pre-differentiation chromatin structure*. Bioessays, 2010. 32(9): p. 791-9.

[31] Newman, A.M. and J.B. Cooper, *Lab-specific gene expression signatures in pluripotent stem cells*. Cell Stem Cell, 2010. 7(2): p. 258-62.

[32] Hong, S.H., et al., *Cell fate potential of human pluripotent stem cells is encoded by histone modifications*. Cell Stem Cell, 2011. 9(1): p. 24-36.

[33] Scott, C.T., et al., *Democracy Derived? New Trajectories in Pluripotent Stem Cell Research*. Cell, 2011. 145(6): p. 820-6.

[34] Lee, H., et al., *Induced pluripotent stem cells in regenerative medicine: an argument for continued research on human embryonic stem cells*. Regen Med, 2009. 4(5): p. 759-69.

[35] Zavazava, N., *Immunity of embryonic stem cell-derived hematopoietic progenitor cells*. Semin Immunopathol, 2011.

[36] Broxmeyer, H.E., *Will iPS cells enhance therapeutic applicability of cord blood cells and banking?* Cell Stem Cell, 2010. 6(1): p. 21-4.

[37] Taylor, C.J., E.M. Bolton, and J.A. Bradley, *Immunological considerations for embryonic and induced pluripotent stem cell banking*. Philos Trans R Soc Lond B Biol Sci, 2011. 366(1575): p. 2312-22.

[38] Kim, J.B., et al., *Pluripotent stem cells induced from adult neural stem cells by reprogramming with two factors.* Nature, 2008. 454(7204): p. 646-50.

[39] Takahashi, K., et al., *Induction of pluripotent stem cells from adult human fibroblasts by defined factors.* Cell, 2007. 131(5): p. 861-72.

[40] Mohamadnejad, M. and E.S. Swenson, *Induced pluripotent cells mimicking human embryonic stem cells.* Arch Iran Med, 2008. 11(1): p. 125-8.

[41] Ang, Y.S., et al., *Stem cells and reprogramming: breaking the epigenetic barrier?* Trends Pharmacol Sci, 2011. 32(7): p. 394-401.

[42] Havlas, V., et al., *[Comparison of chondrogenic differentiation of adipose tissue-derived mesenchymal stem cells with cultured chondrocytes and bone marrow mesenchymal stem cells].* Acta Chir Orthop Traumatol Cech, 2011. 78(2): p. 138-44.

[43] Winter, A., et al., *Cartilage-like gene expression in differentiated human stem cell spheroids: a comparison of bone marrow-derived and adipose tissue-derived stromal cells.* Arthritis Rheum, 2003. 48(2): p. 418-29.

[44] Shafiee, A., et al., *A comparison between osteogenic differentiation of human unrestricted somatic stem cells and mesenchymal stem cells from bone marrow and adipose tissue.* Biotechnol Lett, 2011. 33(6): p. 1257-64.

[45] Riekstina, U., et al., *Embryonic stem cell marker expression pattern in human mesenchymal stem cells derived from bone marrow, adipose tissue, heart and dermis.* Stem Cell Rev, 2009. 5(4): p. 378-86.

[46] Pournasr, B., et al., *In Vitro Differentiation of Human Bone Marrow Mesenchymal Stem Cells into Hepatocyte-like Cells.* Arch Iran Med, 2011. 14(4): p. 244-9.

[47] Witkowska-Zimny, M. and K. Walenko, *Stem cells from adipose tissue.* Cell Mol Biol Lett, 2011. 16(2): p. 236-57.

[48] Mizuno, H., *Adipose-derived stem and stromal cells for cell-based therapy: current status of preclinical studies and clinical trials.* Curr Opin Mol Ther, 2010. 12(4): p. 442-9.

[49] De Toni, F., et al., *Human Adipose-Derived Stromal Cells Efficiently Support Hematopoiesis In Vitro and In Vivo: A Key Step for Therapeutic Studies.* Stem Cells Dev, 2011.

[50] Zhu, M., et al., *[Cell biological study of adipose-derived stem cells].* Nan Fang Yi Ke Da Xue Xue Bao, 2007. 27(4): p. 518-23.

[51] Li, H., et al., *Adipogenic Potential of Adipose Stem Cell Subpopulations.* Plast Reconstr Surg, 2011.

[52] Szoke, K., K.J. Beckstrom, and J.E. Brinchmann, *Human adipose tissue as a source of cells with angiogenic potential.* Cell Transplant, 2011.

[53] Lin, C.S., et al., *Defining adipose tissue-derived stem cells in tissue and in culture.* Histol Histopathol, 2010. 25(6): p. 807-15.

[54] Murohara, T., *Autologous adipose tissue as a new source of progenitor cells for therapeutic angiogenesis*. J Cardiol, 2009. 53(2): p. 155-63.

[55] He, X., et al., *[Morphological characteristics of human adipose-derived stem cells]*. Sheng Wu Yi Xue Gong Cheng Xue Za Zhi, 2011. 28(2): p. 337-41.

[56] Bobbert, M., *Ethical questions concerning research on human embryos, embryonic stem cells and chimeras*. Biotechnol J, 2006. 1(12): p. 1352-69.

[57] Hug, K., *Sources of human embryos for stem cell research: ethical problems and their possible solutions*. Medicina (Kaunas), 2005. 41(12): p. 1002-10.

[58] Hug, K. and G. Hermeren, *Do we Still Need Human Embryonic Stem Cells for Stem Cell-Based Therapies? Epistemic and Ethical Aspects*. Stem Cell Rev, 2011.

[59] Knoepfler, P.S., *Deconstructing stem cell tumorigenicity: a roadmap to safe regenerative medicine*. Stem Cells, 2009. 27(5): p. 1050-6.

[60] Zacharias, D.G., et al., *The science and ethics of induced pluripotency: what will become of embryonic stem cells?* Mayo Clin Proc, 2011. 86(7): p. 634-40.

[61] Volarevic, V., et al., *Human stem cell research and regenerative medicine--present and future*. Br Med Bull, 2011.

[62] Lowry, W.E. and W.L. Quan, *Roadblocks en route to the clinical application of induced pluripotent stem cells*. J Cell Sci, 2010. 123(Pt 5): p. 643-51.

[63] Walia, B., et al., *Induced Pluripotent Stem Cells: Fundamentals and Applications of the Reprogramming Process and its Ramifications on Regenerative Medicine*. Stem Cell Rev, 2011.

[64] Kiefer, J.C., *Primer and interviews: Promises and realities of induced pluripotent stem cells*. Dev Dyn, 2011. 240(8): p. 2034-41.

[65] Zhou, H. and S. Ding, *Evolution of induced pluripotent stem cell technology*. Curr Opin Hematol, 2010. 17(4): p. 276-80.

[66] Amabile, G. and A. Meissner, *Induced pluripotent stem cells: current progress and potential for regenerative medicine*. Trends Mol Med, 2009. 15(2): p. 59-68.

[67] Deng, W., *Exploiting pluripotency for therapeutic gain*. Panminerva Med, 2010. 52(2): p. 167-73.

[68] Baker, D.E., et al., *Adaptation to culture of human embryonic stem cells and oncogenesis in vivo*. Nat Biotechnol, 2007. 25(2): p. 207-15.

[69] Blum, B. and N. Benvenisty, *The tumorigenicity of human embryonic stem cells*. Adv Cancer Res, 2008. 100: p. 133-58.

[70] Enver, T., et al., *Cellular differentiation hierarchies in normal and culture-adapted human embryonic stem cells*. Hum Mol Genet, 2005. 14(21): p. 3129-40.

[71] Yang, S., et al., *Tumor progression of culture-adapted human embryonic stem cells during long-term culture.* Genes Chromosomes Cancer, 2008. 47(8): p. 665-79.

[72] Yuasa, S., et al., *Development and migration of Purkinje cells in the mouse cerebellar primordium.* Anat Embryol (Berl), 1991. 184(3): p. 195-212.

[73] Aoi, T., et al., *Generation of pluripotent stem cells from adult mouse liver and stomach cells.* Science, 2008. 321(5889): p. 699-702.

[74] Ghosh, Z., et al., *Dissecting the oncogenic and tumorigenic potential of differentiated human induced pluripotent stem cells and human embryonic stem cells.* Cancer Res, 2011. 71(14): p. 5030-9.

[75] Gutierrez-Aranda, I., et al., *Human induced pluripotent stem cells develop teratoma more efficiently and faster than human embryonic stem cells regardless the site of injection.* Stem Cells, 2010. 28(9): p. 1568-70.

[76] Zhao, B.C., et al., *Adipose-derived stem cells promote gastric cancer cell growth, migration and invasion through SDF-1/CXCR4 axis.* Hepatogastroenterology, 2010. 57(104): p. 1382-9.

[77] Jeon, B.G., et al., *Characterization and comparison of telomere length, telomerase and reverse transcriptase activity and gene expression in human mesenchymal stem cells and cancer cells of various origins.* Cell Tissue Res, 2011. 345(1): p. 149-61.

[78] Zhang, Y., C.F. Bellows, and M.G. Kolonin, *Adipose tissue-derived progenitor cells and cancer.* World J Stem Cells, 2010. 2(5): p. 103-13.

[79] Zhang, Y., et al., *White adipose tissue cells are recruited by experimental tumors and promote cancer progression in mouse models.* Cancer Res, 2009. 69(12): p. 5259-66.

[80] Catalina, P., et al., *Human ESCs predisposition to karyotypic instability: Is a matter of culture adaptation or differential vulnerability among hESC lines due to inherent properties?* Mol Cancer, 2008. 7: p. 76.

[81] Fu, X. and Y. Xu, *Self-renewal and scalability of human embryonic stem cells for human therapy.* Regen Med, 2011. 6(3): p. 327-34.

[82] Oh, S.K. and A.B. Choo, *Human embryonic stem cells: technological challenges towards therapy.* Clin Exp Pharmacol Physiol, 2006. 33(5-6): p. 489-95.

[83] Vallier, L., *Serum-free and feeder-free culture conditions for human embryonic stem cells.* Methods Mol Biol, 2011. 690: p. 57-66.

[84] Cavallo, C., et al., *Comparison of alternative mesenchymal stem cell sources for cell banking and musculoskeletal advanced therapies.* J Cell Biochem, 2011. 112(5): p. 1418-30.

[85] Kuroda, Y., et al., *Bone Marrow Mesenchymal Cells: How Do They Contribute to Tissue Repair and Are They Really Stem Cells?* Arch Immunol Ther Exp (Warsz), 2011.

[86] Undale, A., et al., *Induction of fracture repair by mesenchymal cells derived from human embryonic stem cells or bone marrow.* J Orthop Res, 2011.

[87] Locke, M., V. Feisst, and P.R. Dunbar, *Concise review: human adipose-derived stem cells: separating promise from clinical need.* Stem Cells, 2011. 29(3): p. 404-11.

[88] Liu, W., et al., *Genetic and epigenetic X-chromosome variations in a parthenogenetic human embryonic stem cell line.* J Assist Reprod Genet, 2011. 28(4): p. 303-13.

[89] Noisa, P. and R. Parnpai, *Technical challenges in the derivation of human pluripotent cells.* Stem Cells Int, 2011. 2011: p. 907961.

[90] Anastasia, L., et al., *Cell reprogramming: expectations and challenges for chemistry in stem cell biology and regenerative medicine.* Cell Death Differ, 2010. 17(8): p. 1230-7.

[91] Takahashi, K. and S. Yamanaka, *Induction of pluripotent stem cells from mouse embryonic and adult fibroblast cultures by defined factors.* Cell, 2006. 126(4): p. 663-76.

[92] Kamata, M., et al., *Live cell monitoring of hiPSC generation and differentiation using differential expression of endogenous microRNAs.* PLoS One, 2010. 5(7): p. e11834.

[93] Gunaratne, P.H., *Embryonic stem cell microRNAs: defining factors in induced pluripotent (iPS) and cancer (CSC) stem cells?* Curr Stem Cell Res Ther, 2009. 4(3): p. 168-77.

[94] Hockemeyer, D., et al., *Genetic engineering of human pluripotent cells using TALE nucleases.* Nat Biotechnol, 2011.

[95] Hoogduijn, M.J., et al., *Immunological aspects of allogeneic and autologous mesenchymal stem cell therapies.* Hum Gene Ther, 2011.

[96] Drukker, M., *Immunological considerations for cell therapy using human embryonic stem cell derivatives.* 2008.

[97] Drukker, M., *Recent advancements towards the derivation of immune-compatible patient-specific human embryonic stem cell lines.* Semin Immunol, 2008. 20(2): p. 123-9.

[98] Zhao, T., et al., *Immunogenicity of induced pluripotent stem cells.* Nature, 2011. 474(7350): p. 212-5.

[99] FDA, *http://www.fda.gov/BiologicsBloodVaccines/CellularGeneTherapyProducts/ApprovedProducts/default.htm.*

Permissions

The contributors of this book come from diverse backgrounds, making this book a truly international effort. This book will bring forth new frontiers with its revolutionizing research information and detailed analysis of the nascent developments around the world.

We would like to thank José A. Andrades, for lending his expertise to make the book truly unique. He has played a crucial role in the development of this book. Without his invaluable contribution this book wouldn't have been possible. He has made vital efforts to compile up to date information on the varied aspects of this subject to make this book a valuable addition to the collection of many professionals and students.

This book was conceptualized with the vision of imparting up-to-date information and advanced data in this field. To ensure the same, a matchless editorial board was set up. Every individual on the board went through rigorous rounds of assessment to prove their worth. After which they invested a large part of their time researching and compiling the most relevant data for our readers. Conferences and sessions were held from time to time between the editorial board and the contributing authors to present the data in the most comprehensible form. The editorial team has worked tirelessly to provide valuable and valid information to help people across the globe.

Every chapter published in this book has been scrutinized by our experts. Their significance has been extensively debated. The topics covered herein carry significant findings which will fuel the growth of the discipline. They may even be implemented as practical applications or may be referred to as a beginning point for another development. Chapters in this book were first published by InTech; hereby published with permission under the Creative Commons Attribution License or equivalent.

The editorial board has been involved in producing this book since its inception. They have spent rigorous hours researching and exploring the diverse topics which have resulted in the successful publishing of this book. They have passed on their knowledge of decades through this book. To expedite this challenging task, the publisher supported the team at every step. A small team of assistant editors was also appointed to further simplify the editing procedure and attain best results for the readers.

Our editorial team has been hand-picked from every corner of the world. Their multi-ethnicity adds dynamic inputs to the discussions which result in innovative outcomes. These outcomes are then further discussed with the researchers and contributors who give their valuable feedback and opinion regarding the same. The feedback is then collaborated with the researches and they are edited in a comprehensive manner to aid the understanding of the subject.

Apart from the editorial board, the designing team has also invested a significant amount of their time in understanding the subject and creating the most relevant covers. They scrutinized every image to scout for the most suitable representation of the subject and create an appropriate cover for the book.

The publishing team has been involved in this book since its early stages. They were actively engaged in every process, be it collecting the data, connecting with the contributors or procuring relevant information. The team has been an ardent support to the editorial, designing and production team. Their endless efforts to recruit the best for this project, has resulted in the accomplishment of this book. They are a veteran in the field of academics and their pool of knowledge is as vast as their experience in printing. Their expertise and guidance has proved useful at every step. Their uncompromising quality standards have made this book an exceptional effort. Their encouragement from time to time has been an inspiration for everyone.

The publisher and the editorial board hope that this book will prove to be a valuable piece of knowledge for researchers, students, practitioners and scholars across the globe.

List of Contributors

Patricia Zuk
Regenerative Bioengineering and Repair Lab, Division of Plastic Surgery, Department of Surgery, David Geffen School of Medicine at UCLA, Los Angeles, USA

Carla Colombo and Valentina Paracchini
Fondazione IRCCS Ca' GrandaOspedale Maggiore Policlinico, Cystic Fibrosis Center, Milan, Italy

Stefano Castellani, Sante Di Gioia and Massimo Conese
Department of Medical and Surgical Sciences, University of Foggia, Foggia, Italy

Annalucia Carbone
Fondazione IRCCS Ca' GrandaOspedale Maggiore Policlinico, Cystic Fibrosis Center, Milan, Italy
Department of Medical and Surgical Sciences, University of Foggia, Foggia, Italy

Hideki Agata
Tissue Engineering Research Group, Division of Molecular Therapy, The Institute of Medical Science, The University of Tokyo, Tokyo, Japan

Razieh Karamzadeh and Mohamadreza Baghaban Eslaminejad
Department of Stem Cell and Developmental Biology, Cell Science Research Center, Royan Institute for Stem Cell Biology and Technology, ACECR, Tehran, Iran

Katsunori Sasaki

Fengming Yue, Hinako Ichikawa, Susumu Yoshie, Akimi Mogi, Shoko Masuda and Tomotsune Daihachiro
Department of Histology and Embryology, Shinshu University School of Medicine, Matsumoto, Nagano, Japan

Sakiko Shirasawa, Mika Nagai and Tadayuki Yokohama
Laboratory for Advanced Health Science, Bourbon Institutes of Health, Bourbon Corporation, Matsumoto, Nagano, Japan

Morikuni Tobita and Hiroshi Mizuno
Department of Plastic and Reconstructive Surgery, Juntendo University School of Medicine, Japan

Vincenzo Vindigni, Giorgio Giatsidis, Francesco Reho, Erica Dalla Venezia, Marco Mammana and Bassetto Franco
Clinic of Plastic Surgery, Department of Surgery, University of Padova, Padova, Italy

Inés Avedillo
Innovaxis Biopharmaceuticals Ltd., Technological Park of Jerez, Jerez de la Frontera, Spain

José M. López-Puerta
Department of Orthopaedic Surgery and Traumatology, Universitary Hospital Virgen del Rocío, Sevilla, Spain
Networking Biomedical Research Center in Bioengineering, Biomaterials and Nanomedicine (CIBER-BBN), University of Málaga, Málaga, Spain

Plácido Zamora-Navas
Networking Biomedical Research Center in Bioengineering, Biomaterials and Nanomedicine (CIBER-BBN), University of Málaga, Málaga, Spain
Department of Orthopaedic Surgery and Traumatology, Universitary Hospital Virgen de la Victoria, Málaga, Spain

Silvia Claros, Gustavo A. Rico-Llanos, José A. Andrades and José Becerra
Networking Biomedical Research Center in Bioengineering, Biomaterials and Nanomedicine (CIBER-BBN), University of Málaga, Málaga, Spain
Laboratory of Bioengineering and Tissue Regeneration (LABRET-UMA), Department of Cell Biology, Genetics and Physiology, Faculty of Sciences, University of Málaga, Málaga, Spain

Bridget M. Deasy
CellStock, Pittsburgh, PA, USA
McGowan Institute for Regenerative Medicine, University of Pittsburgh, Pittsburgh, PA, USA

Jordan E. Anderson
Dept. of Biomedical Engineering, School of Engineering, University of Connecticut, Storrs, CT, USA

Shannon Zelina
CellStock, Pittsburgh, PA, USA

Printed in the USA
CPSIA information can be obtained
at www.ICGtesting.com
JSHW011412221024
72173JS00003B/524

9 781632 412430